SpringerWienNewYork

Bernhard Schaller (ed.)

Imaging of Carotid Artery Stenosis

Springer Wien NewYork

Dr. Bernhard J. Schaller (ed.)

Karolinska Institute, Stockholm, Sweden

This work is subject to copyright.
All rights are reserved, whether the whole or part of the material is concerned, specifically those of translation, reprinting, re-use of illustrations, broadcasting, reproduction by photocopying machines or similar means, and storage in data banks.

Product Liability: The publisher can give no guarantee for all the information contained in this book. This does also refer to information about drug dosage and application thereof. In every individual case the respective user must check its accuracy by consulting other pharmaceutical literature. The use of registered names, trademarks, etc. in this publication does not imply, even in the absence of a specific statement, that such names are exempt from the relevant protective laws and regulations and therefore free for general use.

© 2007 Springer-Verlag/Wien
Printed in Austria

SpringerWienNewYork is part of Springer Science + Business Media
springer.com

Typesetting: Thomson Press Ltd., Chennai, India
Printing: Theiss GmbH, 9431 St. Stefan, Austria

Printed on acid-free and chlorine-free bleached paper
SPIN: 11671961

With 86 (partly coloured) Figures

Library of Congress Control Number: 2006935141

ISBN 978-3-211-32332-8 SpringerWienNewYork

Contents

Introduction 1
(B. J. Schaller, Stockholm, Sweden)

1. Imaging examination techniques of carotid artery 5
    1.1 The pathology of atherosclerosis 7
           (M. P. Dunphy and H. W. Strauss, New York, USA)
    1.2 Correlation of carotid artery pathology and morphology in imaging 19
           (W. S. Kerwin, Seattle, USA)
    1.3 Sonographic evaluation in carotid artery stenosis 35
           (B. K. Lal, New Jersey, USA)
    1.4 Digital subtraction angiography in carotid artery stenosis 41
           (A. Srinivasan and M. Goyal, Ottawa, Canada)
    1.5 Computed tomography imaging in carotid artery stenosis 49
           (M. Berg, R. Canninen and H. Manninen, Kuopio, Finland)
    1.6 Intracerebral imaging and carotid artery stenosis 69
           (K.-O. Lövblad, Geneva, Switzerland)
    1.7 Positron emission tomography imaging in carotid artery stenosis 85
           (C. P. Derdeyn, St. Louis, USA)

2. Specific pathologic problems in carotid artery imaging 103
    2.1 Atherosclerotic plaque characterisation by imaging 105
           (S. P. S. Howarth, J. U. King-Im and J. H. Gillard, Cambridge, UK)
    2.2 Imaging findings in carotid artery dissection 125
           (C. Chaves and G. Lee, Burlington, USA)
    2.3 High suited carotid artery stenosis and imaging 147
           (B. Butz, Regensburg, Germany)
    2.4 Intracranial magnetic resonance and vascular imaging in patients
        with extracranial carotid stenosis 177
           (A. D. Mackinnon, A. D. Platts and D. J. H. McCabe, London, UK)

3. From imaging to therapy in carotid artery stenosis 207
           (K. Bettermann and J. F. Toole, Winston-Salem, USA)

4. Therapy and carotid artery imaging 223

4.1 Imaging of extracranial to intracranial bypass 225
(H. J. N. Streefkerk, C. A. F. Tulleken, J. Hendrikse and C. J. M. Klijn, Nijmegen and Utrecht, The Netherlands)

4.2 Imaging after surgical thrombendarterectomy of the carotid artery 239
(H. Katano and K. Yamada, Nagoya, Japan)

4.3 Imaging after carotid stenting 247
(G. M. Biasi, A. Froio and G. Deleo, Milano, Italy)

5. Imaging in carotid artery stenosis: Prospects to the future 261
(B. J. Schaller and M. Buchfelder, Göttingen, Germany)

List of Authors 273

INTRODUCTION

INTRODUCTION

B. J. Schaller

Department of Neuroscience, Karolinska Institute, Stockholm, Sweden

"The most effective surgery is always that administered by the trained brain and hands of a surgeon" (M. G. Yasargil, 2005)

An adequate and state-of-the-art treatment of atherosclerotic disease of the extra- and intracranial carotid arteries in a patient with an advanced degree of stenosis substantially reduces the risk of subsequent ischemic stroke in patients with recently symptomatic 70 to 99% carotid artery stenosis. The benefit that is to be expected for 50 to 69% symptomatic stenosis, and for asymptomatic stenosis, is more modest [3]. Whether surgical endarterectomy, endovascular stent placement or any other treatment option proves to be the more effective treatment strategy of the narrowed carotid artery has not yet to be demonstrated. In any event, accurate assessment of the degree of luminal narrowing is an important step in the treatment planning. Conventional angiography was generally used to select patients for treatment in the past. However, given the risks of death and disabling stroke due to angiography (1.2% in the Asymptomatic Carotid Atherosclerosis Study [9] versus 1.1% for surgery itself), alternative noninvasive imaging techniques have been sought and investigated during the last years. There are several reasons for such a procedure: (i) the noninvasive methods are safe compared with conventional angiography, which still carries a mortality/morbidity rate of 1.2%, (ii) the noninvasive imaging can be done on an outpatient basis and is clearly preferred by patients and (iii) many physicians believe now that noninvasive imaging is sufficiently sensitive and specific to be used in at least some situations before endarterectomy.

Such new imaging methods necessarily provide more accurate results, and frequent re-evaluation of which methods are most efficacious is appropriate and necessary. The multimodal assessment of the plaque vulnerability involving the combination of biomarkers and these new imaging techniques that also target inflammatory and thrombotic components may be the best prerequisite to better understand the atherothrombotic risk and to be able therefore to better prevent ischemic stroke.

Any such investigation involving multi-technique imaging of the carotid arterial lumen rises the question of how meaningful are the comparisons made between modalities that are sensitive to the luminal area and those that assess the lumen diameter. Magnetic resonance (MR) angiography and computed tomography (CT) angiography provide images of the lumen in cross section, and Doppler sonography provides velocity measurements that are area-dependent, whereas conventional angiography, the historic "gold-standard" technique, is generally interpreted in terms of diameter measures.

Doppler ultrasound techniques are safe and relatively easy to perform, but when compared with angiography, they demonstrate only moderate sensitivity (65 to 87%) and specificity (71 to 91%) for detection of carotid artery stenoses that would be appropriate for surgery [1], [5]. Power Doppler [10] and contrast enhancement [8] are improvements, but ultrasound still cannot reliably differentiate high-grade carotid artery stenosis from occlusion, a critical factor in surgical and also non-surgical decision-making. Transcranial Doppler was limited therefore in the detection of intracranial carotid artery stenoses ("tandem lesions") by a high false positive rate [13], and was not possible in 15 to 20% of patients due to failure of ultrasound to penetrate the skull in the past.

MR angiography (MRA) is increasingly used in the neurovascular evaluation, especially with contrast enhancement [12], and may be improved by high-strength field gradients and high-resolution techniques. CT angiography (CTA) is still not used widely enough to determine its effectiveness and, in any case, can only evaluate a limited segment of cerebral vasculature [6]. Because of its convenience and anatomic imaging qualities, there seems little doubt that CTA will become more widely used to screen for carotid artery stenosis and to assess patients with acute stroke and transient ischemic attacks. Technologic innovations will likely improve its imaging ability.

The choice of imaging strategy is also important in asymptomatic carotid artery disease. There is concern over the generalization of the results of the Asymptomatic Carotid Atherosclerosis Study, given the exemplary perioperative stroke/death rate of 2.3% seen in the trial, 1.2% of which was due to conventional angiography [2], [9]. Quoted surgical complication rates in asymptomatic case series range from 2.5% [7] to 5.6% [11]. Given these higher surgical complication rates seen in real-life clinical practice, the opportunity for patients to benefit from the procedure is further eroded by the inherent risks of angiography. Noninvasive imaging removes this additional risk to patients and may mean that skilled surgeons reach the 3.0% complication rate of stroke/ death suggested by the American Heart Association for carotid endarterectomy to be appropriate for asymptomatic disease [4].

Despite these limitations, there is a growing tendency to rely solely on ultrasound or MRA/CTA in the presurgical assessment of patients with carotid artery stenosis. New and promising imaging techniques are additionally examined. Those capabilities should provide new opportunities for determining those image characteristics of the advanced atherosclerotic lesion that more comprehensively capture the complex nature of disease and more fully identify the true determinants of future neurological risk. The present book tries to give answers and proposals of solutions on some of these questions.

References

[1] Alexandrov A, Brodie DS, McLean A et al.: Correlation of peak systolic velocity and angiographic measurement of carotid stenosis revisited. Stroke 28: 339–342 (1997).

[2] Barnett HJM, Meldrum HE, Eliasziw M: The appropriate use of carotid endarterectomy. Can Med Assoc J 166: 1169–1179 (2002).

[3] Barnett H, Broderick JP: Carotid endarterectomy: another wake-up call. Neurology 55: 746–747 (2000).

[4] Biller J, Feinberg WM, Castaldo JE et al.: Guidelines for carotid endarterectomy. Circulation 97: 501–509 (1998).

[5] Bornstein NM, Chadwick LG, Norris JW: The value of carotid Doppler ultrasound in asymptomatic extracranial arterial disease. Can J Neurol Sci 15: 378–383 (1988).

[6] Brant-Zawadzki M, Heiserman JE: The roles of MR angiography, CT angiography, and sonography in vascular imaging of the head and neck. AJNR 18: 1820–1825 (1997).

[7] Cebul RD, Snow RJ, Pine R et al.: Indictions, outcomes, and provider volumes for carotid endarterectomy. JAMA 279: 1282–1287 (1998).

[8] Droste DW, Jurgens R, Nabavi DG, et al.: Echocontrast-enhanced ultrasound of extracranial internal carotid artery high-grade stenosis and occlusion. Stroke 30: 2302–2306 (1999).

[9] Executive Committee for the Asymptomatic Carotid Atherosclerosis Study (ACAS): Endarterectomy for asymptomatic carotid artery stenosis. JAMA 273: 1421–1428 (1995).

[10] Griewing B, Morgenstern C, Driesner F et al.: Cerebrovascular disease assessed by color-flow and power Doppler ultrasonography. Stroke 27: 95–100 (1996).

[11] Hartmann A, Hupp T, Koch HC et al.: Prospective study on the complication rate of carotid surgery. Cerebrovasc Dis 9: 152–156 (1999).

[12] Rofsky NM, Adelman MA: Gadolinium-enhanced MR angiography of the carotid arteries: a small step, a giant leap? Radiology 209: 31–34 (1998).

[13] Rorick MB, Nichols FT, Adams RJ: Transcranial Doppler correlation with angiography in detection of intracranial stenosis. Stroke 25: 1931–1934 (1994).

IMAGING EXAMINATION TECHNIQUES OF CAROTID ARTERY

Chapter 1.1

THE PATHOLOGY OF ATHEROSCLEROSIS

M. P. Dunphy and H. W. Strauss

Department of Radiology, Memorial Sloan-Kettering Cancer Center, New York, USA

Atherosclerosis is an indolent, chronic arterial disease involving inflammation and thickening of the walls of medium- and large-sized vessels, with potentially-lethal sequelae. An atherosclerotic lesion is an accumulation of lipids and inflammatory cells, within the arterial wall, which becomes more complicated and extensive and deforms the involved artery, with time. Clinically-significant lesions of atherosclerosis typically become manifest after decades of growth and transformation; yet, not all lesions become symptomatic and many end by becoming calcified or fibrotic, with no clinical significance. Atherosclerotic lesions of the carotid arteries begin in infancy [19]. The arterial response that *initiates* atherosclerosis has not been definitively identified [63]. Yet the subsequent natural history of atherosclerosis has been well-characterized. The vascular burden of atherosclerosis increases in volume and extent, over decades, remaining clinically 'silent', while progressing through stages of development, with changes in the morphology and composition of lesions. Atherosclerotic lesions, known in advanced stages as 'atheroma' or 'plaques', may expose 'thrombogenic' substances or become bulging plaques that obstruct blood flow through the carotid, causing local 'hypercoagulability'. Such thrombogenicity and hypercoagulability may provoke the local formation of a blood clot, or 'thrombus', in the lumen of the carotid artery. Thrombi which are so formed may become fragmented, forming 'emboli'. Thromboembolism, or downstream circulation of blood clot fragments, from carotid atheromata, can cause frightening neurological symptoms and permanent damage of the brain, or stroke, when emboli lodge emboli in smaller vessels, blocking blood flow to vital neurological tissues downstream.

Clinicians caring for patients with carotid atherosclerosis are unable to monitor disease-progression or predict the occurrence of sequelae to any reliable degree by physical examination and history alone. Medical imaging modalities, in particular ultrasound and magnetic resonance imaging, have given clinicians the ability to examine the carotid arteries non-invasively [68], to identify and monitor the growth of atherosclerotic lesions, evaluate the adequacy of carotid blood flow, and detect thrombus formation. Regrettably, imaging cannot predict the efficacy of pharmacotherapy or lifestyle-interventions on atheroma; identify patients who will benefit most from invasive carotid procedures (except in limited circumstances [9]); or identify atheroma most likely to provoke a dire vascular event – so-called 'vulnerable' or unstable plaques.

A major goal of non-invasive radionuclide vascular imaging is to supply clinicians with these capabilities. Current medical imaging of carotid atherosclerosis provides information about the morphology of the lesion, while new techniques, interrogating the cellular composition of the lesions, are likely to identify factors that promote plaque instability.

Atherogenesis

The *response to injury hypothesis* [51], [32] proposes that an injury to the endothelium exposes the underlying vessel wall, triggering a vascular response which, rather than being reparative, results in an atherosclerotic lesion. The precise nature of this initial dys-response, the ultimate cause of atherosclerosis, or atherogenesis, remains a mystery. Yet the formation and propagation of atherosclerotic lesions, is increasingly well-understood to involve dyslipidemia and inflammation [32], [14].

Atherosclerosis is common, detected even in the arteries of healthy young people, in their second or third decade of life [36], and has even been found in the newborns of hyperlipidemic mothers. Yet atherosclerosis does not manifest itself clinically until much later in life. The symptoms are due to decreased perfusion distal to the atheroma, due to the flow limiting stenosis in a major vessel such as a carotid or coronary artery, or to a pathological expansion of the diameter of an affected segment of artery, as in abdominal aortic aneurysms (AAAs). These two types of arterial 'remodeling' can overlap, as, for example, an outward enlargement of coronary lesions precedes narrowing of the lumen [20] in atherosclerosis of the heart. Atheromata develop in stages, with years of silent progression leading up to an event, such as a transient ischemic attack or stroke. In the early stages, atheromata accumulate lipids, such as low-density lipoproteins (LDL), between the endothelium and intima/media of the vessel. The endothelium is a single layer of cells, which lines the inner surface of blood vessels. The endothelial cells communicate with other cells in important ways, as will be discussed.

Traditionally, lipids are thought to enter atherosclerotic lesions by diffusion from the lumen, diffusing through the inner layers of the vascular wall. Yet, atheroma may also gather lipids from the vasculature of the vessel itself, the *vasa vasorum*. In growing atherosclerotic lesions, the number of vessels in the vasa vasorum is increased, in response to the inflammation in the lesion, and these proliferating vasa are fragile and permeable. These fragile vessels can rupture, leading to intramural hemorrhage, or may allow small amounts of plasma and red cells to extravasate. When this occurs, the plasma membranes of the extravasated erythrocytes provide atheromata with a rich source of additional lipids and cholesterol [29], leading to further growth of the lesion. Inflammation caused by the atheroma leads to macrophage recruitment. The macrophages attempt to ingest and digest the lipid, which leads to increased metabolism on the part of the cells, and creation of a local environment conducive to oxidation of LDL in the area. While non-oxidized LDL cholesterol is a normal component of the arterial wall, oxidized LDL is extremely irritating, contributing to local inflammation in the lesion.

Oxidized molecules accumulate in atheroma, often in association with an undersupply of antioxidants in the microenvironment [59], [35]. The excess of oxidants in vascular cells puts an 'oxidative stress' on the vessel wall which promotes atherosclerosis by impairing endothelial cell function and oxidizing LDL [59], [35].

The hostile microenvironment of inflammatory cells provokes the overlying endothelium to release cytokines and growth factors which stimulate the growth of smooth muscle cells (SMCs), degrade the extracellular matrix of the atheroma, and invite additional inflammatory cells into the lesion, from the blood. As lipid-laden macrophages, or 'foam cells', accumulate and SMC proliferation continues, the atheroma grows.

Predispositions to atherosclerosis

Patients with a family history of atherosclerotic disease are at higher risk of developing significant atherosclerotic disease, and several genes have been associated with worse manifestations of atherosclerosis [18]. The genes which transmit a heritable trait of susceptibility to worse forms of atherosclerosis do not follow simple Mendelian patterns, and atherosclerotic susceptibility is likely the result of multiple genes. For example, progression of atherosclerotic lesions is associated with 'remodeling' of the microenvironment of the lesion, including degradation of the extracellular matrix, by the family of matrix metalloproteinases (MMPs). Abnormal polymorphisms in the genes for MMPs-3 and -9 have been identified, in patients suffering from more severe atherosclerosis. Similarly, a large number of genes control plasma levels of lipids, such as LDL cholesterol, HDL cholesterol, triglycerides and lipoprotein (a) (reviewed by [4]) which, typically in conjunction with diet, can play key roles in atherogenesis. Preliminary research into genetic alterations affecting inflammatory biomolecules, such as CRP, various interleukins, chemokines and Toll-like receptors (reviewed by [4]) suggest a heritable risk in the inflammatory component of atherosclerosis, as well.

Gene therapy is being explored to correct the imbalances of gene expression at sites of disease or at one or more organ sites to effect systemic changes. For example, in carotid atherosclerosis, local gene transfer to the arterial wall may be employed to inhibit restenosis after carotid vascular interventions, or stabilize vulnerable plaques; or gene transfer may seek to produce systemic changes in lipoprotein metabolism, for example, by targeting metabolic genes in the liver.

Recent research implicates the aging of the endothelial layer in the progression of atherosclerosis. Endothelium is subject to injury and must be able to replace lost endothelial cells. Recent data suggests that, as people age, endothelium becomes *senescent*, losing its ability to regenerate after injury. This observation adds a maladaptive healing *response* to injury as an age-related cause of atheroma.

Young blood vessels reconstitute defects in the endothelial layer through the formation of new endothelial cells by *proliferation* of neighboring vascular endothelial cells, or the recruitment of endothelial progenitor cells (EPCs) which circulate in the bloodstream after being formed in the bone marrow. During life, endothelial cells and the marrow precursors are called upon to divide, creating new (duplicate) cells. With each cell division, the length of chromosomal telomeres becomes shorter, called *telomeric attrition*. Telomeres are repetitive nucleotide sequences found at the end of chromosomes, crucial for DNA replication and stability. The more often an endothelial cell divides, the more its chromosomal telomeres shorten. Radioautographic studies show a higher rate of turnover of endothelial cells overlying atherosclerotic lesions than cells in normal endothelium. Once telomere length shortens to a critical threshold, endothelial cells will no longer divide, a state known as *senescence*. Senescent endothelial cells have been found covering plaques, in autopsy studies of adults [39].

Endothelial senescence likely plays an important role in progression of disease but is unnecessary for the initiation of atheroma since fatty streaks can be found in the aortae and carotid arteries of healthy infants [19], before telomere attrition would reasonably occur. However, injury to the endothelium accelerates endothelial senescence and, therefore, may contribute to the development of carotid atherosclerosis in younger patients exposed, for example, to carotid balloon injury or neck irradiation. Progression of atherosclerosis, in the aged, is also associated with changes in sex hormones, in both men and women.

The prevalence and extent of atheromata is increased by cigarette-smoking [37], hypertension, diabetes, and specific genetic diseases [4]. In carotid atherosclerosis, cigarette-smoking has been shown to increase intralesional macrophage content, with an associated increase in intralesional inflammatory enzymes (i.e., macrophage-derived metalloelastase) which degrade vascular tissue.

Morphology

Atherosclerotic lesions have traditionally been analyzed in terms of histology; the progression of a plaque is commonly-rated according to its histological structure and composition [65]. In youth, atherosclerotic lesions are frequently composed of 'fatty streaks' [10]; the prevalence of such lesions plateaus after the first three or four decades of life, whereas raised plaques, more advanced forms of atherosclerosis, continue to accumulate until the end of life. An 'advanced' atherosclerotic lesion is commonly called either an 'atheroma', after the Greek words *athere*, for 'porridge', and *oma*, for tumor (referring to the swollen appearance of the lesion,) or a plaque, denoting its raised morphology (see discussion of atherosclerosis terminology below). A formal definition of an 'advanced' atherosclerotic lesions has been given as one in which in the layer of the blood vessel wall immediately adjacent to the vascular lumen, or *intima*, has become thickened and disorganized and the artery deformed [62]. Plaques are often associated with complications, on or immediately beneath the luminal surface, in the 'cap' of the lesion, such as fissures, ulcerations, and ruptures (*see below*). Deposits of hematoma, or intraplaque hemorrhage, and thrombosis may become incorporated into plaques as fibromuscular tissue [65].

The American Heart Association (AHA) proposed a formal system of histological classification, of early versus advanced atherosclerotic lesions, using a numerical nomenclature (see Fig. 1), and recommended the use of such classifications as "histological 'templates' for images of lesions... obtained with a variety of invasive and noninvasive techniques" [65].

The arrangement of lesion-types, from I to VIII, is intended to reflect the natural history of atherosclerosis and distinguishes lesions associated with adverse clinical manifestations (types IV–VIII) from lesions without such potential (types I–III) [62]. In what is generally-regarded as early forms of atherosclerosis (types I–III) [63], endothelial injury exposes the intima to deposition of a small amount of lipids, inciting a local inflammatory reaction populated by macrophages. In early-stage lesions endothelial integrity is usually intact, although, in animal models of aggressive atherosclerosis, it can be focally-disrupted, with platelets bound to exposed foam cells [12], [13]. The endothelium overlying lesions undergoes other changes, even at early stages, including a loss of alignment to blood flow, increase in stress fiber content, and an increased susceptibility to adherence by circulating leukocytes, thought to be due to increased endothelial expression of specific adherence molecules like vascular cell adhesion molecule-1 (VCAM-1).

Injury exposes the vessel wall to the deposition of circulating lipids. Infiltrating macrophages ingest the lipid deposits, becoming *foam cells*, and secrete growth factors and pro-inflammatory molecules (eg, matrix metalloproteinases, and possibly myeloperoxidase [38]) that perpetuate and amplify local inflammation, e.g., by oxidation products (see below). Initially, atheromata are no more than yellow dots (type I) on the vascular surface, composed of foam cells. As foam cell groups expand into layers (type II), sometimes visible as streaks, smooth muscle cells begin accumulating lipids, mostly cholesterol esters, though a surplus of lipid-free macrophages are present. Mast cells and T-lymphocytes also arrive, but in far fewer numbers. In 'pre-atheroma' (type III) lesions, lipid begins accumulating in small 'pools', outside of cells, but not to a large extent; and the lipids are of a different mixture than in prior stages, including more free cholesterol [60].

The term 'atheroma' is commonly used to refer to all advanced lesions (types IV–VIII) which are distinguished by (1) accumulations of lipid, cells, and/or matrix components, including minerals; (2) intimal disorganization, repair, and thickening; and (3) deformity of the arterial wall [62]. 'Atheroma' originally referred to the type IV lesion, which has a large 'core' of confluent extracellular lipid pools. **Type IV** atheromata expand by growth of the lipid core, but usually away from the lumen, so-called Glagovian expansion [20]. This type of lesion rarely occludes blood vessels [65]. The type IV atheroma has a normal '*cap*' – i.e., intimal tissue found between lesion and endothelium is normal [64]; though the cap can be relatively-thick, at characteristic arterial sites, as an adaption to mechanical forces, its composition is that of normal intimal tissue. Yet inflammatory macrophages are abundant, in the periphery of type IV atheromata. The

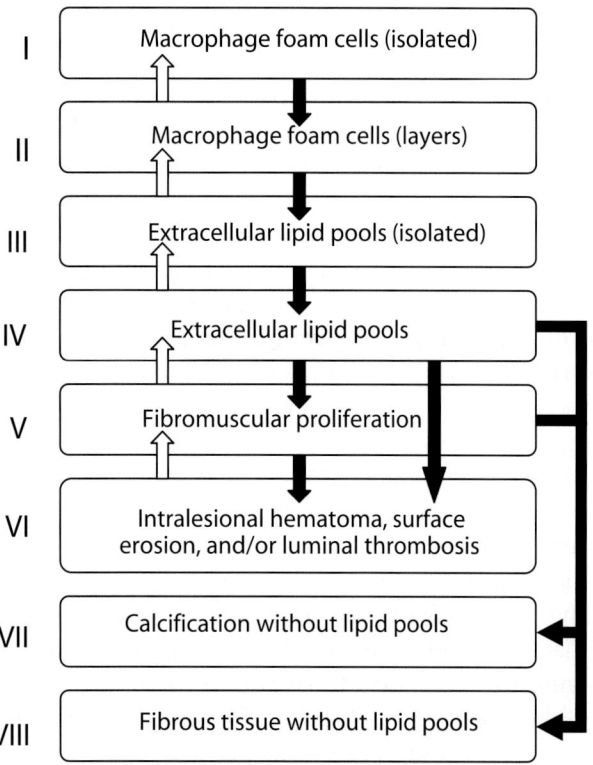

Fig. 1. An outline showing the AHA-recommended numerical classification of atherosclerotic lesions, with roman numerals and predominant histological characteristic(s). Arrows indicate possible changes in the histology of atherosclerotic lesion at different stages. Modified from [65].

integrity of the cap is important, since 'fissures', 'ulcerations', or 'ruptures' of the cap can provoke vascular thrombosis [74]. Thinning of the cap is also more frequent in symptomatic than in asymptomatic carotid plaques [5]. Having well-maintained caps, type IV atheromata are rarely associated with vascular events [65], unless type IV lesions become type VI lesions (see below). **Type V** lesions, once called 'fibroatheroma' are distinguished by an increased amount of smooth muscle cells, in the intima, and fibrous tissue, mostly notably in the cap, with persistence of a fatty lesion core. The fibromuscular tissue arises during repairs of intima from damage caused by the extracellular lipids or thrombotic deposits. The term 'plaque' was initially intended to denote the fibrous cap of type V lesions [62]; however, like 'atheroma', 'plaque' has become indiscriminately-used to refer to all types of advanced atherosclerotic lesions. Repeated repair episodes are the presumed cause of multi-layered (type V) lesions. As each new layer forms, the tough fibrous tissue of underlying plaque-layers forces the lesion to expand by growing into the lumen of the artery. The layer outside of the intima, the media, and the outermost vascular layer, the adventitia, both demonstrate changes, in composition, in type V lesions. For example, the smooth muscle cells are disorganized, in the media, and both the media and adventitia accumulate inflammatory cells, including macrophages, lymphocytes, and, sometimes, mast cells. The lipid pool may persist, in type V lesions, or be absent, though inflammatory cells persist regardless. For the first time, calcifications are sometimes seen. A **type VI**, or complicated, lesion is marked by the occurrence of (1) erosions or fissures on the surface of the lesion, whether superficial, involving only the endothelium, or deep, down to the lipid core; (2) hematoma, blood collections within the lesion, which may form by tears in the surface of the lesion and/or rupture of lesional microvessels formed during angiogenesis (see below) [1], [47]; and/or (3) thrombosis, on the surface of the lesion, which can be microscopic or grossly-visible [7]. Type VI is the lesion-type most often associated with clinical manifestations, including lethal ones [65]; hemorrhage-laden type VI lesions are likely to increase in volume, expand their necrotic lipid cores, and develop recurrent intralesional hemorrhages, from year to year [67]. As lesions become advanced, apoptotic cells begin accumulating, particularly around the necrotic lipid core [24], [27], [69]. In part, apoptotic cell-accumulation can be attributed to the increasing oxidative stress, in advanced lesions, which interferes with the phagocytosis and clearing functions of infiltrating macrophages [58].

As illustrated in Fig. 1, type VI lesions arise from lesions of either type IV or type V. A type VI lesion can worsen, leading to thrombotic occlusion of the carotid artery, or repair itself, becoming a type V lesion. Not all type VI lesions have acute consequences or will necessarily become clinically-manifest, nor are such lesions even uncommon in the arterial tree; for example, type VI lesions have been found in young adults [61] and in the aortae of 38% of adults below the age of 60 years [7]. Yet, in carotid atherosclerosis, plaque disruption is associated with symptomatic disease, even between lesions with similar degrees of stenosis [5].

Should the lipid core of a type IV–VI lesion regress, either calcification (**type VII**, or calcific, lesion) or fibrous tissue (**type VIII**, or fibrotic, lesion) will predominate, replacing normal intimal tissue [61]. Lastly, the histology of a specific atherosclerotic lesion most often varies, along its extent (e.g., a lesion may demonstrate type II features, in one area, and type V, in another); yet, in pathology, atherosclerotic lesions are classified according to the most advanced and clinically-significant intralesional histology present.

Causes of plaque 'vulnerability'

Acute vascular events associated with atheroma do not require exposure of thrombogenic substances, since thrombi may form on the surface of lesions with intact endothelium. The hypothesized etiology of thrombosis in such cases is a focal change in blood flow secondary to deformity of the vessel overlying a lesion. Thrombotic occlusion tended to occur at flow dividers and locations of arterial angulation [66], suggesting a role for shear stress in thrombosis or underlying intimal disruption and hematoma and a reason for the predilection of atherosclerosis at the carotid bifurcation [45]. Another factor in the development of a clinical event is the patients likelihood of forming a thrombus. This concept of 'vulnerable blood' (an integral component of the vulnerable patient), proposed by Naghavi et al. [42] suggests that some patients are more likely to form an obstructive thrombus following a triggering event.

In 1995, Stary et al. summarized evidence implicating numerous biological elements leading to disruption of the intima, particularly macrophages, which release proteolytic enzymes. This disruption can result in coronary spasm and structural weakness particularly in lesions with a high concentration of foam cells [48] and shear stress [20].

Immune components of atherosclerosis

There is a growing body of evidence linking inflammation and atherosclerosis [21]. Many reports [8], [30], [71], [3], [72], [26], [34], [40] have correlated inflammation in the cap and shoulder of the atherosclerotic lesion with plaque disruption and consequent acute thrombotic complications. The concentration of active inflammatory cells is higher in ruptured plaques than in asymptomatic carotid plaques, with similar degrees of stenosis, and carotid plaques with greater concentrations of foam cells are more likely to be symptomatic [5]. In the coronary arteries, plaques usually rupture at sites where the circumferential stress is high [48] and where the plaque has been weakened as a result of a local inflammatory reaction [40], [73]. The association between inflammation and the progression of atherosclerotic lesions, specifically in the carotid arteries, is supported by associations with serum markers [56].

Apart from inflammation within the cap, it has been proposed [30], [71], [30], [28] that adventitial inflammation and neovascularization contribute to plaque instability, by thinning the medial layer of coronary artery segments, with resultant 'compensatory enlargement'. Compensatory enlargement can be seen, teleologically, as a means of preserving the patency of the vessel lumen; yet disrupted plaques are found in areas of compensatory enlargement [20], [46], [75], [57]. Rupture of the internal elastic lamina, allowing expansion of the atherosclerotic process into the tunica media, is a recognized feature of complex atherosclerotic plaques [34], [31].

Inflammatory cells in the plaque secrete a variety of vascular growth factors, which promote the growth of *vasa vasorum* to meet the metabolic needs of the inflammatory cells [31], [41], [22] (see below).

In addition to macrophages, mast cells and T-lymphocytes [49] are present, in atherosclerotic lesions, but far less prevalent. Leukocytes which infiltrate the vessel wall at sites of inflammation and populate atherosclerotic lesions are drawn from the circulation. The recruitment of circulating leukocytes begins with a leukocyte responding to increased adhesion molecule expression on the endothelium. Different cellular adhesion molecules (CAMs) mediate this process, depending on the type of tissue and type of inflammation. Most notably, the endothelium expresses P- and E-selectin, the latter also being known endothelial-leukocyte adhesion molecule-1 (ELAM-1); the endothelial selectins interact with α4-integrin receptors on some leukocytes to cause the leukocyte tethering and rolling phenomenon. Well-characterized molecules which regulate adhesion include VCAM-1 and ICAM-1. Circulating forms of VCAM-1, ICAM-1 and E-selectin are present in plasma, for unknown reasons.

Other components of the immune system also have roles in atherosclerosis. Deposition of complement complexes, including C5b-9, increases, with progression of atherosclerotic lesions. Lipoproteins, including free cholesterol, that become trapped within the vessel wall are capable of activating complement pathways. Lipoproteins, particularly LDL, are modified by proteases and cholesteryl esterases when 'trapped' within the vessel wall. The modified lipoproteins activate complement pathways for the physiological purpose of recruiting innate immune responses to remove the trapped lipoproteins and bind C-reactive protein (CRP), from the circulation. CRP, which is made by the liver, regulates complement activation when bound to trapped lipids and, in the circulation, likely interferes with the reparative functions of endothelial progenitor cells [17].

Lastly, autoimmune cross-reactivity, between antigens of pathogens and homologous human antigens in the vascular wall (e.g., the 60 kDa heat shock protein of *Chlamydia pneumoniae*) may be another means of provoking immune-mediated atherosclerosis.

The redox balance

The accumulation of *oxidants* in atherosclerotic lesions damages the vascular wall by increasing lesion-inflammation, through lipid oxidation and production of toxic molecules, such as hydroxyl radicals ($\cdot$OH) and other 'reactive species' [59]. Others [76] have also proposed reductive stress, the excessive accumulation of molecular *reductants*, as another cause of vascular damage, particularly in association with diabetes.

Angiogenesis

Vasa vasorum feed the outer layers of blood vessels, which are too distant from the vascular lumen to receive nutrition by direct diffusion through the intima. Similar to other pathological conditions (most notably neoplastic tumor formation [25]) the *vasa vasorum* are stimulated to grow by the atheroma itself [22]. This *angiogenesis* is vital for the progression of atheromata [41]. As observed by Judah Folkman [16], it is an interesting fact that patients with Down Syndrome (trisomy 21) do not develop clinically-significant atherosclerosis, despite living to relatively-advanced ages [6]. This resistance to atherosclerosis may be attributable to the presence of three copies of a gene on chromosome 21, which provide Down Syndrome patients with high serum levels of endostatin [77], an inhibitor of angiogenesis. This observation suggests that a pathological form of angiogenesis plays a significant role in the progression of atherosclerosis.

Pathological angiogenesis yields a dense net of deformed and leaky microvessels, without any obvious organization [25]. Such *vasa* may allow erythrocytes, with lipid-rich plasma membranes to *extravasate* into atheromata [29]. Moreover, angiogenic microvessels, in atheromata, are weak and prone to rupture (i.e., the formation of type VI lesions) and are implicated in plaque instability [29], [1].

Endothelium regulates the migration of smooth muscle cells (SMCs), in normal angiogenesis [15]. As endothelial cells form a new lumen, SMCs migrate, according to a gradient of endothelial signals [55], [33], to surround the vessels and establish a mature vasculature. In dys-angiogenesis, a disarray of signal-gradients from endothelial cells may account for the disorganized migration of SMCs into the media and adventitia, as seen in type V lesions [18]. Similarly, migration of SMCs into the cap of plaques may represent a dys-angiogenic phenomenon, related to endothelial signaling.

The role of lymphatic function and lymphangiogenesis, in atherosclerosis, has rarely been studied [43]. Nakano et al. [43] presented evidence, in one of the rare studies, that lymphatic drainage from plaques may be poor. Lymphatic vessels are responsible for draining inflammatory cells; as such, impaired lymphatic function may directly amplify atherosclerotic inflammation. Indirectly, poor lymphatic function could hypothetically lead to the accumulation of interstitial fluid and proteins, which may further derange healing in the tissue microenvironment.

Thrombosis and blood elements in atherosclerosis

Circulating endothelial progenitor cells (EPCs) have a reparative role in vascular biology. In addition to the known hemostatic and thrombotic functions of platelets, studies now reveal a pro-inflammatory role for platelets in atherosclerosis. Platelets carry granules laden with immune-signaling molecules. When passing over endothelium overlying inflamed plaques, platelets are activated to release platelet microparticles (PMPs); PMPs, scattered over the endothelium, also secrete granular contents, including RANTES, or the 'regulated on activation normal T cell expressed and secreted' molecule. RANTES is detectable on the luminal surface of atherosclerotic human carotid arteries. RANTES, when scattered over the atherosclerotic endothelium, by platelets, promotes monocyte infiltration into the vascular wall. PMPs also express various adhesion molecules.

Though PMPs promote atheromatous inflammation, PMPs also contact hematopoietic stem-progenitor cells (HSPCs), which help repair the endothelium. HSPCs that contact platelets subsequently display PMP-derived molecules which enhance the adhesion of HSPCs to the endothelium, suggesting a mechanism for EPC homing, during endothelial regeneration.

Conclusions on carotid atherosclerosis

Carotid atherosclerosis is a chronic disease of the carotid arteries, with potentially-life threatening acute complications, particularly stroke. Atheromata can become clinically-evident either by the growth of the lesion within the vascular wall, until blood flow through the lumen is obstructed, and/or by provoking thrombo-emboli, with or without blood flow obstruction, by exposing the bloodstream to thrombogenic substances within the lesion.

In response to injury, inflammation may moderate the healing of the vessel wall, as in other tissues. In atherogenesis, the vascular healing process goes awry. Atheromata are made by insudates of inflammatory cells and inflammants, particularly lipids, and, in advanced lesions, by the hyperplasia of vascular tissue. Inflammatory cells and molecules are drawn into atherosclerotic lesions both through the intima and outer layers of the vessel wall. The internal microenvironment of the atheroma is a haywire network of cell signaling and a poisoned atmosphere, with oxidants which derange inflammatory and endothelial cells. Vascular inflammation can perpetuate itself, by stimulating the (mal)formation of new, incompetent *vasa vasorum* which spill inflammatory cells and substances into the lesion. If the vessel wall fails to heal, after decades, then the endothelium loses its capacity for further self-repair; such endothelial *senescence* opens the intimal door to tissue inflammants.

Yet not all carotid atheromata become clot-provoking lesions. Some resolve into silent fibrotic or calcific scars. The incidence and fate of nascent atheromata are determined at all levels, even beyond the plaque itself, reflecting a profile of the whole patient, from genetics, cellular events, and *blood biochemistry* [70], to patient diet and behavior. For example, the 'vulnerable patient' and the patient who is less or not vulnerable to a stroke may, theoretically, have identical plaques, but one patient is 'vulnerable' because his or her *blood* has a composition with a greater predisposition to clotting, when exposed thrombogenic factors within the plaque. As such, other non-imaging clinical tests, particularly serum analyses, will play a great role, in risk-stratifying patients with carotid atherosclerosis.

The character of the plaque is a key to distinguishing the vulnerable patient, as carotid symptoms and events are associated with specific plaque characteristics. The concentration of inflammation in the cap and rupture of malformed vessels frequently mark the 'vulnerable plaque'. Noninvasive imaging has begun to provide physicians with the ability to detect and measure the plaque features which precipitate carotid stroke, on anatomical and biochemical levels, as subsequent chapters will discuss.

Medical imaging of atherosclerosis by scintigraphy

In the past contrast angiography of the carotid and cerebral vessels was the norm to objectively evaluate the degree of carotid stenosis. Today less invasive approaches, such as duplex Doppler ultrasound and magnetic resonance angiography are routinely performed to determine the severity of carotid lesions. These techniques will be discussed in detail in subsequent chapters.

In addition to these anatomic techniques, nuclear medicine approaches are being developed to specifically identify and characterize plaques. The *in vivo* biodistribution of administered radiopharmaceuticals can be visualized by *scintigraphy*. Radiopharmaceuticals used in single photon emission computed tomography (SPECT) and positron emission tomography (PET) differ by the types of radioactivity emitted. Radiopharmaceuticals used in SPECT emit gamma rays, which are physically-identical to X-rays (X-rays and gamma rays only differ in how they are created). In PET, radiopharmaceuticals release positrons, which are the antimatter of electrons. A positron will travel a very short distance in tissue (typically 1–3 millimeters) before encountering an electron. The mass of the positron and electron is converted into pure energy (in a demonstration of Einstein's formula $E = mc^2$). The energy from this 'annihilation reaction' splits, forming two gamma rays traveling in opposite directions. In general, PET is superior to SPECT, in terms of the image detail, or spatial resolution, that is possible. The strength of the signal from PET radiopharmaceuticals is also better (i.e., improved sensitivity), because the gamma rays are of a much higher energy and do not get absorbed by the body as much as the lower-energy photons typically emitted by SPECT radiopharmaceuticals.

Nuclear imaging of atherosclerosis can be categorized as direct or indirect. Direct methods of imaging atherosclerosis involve scintigraphic visualization of radiolabeled biomolecules that can accumulate within atheroma [23]. Indirect methods have dominated myocardial and brain blood flow measurements by depicting the altered distribution of perfusion in the downstream tissue.

Since carotid endarterectomy (CEA) reduces the risk of stroke in symptomatic patients with a lesion causing a severe (>70%) stenosis [2], it is important to objectively evaluate the carotid vessels of patients with symptoms. The risks associated with CEA are not insignificant and the prevalence of surgical complications has likely been underestimated by even the most notable trials [52]. It is, of course, imperative, therefore, to identify patients with the most favorable risk:benefit ratio, before undertaking carotid surgery. Yet US is incapable of this task, in asymptomatic patients with severe carotid stenosis [11] and in symptomatic patients with moderate carotid stenosis [53]. Radiotracer techniques may have a role in the management of carotid artery disease, particularly if the images provide information on the vulnerability of an individual plaque to rupture.

Scintigraphic visualization of atherosclerotic elements: feasibility of nuclear imaging

Factors which hinder the ability of scintigraphy (including PET) to visualize activity within a carotid atheroma include (1) lesion size, (2) background activity, (3) biological flux or density of the specific target of a tracer, and (4) motion artifact.

Size

As of 2006, the overall spatial resolutions of state-of-the-art clinical PET and SPECT cameras are roughly 4- and 7-mm respectively. This fact might discourage one, at first, from attempting to detect a lesion within the thin walls of the vasculature. Yet the ability of scintigraphic cameras to detect lesions depends not only upon spatial resolution and contrast, as in X-ray computed tomography (CT), but also upon the intensity of the signal. If a particular radiotracer accumulates in a lesion, the lesion becomes a 'focus' of radioactivity, emitting rays like a star in the night sky. Though scintigraphy may not have the resolving capacity to separate the signal from two tiny, adjacent lesions, or *foci*, scintigraphy can detect the strength of the signal(s). Macrophages utilize circulating glucose as a substrate for metabolism. When positron emission tomography is performed with an intravenous injection of the radiolabeled glucose analog ^{18}F fluorodeoxyglucose (FDG), these lesions can be seen on the scan as foci of increased tracer concentration in the artery. For vascular lesions, which are much smaller than the spatial resolution of the scintigraphic cameras, the strength of the signal that is measured will actually be the average of the lesion signal-strength and any other activity nearby, a problem known as 'partial-volume averaging'. So, for example, if the activity in a millimeter-sized lesion is very high, but the background is very low, partial volume averaging will make the activity appear dimmer than it truly is. In atherosclerosis, however, the boundaries of vulnerable plaques can be defined by the extent of the pathogenetic milieu forming the plaque, upon which scintigraphy focuses, rather than the just the anatomy of the plaque itself, as imaged by other modalities. For example, atherosclerotic inflammation may involve the intima, perivascular adventitia or extend even into underlying tissues [30], [44]. Thus, in some cases, the pathobiological area of vulnerable plaques may actually approach the area required for accurate, quantitative imaging by scintigraphy.

The feasibility of scintigraphic detection of metabolic activity in carotid atheroma, despite such hurdles, has been validated by the work of Rudd et al. [54] who performed preoperative FDG PET imaging in patients scheduled for endarterectomy. The tracer concentration in the image was confirmed by lesion histopathology. Although no clinical study has yet validated the prognostic significance of any scintigraphic marker of atherosclerosis, prospective studies are in progress.

References

[1] Barger AC et al.: Hypothesis: vasa vasorum and neovascularization of human coronary arteries. A possible role in the pathophysiology of atherosclerosis. N Engl J Med 310: 175–177 (1984).

[2] Beneficial effect of carotid endarterectomy in symptomatic patients with high-grade carotid stenosis. North American Symptomatic Carotid Endarterectomy Trial Collaborators. N Engl J Med 325: 445–453 (1991).

[3] Boyle JJ: Association of coronary plaque rupture and atherosclerotic inflammation. J Pathol 181: 93–99 (1997).

[4] Cambien F: Coronary Heart Disease and Polymorphisms in Genes Affecting Lipid Metabolism and Inflammation. Curr Atheroscler Rep 7: 188–195 (2005).

[5] Carr S et al.: Atherosclerotic plaque rupture in symptomatic carotid artery stenosis. J Vasc Surg 23: 755–765; discussion 765–766 (1996).

[6] Chadefaux B et al.: Is absence of atheroma in Down syndrome due to decreased homocysteine levels? Lancet 2: 741 (1988).

[7] Chandler A, Pope J: Arterial thrombosis in atherogenesis: a survey of the frequency of incorporation of thrombi into atherosclerotic plaques., in Blood and Arterial Wall in Atherogenesis and Arterial Thrombosis (Hautvast J, Hermus R, Van der Haar F, eds). EJ Brill: Leiden, Netherlands. 112–118 (1975).

[8] de Boer OJ et al.: Leucocyte recruitment in rupture prone regions of lipid-rich plaques: a prominent role for neovascularization? Cardiovasc Res 41: 443–449 (1999).

[9] Easton JD: Chapter 349. Cerebrovascular Diseases. In: Harrison's Online (Kasper DL et al., eds) McGraw-Hill (2005).

[10] Eggen DA, Solberg LA: Variation of atherosclerosis with age. Lab Invest. 18: 571–579 (1968).

[11] Endarterectomy for asymptomatic carotid artery stenosis. Executive Committee for the Asymptomatic Carotid Atherosclerosis Study. JAMA 273: 1421–1428 (1995).

[12] Faggiotto A, Ross R, Harker L: Studies of hypercholesterolemia in the nonhuman primate. I. Changes that lead to fatty streak formation. Arteriosclerosis 4: 323–340 (1984).

[13] Faggiotto A, Ross R: Studies of hypercholesterolemia in the nonhuman primate. II. Fatty streak conversion to fibrous plaque. Arteriosclerosis 4: 341–356 (1984).

[14] Faxon DP et al.: Atherosclerotic Vascular Disease Conference: Writing Group III: pathophysiology. Circulation 109: 2617–2625 (2004).

[15] Folkman J, D'Amore PA: Blood vessel formation: what is its molecular basis? Cell 87: 1153–1155 (1996).

[16] Folkman J: Endogenous angiogenesis inhibitors. Apmis 112: 496–507 (2004).

[17] Fujii H, Li SH, Szmitko PE et al.: C-Reactive Protein Alters Antioxidant Defenses and Promotes Apoptosis in Endothelial Progenitor Cells. Arterioscler Thromb Vasc Biol (E-publ. on Aug. 24, 2006).

[18] Gargalovic PS, Imura M, Zhang B et al.: Identification of inflammatory gene modules based on variations of human endothelial cell responses to oxidized lipids. Proc Natl Acad Sci USA 103(34): 12741–12746 (2006).

[19] General findings of the International Atherosclerosis Project. Lab Invest 18: 498–502 (1968).

[20] Glagov S et al.: Compensatory enlargement of human atherosclerotic coronary arteries. N Engl J Med 316: 1371–1375 (1987).

[21] Hansson GK, Libby P: The immune response in atherosclerosis: a double-edged sword. Nat Rev Immunol. 6(7): 508–519 (2006).

[22] Inoue M et al.: Vascular endothelial growth factor (VEGF) expression in human coronary atherosclerotic lesions: possible pathophysiological significance of VEGF in progression of atherosclerosis. Circulation 98: 2108–2116 (1998).

[23] Isobe S, Tsimikas S, Zhou J et al.: Noninvasive imaging of atherosclerotic lesions in apolipoprotein E-deficient and low-density-lipoprotein receptor-deficient mice with annexin A5. J Nucl Med 47(9): 1497–1505 (2006).

[24] Isner JM et al.: Apoptosis in human atherosclerosis and restenosis. Circulation 91: 2703–2711 (1995).

[25] Jain RK: Molecular regulation of vessel maturation. 9: 685–693 (2003).
[26] Kaartinen M et al.: Mast cell infiltration in acute coronary syndromes: implications for plaque rupture. J Am Coll Cardiol 32: 606–612 (1998).
[27] Kockx MM et al.: Distribution of cell replication and apoptosis in atherosclerotic plaques of cholesterol-fed rabbits. Atherosclerosis 120: 115–124 (1996).
[28] Kohchi K et al.: Significance of adventitial inflammation of the coronary artery in patients with unstable angina: results at autopsy. Circulation 71: 709–716 (1985).
[29] Kolodgie FD et al.: Intraplaque hemorrhage and progression of coronary atheroma. N Engl J Med 349: 2316–2325 (2003).
[30] Laine P et al.: Association between myocardial infarction and the mast cells in the adventitia of the infarct-related coronary artery. Circulation 99: 361–369 (1999).
[31] Libby P et al.: Macrophages and atherosclerotic plaque stability. Curr Opin Lipidol 7: 330–335 (1996).
[32] Libby P: Inflammation in atherosclerosis. Nature 420: 868–874 (2002).
[33] Liu Y et al.: Edg-1, the G protein-coupled receptor for sphingosine-1-phosphate, is essential for vascular maturation. J Clin Invest 106: 951–961 (2000).
[34] Mach F et al.: Reduction of atherosclerosis in mice by inhibition of CD40 signalling. Nature 394: 200–203 (1998).
[35] Madamanchi NR Vendrov A, Runge MS: Oxidative stress and vascular disease. Arterioscler Thromb Vasc Biol 25: 29–38 (2005).
[36] McGill HC Jr et al.: Association of Coronary Heart Disease Risk Factors with microscopic qualities of coronary atherosclerosis in youth. Circulation 102: 374–379 (2000).
[37] McGill HC Jr et al.: Effects of nonlipid risk factors on atherosclerosis in youth with a favorable lipoprotein profile. Circulation 103: 1546–1550 (2001).
[38] McMillen TS, Heinecke JW, Leboeuf RC: Expression of Human Myeloperoxidase by Macrophages Promotes Atherosclerosis in Mice. Circulation 11: 2798–2804 (2005).
[39] Minamino T et al.: Endothelial cell senescence in human atherosclerosis: role of telomere in endothelial dysfunction. Circulation 105: 1541–1544 (2002).
[40] Moreno PR et al.: Macrophage infiltration in acute coronary syndromes. Implications for plaque rupture. Circulation 90: 775–778 (1994).
[41] Moulton KS et al.: Inhibition of plaque neovascularization reduces macrophage accumulation and progression of advanced atherosclerosis. Proc Natl Acad Sci USA 100: 4736–4741 (2003).
[42] Naghavi M et al.: From vulnerable plaque to vulnerable patient: a call for new definitions and risk assessment strategies: Part II. Circulation 108: 1772–1778 (2003).
[43] Nakano T et al.: Angiogenesis and lymphangiogenesis and expression of lymphangiogenic factors in the atherosclerotic intima of human coronary arteries. Human Pathology 36: 330–340 (2005).
[44] Okamoto E et al.: Perivascular inflammation after balloon angioplasty of porcine coronary arteries. Circulation 104: 2228–2235 (2001).
[45] Orr AW, Ginsberg MH, Shattil SJ et al.: Matrix-specific Suppression of Integrin Activation in Shear Stress Signaling. Mol Biol Cell (E-publ. on Aug. 23, 2006).
[46] Pasterkamp G et al.: Relation of arterial geometry to luminal narrowing and histologic markers for plaque vulnerability: the remodeling paradox. J Am Coll Cardiol 32: 655–662 (1998).
[47] Paterson J: Vascularization and hemorrhage of the intima of arteriosclerotic coronary arteries. Arch Pathol 22: 313–324 (1936).
[48] Richardson PD, Davies MJ, Born GV: Influence of plaque configuration and stress distribution on fissuring of coronary atherosclerotic plaques. Lancet 2: 941–944 (1989).
[49] Robertson AK, Hansson GK: T Cells in Atherogenesis. For Better or For Worse? Arterioscler Thromb Vasc Biol (E-publ. on Sept. 14, 2006).
[50] Ross R, Glomset JA: The pathogenesis of atherosclerosis (second of two parts). N Engl J Med 295: 420–459 (1976).
[51] Ross R: The pathogenesis of atherosclerosis: a perspective for the 1990s. Nature 362: 801–809 (1993).
[52] Rothwell PM, Goldstein LB: Carotid Endarterectomy for Asymptomatic Carotid Stenosis: Asymptomatic Carotid Surgery Trial. Stroke 35: 2425–2427 (2004).
[53] Rothwell PM et al.: Endarterectomy for symptomatic carotid stenosis in relation to clinical subgroups and timing of surgery. Lancet 363: 915–924 (2004).
[54] Rudd JH et al.: Imaging atherosclerotic plaque inflammation with [18F]-fluorodeoxyglucose positron emission tomography. Circulation 105: 2708–2711 (2002).
[55] Sato TN: A new role of lipid receptors in vascular and cardiac morphogenesis. J Clin Invest 106: 939–940 (2000).
[56] Schillinger M et al.: Inflammation and Carotid Artery—Risk for Atherosclerosis Study (ICARAS). Circulation 111: 2203–2209 (2005).
[57] Schoenhagen P et al.: Extent and Direction of Arterial Remodeling in Stable Versus Unstable Coronary Syndromes: An Intravascular Ultrasound Study. Circulation 101: 598–603 (2000).
[58] Schrijvers DM et al.: Phagocytosis of Apoptotic Cells by Macrophages Is Impaired in Atherosclerosis. Arterioscler Thromb Vasc Biol 25: 1256–1261 (2005).

[59] Schulze PC, Lee RT: Oxidative stress and atherosclerosis. Curr Atheroscler Rep 7: 242–248 (2005).
[60] Small DM: George Lyman Duff memorial lecture. Progression and regression of atherosclerotic lesions. Insights from lipid physical biochemistry. Arteriosclerosis 8: 103–129 (1988).
[61] Stary H: Atlas of Atherosclerosis Progression and Regression. 1999, New York/London: Parthenon Publishing.
[62] Stary HC et al.: A definition of advanced types of atherosclerotic lesions and a histological classification of atherosclerosis. A report from the Committee on Vascular Lesions of the Council on Arteriosclerosis, American Heart Association. Circulation 92: 1355–1374 (1995).
[63] Stary HC et al.: A definition of initial, fatty streak, and intermediate lesions of atherosclerosis. A report from the Committee on Vascular Lesions of the Council on Arteriosclerosis, American Heart Association. Circulation 89: 2462–2478 (1994).
[64] Stary HC et al.: A definition of the intima of human arteries and of its atherosclerosis-prone regions. A report from the Committee on Vascular Lesions of the Council on Arteriosclerosis, American Heart Association. Arterioscler Thromb 12: 120–134 (1992).
[65] Stary HC: Natural history and histological classification of atherosclerotic lesions: an update. Arterioscler Thromb Vasc Biol 20: 1177–1178 (2000).
[66] Taeymans Y et al.: Quantitative angiographic morphology of the coronary artery lesions at risk of thrombotic occlusion. Circulation 85: 78–85 (1992).
[67] Takaya N et al.: Presence of Intraplaque Hemorrhage Stimulates Progression of Carotid Atherosclerotic Plaques. A High-Resolution Magnetic Resonance Imaging Study. Circulation 111: 2768–2775 (2005).
[68] Tardif JC, Heinonen T, Orloff D, Libby P: Vascular biomarkers and surrogates in cardiovascular disease. Circulation 113(25): 2936–2942 (2006).
[69] Tedgui A, Mallat Z: Apoptosis as a determinant of atherothrombosis. Thromb Haemost, 86: 420–426 (2001).
[70] Tivesten A, Hulthe J, Wallenfeldt K et al.: Circulating Estradiol is an Independent Predictor of Progression of Carotid Artery Intima-Media Thickness in Middle-Aged Men. J Clin Endocrinol Metab (E-publ.on Aug. 29, 2006).
[71] van der Wal AC, Becker AE, Das PK: Medial thinning and atherosclerosis—evidence for involvement of a local inflammatory effect. Atherosclerosis 103: 55–64 (1993).
[72] van der Wal AC et al.: Recent activation of the plaque immune response in coronary lesions underlying acute coronary syndromes. Heart 80: 14–18 (1998).
[73] van der Wal AC et al.: Site of intimal rupture or erosion of thrombosed coronary atherosclerotic plaques is characterized by an inflammatory process irrespective of the dominant plaque morphology. Circulation 89: 36–44 (1994).
[74] Virmani R et al.: Lessons from sudden coronary death: a comprehensive morphological classification scheme for atherosclerotic lesions. Arterioscler Thromb Vasc Biol 20: 1262–1275 (2000).
[75] von Birgelen C et al.: Size of emptied plaque cavity following spontaneous rupture is related to coronary dimensions, not to the degree of lumen narrowing. A study with intravascular ultrasound in vivo. Heart 84: 483–488 (2000).
[76] Williamson JR, Kilo C, Ido Y: The role of cytosolic reductive stress in oxidant formation and diabetic complications. Diabetes Res Clin Pract 45: 81–82 (1999).
[77] Zorick TS et al.: High serum endostatin levels in Down syndrome: implications for improved treatment and prevention of solid tumours. Eur J Hum Genet 9: 811–814 (2001).

Chapter 1.2

CORRELATION OF CAROTID ARTERY PATHOLOGY AND MORPHOLOGY IN IMAGING

W. S. Kerwin

Department of Radiology, University of Washington, Seattle, USA

Introduction

The carotid artery is the dominant imaging target for non-invasive assessment of vessel wall morphology in atherosclerotic disease. In part, this arises from the clinical importance of the carotid artery in stroke prevention. Stroke is the third leading cause of death worldwide [45] and carotid atherosclerosis is thought to be the leading cause of embolic stroke. Additionally, stroke survival, estimated at greater than 75% in the United States [5], results in a massive disability burden costing billions of dollars per year. Surgical revisions of the carotid artery are the most common procedure for any vascular territory outside of the coronary arteries. In the United States alone, some 140,000 carotid endarterectomies are performed annually to remove the diseased neointimal layers of the artery. Clearly, diagnostic procedures affecting the treatment of carotid atherosclerosis can have a profound effect on patient survival, quality of life, and healthcare costs.

Additionally, several issues of expedience have contributed to the rise of the carotid artery as an imaging target for assessing vessel wall morphology. First, the relatively large size of the carotid artery, its proximity to the skin surface, and its isolation from rapidly moving structures, such as the heart, greatly simplifies the imaging procedure. Second, the site of the disease at the point where the common carotid artery bifurcates into internal and external carotid arteries is highly predictable. Third, the frequency of elective CEA permits histological validation of pre-surgery imaging results. Thus, the carotid artery serves as a logical test bed for imaging procedures that may ultimately have applicability in other vessels, notably the coronary arteries.

The purpose of this chapter is to establish the important pathological targets for imaging the carotid artery wall and summarize the state of the art of in vivo imaging techniques for these targets. To understand the implications of these results, it is important to understand the range of applications of the techniques, which go beyond diagnostics alone. Once these applications have been summarized, the chapter will address the specific pathology of lesion progression appropriate for imaging. The demonstrated capabilities of various established and emerging techniques for imaging carotid wall pathology are then presented. Finally, the use of these techniques in several clinical trials is reviewed.

Applications of carotid wall imaging

Establishing new clinical guidelines

The fundamental goal in carotid wall imaging is to provide better risk stratification for patients with advanced carotid atherosclerosis. Currently stroke risk secondary to carotid atherosclerosis is assessed via stenosis measurements and patient symptoms. Studies such as the European Carotid Surgery Trial [19], North American Symptomatic Carotid Endarterectomy Trial [53] and Asymptomatic Carotid Atherosclerosis Study [1] have all demonstrated an increased risk of stroke in subjects with increasing carotid stenosis. These studies demonstrated a reduction in stroke risk as a result of CEA for subjects with >60% stenosis and no neurological symptoms, and for subjects with >50% stenosis and recent transient ischemic attacks or amaurosis fugax [6], [57]. These cutoff values for stenosis in asymptomatic and symptomatic carotid disease have been adopted as guidelines indicating the need for CEA.

The guidelines, however, remain controversial and actual patient selection varies by practice. The clinical benefit of CEA is also highly dependent on the surgeon's rate of complications, dropping by 20–30% for each 2% rise in the rate of complications [4], [24]. For asymptomatic patients, CEA is only recommended if performed by surgeons having individual rates of morbidity/mortality less than 3% [22]. Furthermore, a combined analysis of the results from several clinical trials indicates that the number of surgeries necessary to prevent a single stroke within two years after CEA ranges from 8 to 83, depending on patient symptoms and the degree of luminal stenosis [24]. Finally, by some estimates, 10% of all endarterectomies are performed for inappropriate reasons [27]. These data suggest that the ability to stratify risk within the group of patients having high-grade stenosis could eliminate unnecessary surgeries.

On the other hand, patients with stenosis near 50% who do not meet the guidelines for surgery face the knowledge that they have a five year stroke risk approaching 5% [19]. These subjects are not candidates for surgical intervention because complication rates equal or exceed the stroke risk. These individuals would benefit from diagnostic techniques that identify subgroups with elevated risk of stroke.

Finally, the emergence of stenting as a viable alternative to CEA has opened the door to new risk factors in clinical decisions. Currently, stenting is widely accepted for patients considered high-risk surgical candidates [77]. Amongst all patients with high-grade stenosis, however, the relative performance of stenting versus CEA is uncertain. In all likelihood, certain subgroups will respond better to one procedure or another.

The logical target for identifying patients with significant stenosis who nevertheless have low-risk plaques, patients with moderate stenosis and high-risk plaques, or patients who would benefit from stenting is the atherosclerotic lesion itself. In this case, the goal is to identify the features of plaque morphology that lead to higher risk of stroke. Lesions exhibiting high-risk features are conceptually referred to as "vulnerable plaque" [67].

Systemic disease evaluation

The accessibility of the carotid artery for imaging has led to an additional goal in the assessment of carotid wall morphology. The carotid artery may offer a snapshot of the state of atherosclerotic disease throughout the body. For example, morphological features of a carotid lesion may correlate with the existence of high-risk lesions in the coronary arteries. Systemic treatment could thus be indicated by local features. Conceptually, this represents the transition from the idea of vulnerable plaque to a "vulnerable patient" [52].

An important consideration in assessing the systemic implications of carotid wall morphology is that some features of the vulnerable plaque may not translate to plaque vulnerability elsewhere in the body. The goal in this case is to identify the specific features of carotid disease that do.

Natural history and clinical trials

A third goal in assessing carotid morphology by imaging is to serially monitor changes in the disease. Much of the natural history of atherosclerotic lesions has been pieced together from autopsy specimens. Culprit lesions implicated in stroke and heart attack have been examined to determine the probable features of plaques that precipitate thrombosis and embolization. Additionally, lesions of different apparent ages have been pieced together into hypothesized pathways of progression. Without the ability to image individual plaques non-invasively, however, these pathways and features of culprit lesion have not been evaluated prospectively.

Some additional evidence has been provided by animal models of atherosclerosis. After genetic modification, arterial injury, or diet modification, numerous animal models develop lesions similar to human atherosclerosis. Given the controlled timelines involved in animal experiments, animal models have been used to better delineate the sequence of events in human disease. However, animal models generally develop lesions that differ from human lesions in many aspects. Additionally, histological study of animal lesions precludes serial studies of lesions within the same animal.

Non-invasive, serial imaging provides the unique opportunity to use both human and animal subjects to test theories of progression or therapeutic effects on plaque prospectively. In this case, the goal is to identify a given feature of interest relevant to the study or trial. For example, a lipid-lowering drug might be evaluated in terms of its effect on plaque lipid content. The ability to image human carotid plaque morphology makes this artery an attractive target for such studies.

Carotid plaque pathology

Early lesions

The normal carotid artery consists of three layers, the intima, media, and adventitia. The intima is the layer adjacent to the lumen and in humans consists of smooth muscle cells, proteoglycan-rich extracellular matrix, and a layer of endothelial cells lining the lumen surface. The next layer, the media, is separated from the intima by the internal elastic lamina and is composed of multiple bands of elastin interspersed with smooth muscle cells. Between the media and adventitia is another thick band of elastic called the external elastic lamina. The adventitia covers the outer surface of the vessel and provides thin strands of connective tissue to anchor the artery to surrounding structures. Under normal conditions the adventitia contains the vaso vasorum, the small blood vessels that supply blood to the artery wall, smooth muscle cells and macrophages.

Initiation of the carotid atherosclerotic plaque begins with adaptive intimal thickening and development of fatty streaks in the intima. These nascent lesions consist of lipid-containing macrophages called foam cells, smooth muscle cells, and lymphocytes. Lipid, in early lesions is distributed in the extracellular matrix with foci of fat-filled macrophages and smooth muscle cells. Such lesions correspond to the type I and II lesions in coronary arteries [9].

In general, the first lesions that are clearly identifiable by non-invasive imaging are the type III lesions that have extracellular lipid pools below layers of foam cells. From an imaging perspective, these lesions are of most interest for investigating the natural history of the disease, or the therapeutic response of early lesions. Imaging may also serve as a screening tool to identify appropriate subjects for aggressive, early therapy.

Advanced lesions

Type IV, V, and VI lesions are characterized by the appearance of a fibrous cap separating the lipid/necrotic core of the plaque from the lumen. Type IV and V lesions are distinguished by the transition of the fibrous cap from one consisting primarily of proteoglycan and smooth muscle cells into a thicker collagen-rich cap in the latter type. Type VI lesions (Fig. 1) are characterized by disruption of the plaque leading to fibrous cap rupture, intraplaque hemorrhage, and/or luminal thrombi. Type VII lesions are predominately calcified, and Type VIII lesions consist of thickened, reparative fibrous connective tissue with an absence of necrotic cores or calcifications [10]. Lesions Type IV thru VI are of considerable importance in imaging with the goal of identifying them prior to clinical events.

Vulnerable lesions

Diagnostic imaging of carotid artery walls seeks to identify features of the "vulnerable plaque". Vulnerable plaque is defined as an atherosclerotic lesion that poses increased risk of causing thrombo-embolic events. Histological studies in various vascular beds have established that plaque tissue composition and distribution may strongly influence its clinical course. For example, a thin fibrous cap covering a large lipid-rich necrotic core appears to be a clear marker of vulnerable plaque. The thinning fibrous cap indicates weakened structural integrity and possible future rupture leading to an embolic event. Furthermore, in a landmark study based on coronary autopsy specimens, ruptured fibrous cap, calcium nodules and endothelial erosion were highly associated with sudden cardiac death [67].

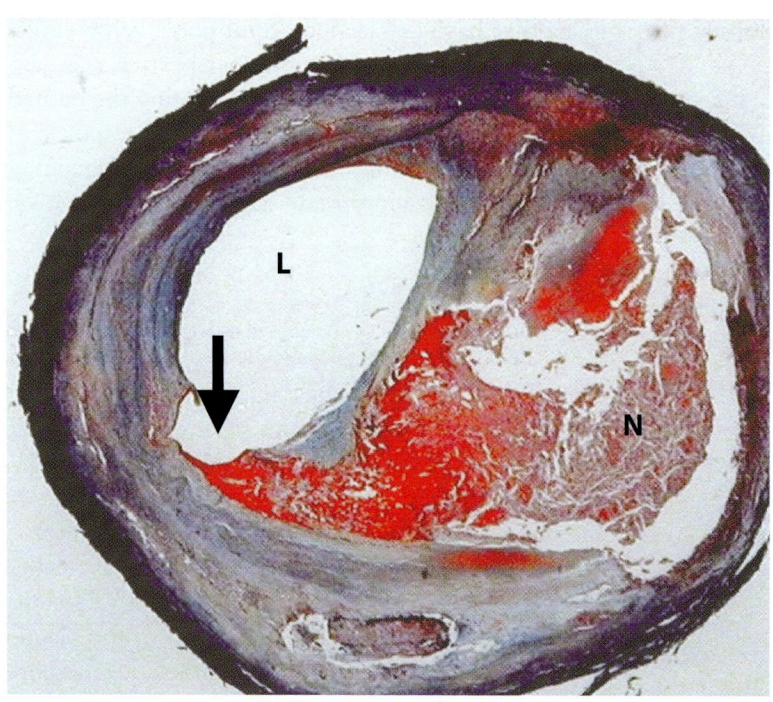

Fig. 1. Cross-section of a type VI plaque specimen from carotid endarterectomy stained with Movat's pentachrome. A rupture (arrow) of the blue fibrous cap has occurred exposing the thrombogenic lipid-rich necrotic core (N) to the lumen (L). Resultant intraplaque hemorrhage appears red.

Studies of the carotid arteries have confirmed that similar plaque features lead to brain ischemic symptoms. Specifically, thinned and ruptured fibrous caps are significantly more common in patients with symptomatic carotid arteries [11]. Other features of carotid plaques associated with patient symptoms are ulceration, luminal thrombus in conjunction with ulceration, the presence of large neovessels, and foam cell infiltration into the fibrous cap [20], [47], [11].

Experimental results in imaging

Ultrasound

Because the carotid bifurcation lies close to the surface of the neck, without overlying bony structures or air spaces, trans-cutaneous B-mode ultrasound has been a very effective tool for evaluating carotid disease. Aside from the utility of Doppler ultrasound to measure carotid stenosis, B-mode ultrasound provides detailed information regarding carotid wall morphology (Fig. 2).

A leading application of carotid ultrasound is the measurement of intima-media thickness (IMT).

As shown in Fig. 2, distinct echoes occur at the boundaries between the lumen and intima and between the media and adventitia. The average distance between these echoes is the IMT, which serves as a measurement of the degree of diffuse intimal thickening. By comparing the distance between these lines to various histological measurements in the aorta and carotid arteries, Pignoli et al. [56] demonstrated that this distance did correspond to the combined thickness of the intima and media. Further evaluations showed that this measurement could be made accurately at the far wall [74] and that IMT does appear to represent atherosclerosis as opposed to a general response to changes in shear and tensile stress [7].

Also evident in Fig. 2 is a significant plaque distal to the region where IMT is measured. Such plaques range in appearance from echolucent to hyperechoic which has led to efforts to characterize plaque composition based on echogenicity. These studies have divided echogenicity into two [30], four [25], or six [60] subjective categories as well as investigating direct measures of echogenicity [65], [71]. Comparisons of echogenicity to histological samples has generally found that echolucent plaques are

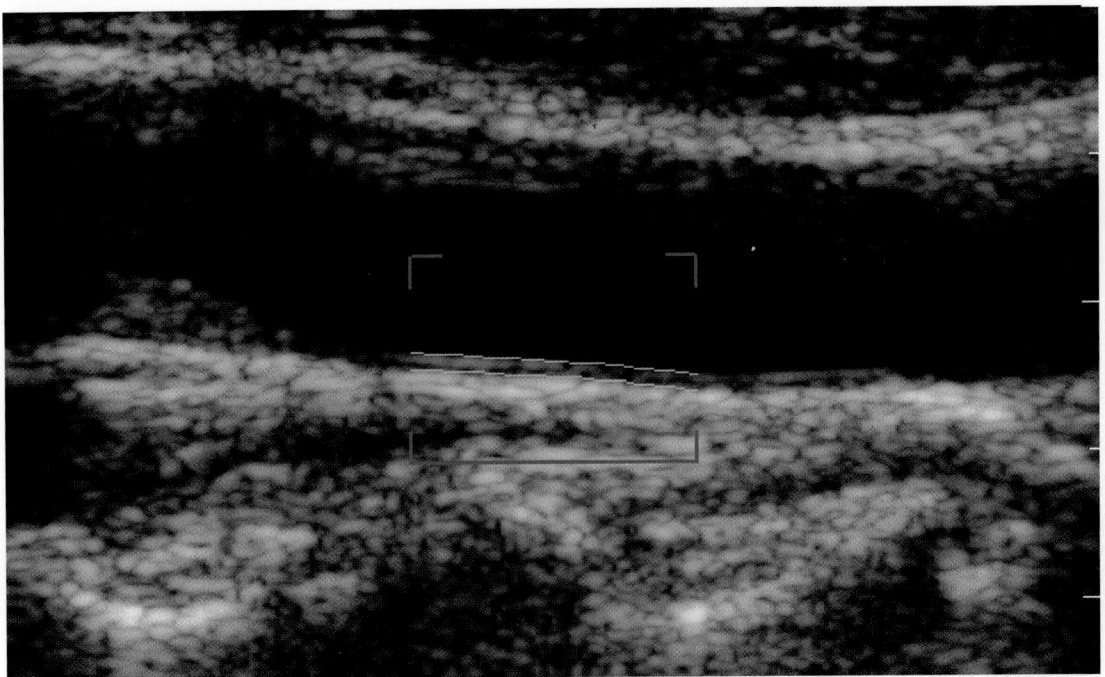

Fig. 2. Longitudinal B-mode ultrasound image of a carotid artery with a large atherosclerotic plaque (arrow) and demonstrating intima-media thickness (IMT) measurement. A region (box) of the common carotid artery proximal to the plaque is selected and echoes corresponding to the intimal and medial boundaries are detected (lines). The average distance between these lines is IMT.

likely to contain intraplaque hemorrhage and other soft plaque materials. Wilhjelm et al. [71] further showed that the mean gray scale value of the plaque by B-mode ultrasound is significantly correlated with decreasing amounts of soft plaque materials ($r = -0.42$). Hatsukmai et al. [30] demonstrated that the echolucent region could be localized within the plaque to identify the quadrant containing the soft plaque features. This study also found a prevalence of speckled calcification and foam cells in echolucent regions in addition to intraplaque hemorrhage and necrosis.

Hyperechoic regions in carotid plaques are associated with fibrous tissue. In a recent study, the thickness of the hyperechoic plaque region adjacent to the lumen was shown to agree well with histologically measured cap thickness [17].

B-mode ultrasound is attractive because the imaging procedure is relatively simple. However, B-mode ultrasound provides limited view angles for imaging plaques. Furthermore, plaque appearance can vary with the view angle and calcifications can cause shadow artifacts that obscure deeper plaque structures [54]. To some extent, these limitations are addressed by 3D imaging techniques [78], [61].

CT

X-ray computed tomography (CT) is another effective technology for visualizing plaque morphology. In CT angiograms used to measure carotid stenosis clinically, calcifications are clearly visible (Fig. 3). The presence of high density regions within the carotid wall has been definitively linked to calcifications. Furthermore, the amount of calcification visible by CT has been shown to correlate with the percent stenosis in the carotid [48] and with reduced inflammatory content of the vessel wall [62].

In addition to being sensitive to calcified content, CT has also shown promise for identifying other components within carotid plaque. Walker et al. [69] showed that decreasing tissue density was associated with increasing plaque lipid content. Fi-

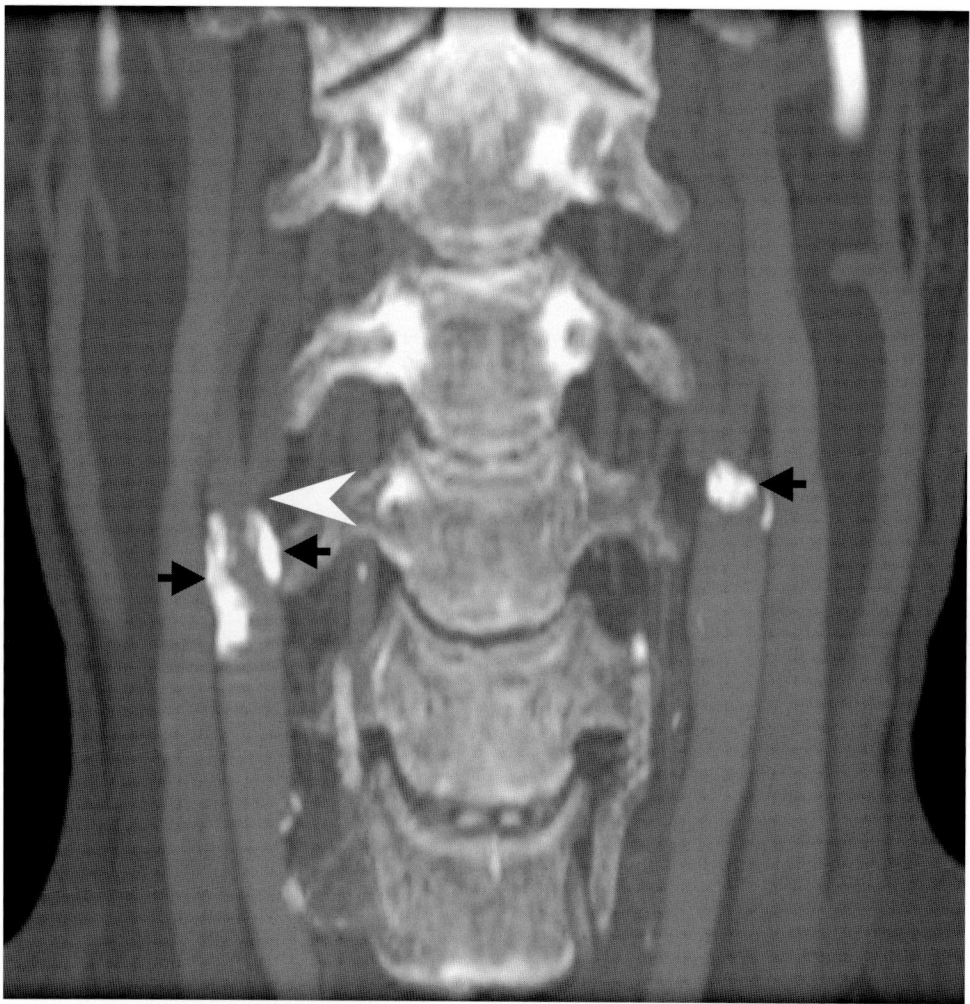

Fig. 3. Maximum intensity projection (MIP) X-ray Computed Tomography image of the carotid vasculature showing large areas of calcification (arrows) in the left and right carotid arteries. A significant stenosis of the right carotid artery is indicated by an arrowhead.

brous plaques have been shown to yield densities similar to soft tissues [54].

An important advantage of CT is its ability to yield absolute measures of tissue densities in terms of Hounsfield units. This permits consistent thresholds to be defined for characterizing plaque content. Disadvantages of CT include the use of ionizing radiation and nephrotoxic contrast agents.

MRI

Magnetic resonance imaging (MRI) has been most thoroughly investigated for its ability to characterize plaque morphology. MRI is uniquely able to tune the acquisition to increase sensitivity to specific physical characteristics of the tissue. Images can be specifically weighted to highlight regional proton density, magnetic relaxation time constants T1 and T2, flowing blood, or uptake of injected contrast agents. Images with each of these contrast weightings are analyzed together to provide a comprehensive picture of plaque composition (Fig. 4).

The use of black-blood imaging techniques, particularly T1-weighted double inversion recovery techniques, allows clear delineation of the vessel wall boundaries (inner and outer) in cross-sectional images of the carotid. The areas of individual slices can

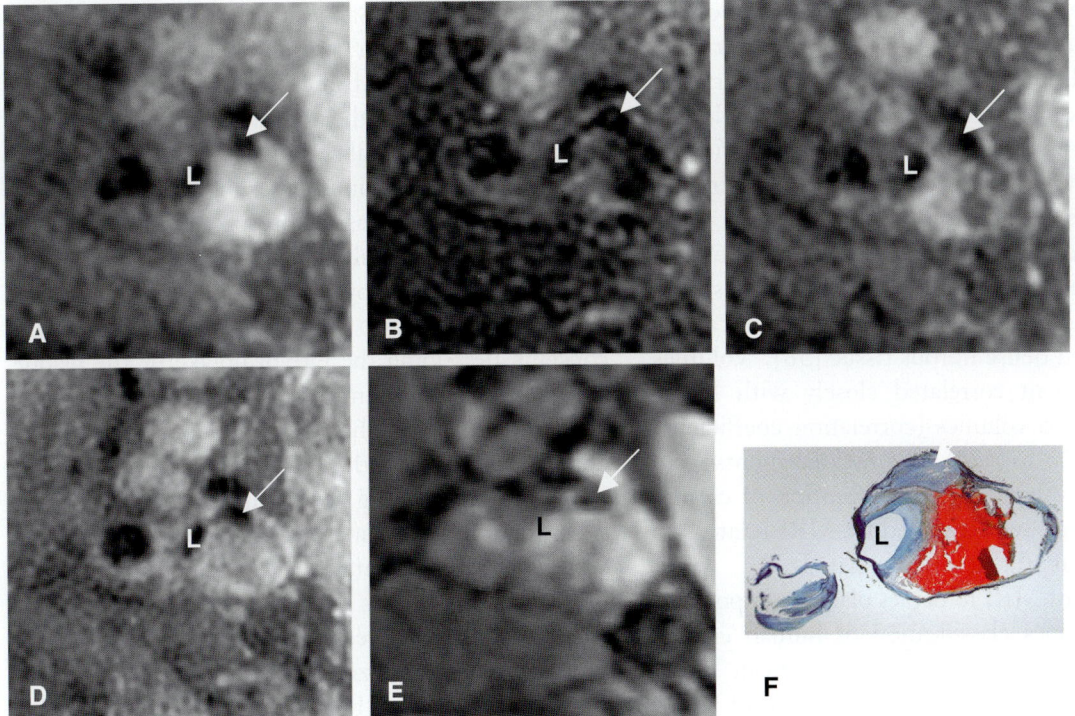

Fig. 4. Axial, multiple-contrast-weighting magnetic resonance images of an atherosclerotic carotid artery distal to the bifurcation with corresponding histology. Images are **a** T1-weighted, **b** T2-weighted, **c** proton-density-weighted, **d** contrast-enhanced T1-weighted, **e** time-of-flight, **f** histology stained with Movat's pentachrome. The lumen of the internal carotid artery is indicated by an "L" and a region of calcification is indicated by an arrow. The large hemorrhagic core (red) leads to bright signal on T1-weighted and time-of-flight images.

be combined into a total wall volume using Simpson's rule. This wall volume has been shown to correlate with plaque volume measured ex vivo with a correlation coefficient of 0.92 [44]. Additionally, this measurement is highly reproducible, with an error standard deviation under 6% [35].

Besides the ability of MRI to depict vessel boundaries, it is also able to depict substructures of the plaque. Using a bright-blood, 3D-time-of-flight imaging technique, Hatsukami et al. [31] showed that a hypointense band adjacent to the lumen indicates a thick (>0.25 mm) fibrous cap and that communication of a bright plaque interior with the lumen is indicative of a fibrous cap rupture. Agreement between the MR findings and histological state of the fibrous cap showed a Kappa value of 0.83. The addition of information from black-blood sequences to the fibrous cap evaluation was further shown to aid in discriminating juxtaluminal calcification and flow artifacts [49]. By comparing MRI findings to histology, this study showed a sensitivity of 0.81 and a specificity of 0.90 for identifying an unstable cap in vivo

MRI is also able to detect the soft plaque components underlying the fibrous cap by their unique combinations of intensities under different contrast weightings. Especially apparent by MRI is a high signal on T1-weighted imaging corresponding to soft plaque components (necoritc core or hemorrhage), which can be identified with a sensitivity of 85% and a specificity of 92% [80]. Hyperintensity is especially apparent in the event of intraplaque hemorrhage, which led to the development of direct thrombus imaging [50]. Chu et al. [12] showed that subsequent breakdown of the hemorrhage components leads to characteristic changes in signal intensity that allow hemorrhage to be classified as fresh, recent, or old. Comparison with histology showed that these stages could be identified with a Cohen's Kappa equal to 0.7. In another study, hemorrhage was subdivided into cases where the hemorrhage did, or did not directly communicate with the lumen [34]. Direct communication implies a disruption of the fibrous cap and was differentiated from intraplaque hemorrhage with an accuracy of 96%.

MRI is also capable of quantifying components of the plaque. In a recent study, carotid plaques were divided into regions of necrotic core, calcification, loose matrix, and dense fibrous tissue [58]. Volumes of each component correlated closely with histologically measured volumes (correlation coefficients ranging from 0.55 to 0.74). The measurements were statistically equivalent with the exception of calcification, which was overestimated by MRI relative to histology, but was still closely correlated.

The ability of MRI to depict plaque composition in vivo also enables classification of human carotid atherosclerotic plaque according to American Heart Association (AHA) classifications. In a recent study, cross sectional images were classified into types I/II, III, IV/V, VI, VII, and VIII. With the exception of types I/II and VIII, which were under-represented in the study, all classifications predicted histological classifications with sensitivities and specificities exceeding 80%. For all classifications, MRI and histology showed good agreement, with Cohen's $\kappa = 0.74$ [10].

Further delineation of plaque composition may be facilitated by contrast enhanced (CE) MRI using gadolinium-based contrast agents. In parallel investigations, Yuan et al. and Wasserman et al. showed that comparison of pre- and post-CE MRI improves differentiation of necrotic core from fibrous tissue [81], [70]. In the latter study, CE MRI helped discriminate fibrous cap from lipid core with a contrast-to-noise ratio as good as or better than that with T2-weighted images but with approximately twice the SNR. These findings provide quantitative evidence that CE MRI is a viable tool for in vivo study of atherosclerosis and can be used in combination with other contrast weightings to identify plaque composition.

Gadolinium-enhanced MRI also provides information regarding plaque inflammatory characteristics, including in-growth of neovasculature and macrophages. In a kinetic analysis of dynamic CE MRI from 16 subjects with carotid atherosclerosis, Kerwin et al. [40] compared the fractional blood volume measured by MRI to the area of neovasculature in corresponding histological specimens. A correlation coefficient of 0.80 was found suggesting that dynamic CE MRI provides a means for prospectively studying the link between neovasculature, inflammation, and plaque vulnerability. In a follow-on study, plaque macrophage content was shown to be associated with the transfer constant, describing the rate of uptake by the plaque. A correlation coefficient of 0.76 was observed [41].

Although MRI has tremendous capabilities for characterizing carotid plaque, most information is derived by combining several images, with different contrast weightings or from time-series images. The complexity of the data is the biggest limitation for MRI, and it requires specialized analysis tools and streamlined procedures for image review. To assist in the analysis, specialized algorithms for registration of carotid MRI have been proposed [38], [39]. Additionally, methods for automated segmentation of the plaque into constituent components are under development. For the most part, these studies have focused on ex vivo imaging experiments, with established segmentation procedures [63], [13], [33]. Recent experiments in vivo show that more specialized segmentation procedures that overcome the limitations of in vivo imaging are able to identify many of the principle plaque components [23], [43]. Delineation of the wall itself has been facilitated by active contour techniques for boundary detection [79], [28], [29]. Finally, these features have been combined into integrated processing packages, such as CASCADE (Fig. 5 [75]).

Novel imaging techniques

The utility of basic contrast agents in MRI has led to several investigations of contrast agents that target specific plaque features. In MRI, ultra-small particles of super-paramagnetic iron oxides (USPIOs) have been shown to be macrophage-specific [42]. USPIOs may thus aid in the detection and measurement of plaque inflammation by leading to signal decreases in MRI. Other MRI agents are specifically being

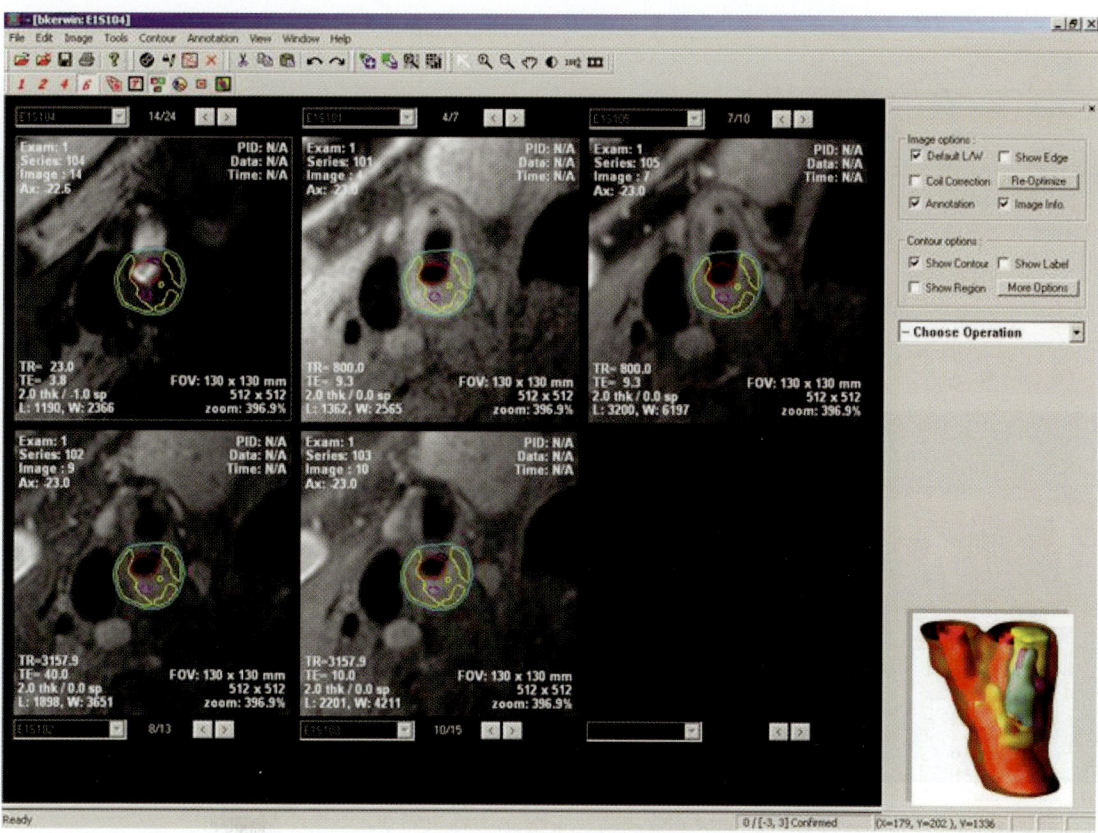

Fig. 5. The CASCADE interface for computer-aided evaluation of carotid MRI.

targeted to bind to fibrin [21], [72], which may facilitate rapid screening for the presence of fibrin-rich clot material in the carotid artery and other vessels. Another target that has been proposed for plaque imaging is $\alpha_v\beta_3$-integrin, which is expressed in the vascular wall and is associated with angiogenesis [73].

Similar efforts have been made in nuclear medicine, using radioisotopes to mark the presence of agents bound to specific receptors [66]. In an ex vivo carotid experiment, platelets tagged with (111)In showed promise for identifying plaque thrombosis [46].

A final notable imaging technology for characterizing plaque morphology is optical coherence tomography (OCT). Unlike the non-invasive or minimally invasive procedures detailed in the remainder of this chapter, OCT requires catheterization. The benefit of OCT, however, is a level of resolution on the order of microns, which is unattainable by the other techniques. OCT may thus be uniquely capable of observing the condition, thickness, and cellular composition of the fibrous cap. One study investigating this possibility showed that plaques could be subdivided into fibrous, fibrocalcific, and lipid-rich categories based on signal characteristics [76]. For example, fibro-calcific plaques (Fig. 6) showed a distinct boundary between a signal-rich fibrous layer and a signal-poor calcified region. OCT has also been shown to produce higher signal variability in fibrous caps with elevated macrophage composition [62].

Clinical use of carotid wall imaging

Assessment of plaque vulnerability

The ultimate goal of imaging carotid plaque morphology is to characterize structures associated with

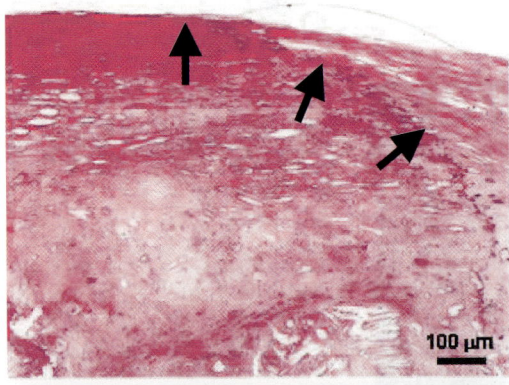
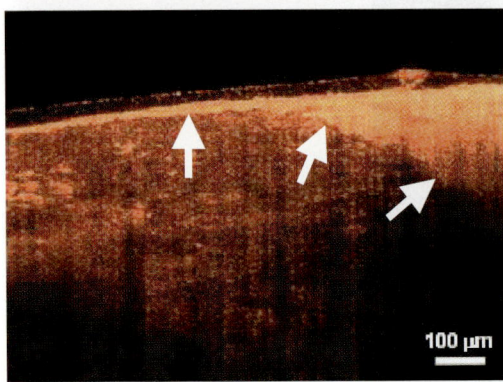

Fig. 6. Ex vivo optical coherence tomography (OCT) image of a carotid plaque (bottom) with corresponding histology (top). The boundary (arrows) between the cellular, fibrous cap and a calcified interior evident in histology is also clearly evident in the OCT image (Courtesy Xingde Li, University of Washington, Department of Bioengineering).

vulnerable plaque. For this purpose, studies are needed that identify associations between validated imaging targets and patient outcome. To date, however, most studies have focused on retrospective studies of plaques known to have caused recent symptoms.

Fibrous cap characteristics assessed by MRI or Ultrasound have been especially important for predicting prior symptoms. In an MRI study, fibrous caps appearing ruptured were 23 times more likely to be associated with symptomatic patients as fibrous caps appearing intact and thick [82]. Ultrasound measurements of mean cap thickness were shown to have an area under the receiver operating characteristic curve of 0.88, implying high sensitivity and specificity for identifying symptomatic patients [17].

Internal plaque composition is also important in determining the likelihood of patient symptoms. Intraplaque hemorrhage identified by echolucent regions in ultrasound or bright signal on T1-weighted MRI has been shown to associate with prior patient symptoms [37], [23], [51]. Percent plaque calcification detected by CT, on the other hand, has been shown to be associated with reduced likelihood of patient symptoms [62].

Fewer studies have been done prospectively and, to date, only using ultrasound. Carotid IMT has been shown to predict myocardial infarction and stroke, with odds ratios of approximately 1.4 for each 0.16 mm increase in IMT [8]. However, the marginal improvement including IMT in addition to traditional risk factors is not considered effective for screening [16]. Echolucency has also emerged as a predictor of future strokes in patients with prior symptoms, but not asymptomatic patients [26]. Ongoing studies will determine which if any of the plaque morphological characteristics can be used as a viable clinical variable.

Clinical trials

The near term application of these techniques in patients will likely remain in the assessment of therapeutic response by directly measuring plaque progression or regression. Numerous studies have utilized IMT measured by ultrasound to assess the response of the carotid artery to pharmacological agents [15], [18], [36], [32]. MRI has been used to a lesser extent, but offers the possibility of assessing changes not only in wall morphology, but also plaque composition [83], [14], [3]. MRI has also been used to investigate ethno-racial differences in carotid plaque, that may lead to new therapies or lifestyle guidelines in treating atherosclerosis [59].

Future of carotid wall imaging

Despite the considerable success in imaging carotid plaque morphology and the correlation with histology, the techniques in this chapter remain largely constrained to research applications. The main hurdle remaining is to demonstrate a prospective link between plaque morphology by imaging and outcome. To some extent, this link has been established for IMT measurements by B-mode ultrasound. Risk of future heart attack and stroke increases with higher IMT. However, IMT has not demonstrated sufficient specificity to greatly alter individual patient management. Furthermore, reductions in IMT have not been shown to independently reduce overall patient risk. Thus, IMT has not been accepted as a surrogate endpoint for clinical trials. Other methods outlined in this chapter are further from clinical acceptance. Thus, much of the near-term work in this field will focus on prospective studies that will establish which methodologies are clinically meaningful.

Take-home message

This chapter reviewed the abilities of various in vivo imaging techniques to resolve morphological features of the atherosclerotic carotid artery. The focus was on correlations between *in vivo* imaging results and *ex vivo* pathology. MRI, ultrasound, and CT have all been shown to provide detailed information regarding certain aspects of the plaque. The most suitable method for a given application depends on the requirements and constraints inherent in the application. MRI generally offers the widest range of sensitivities to various plaque features and components, but also involves a more complicated imaging procedure than CT or ultrasound. In contrast, CT and ultrasound offer simpler imaging procedures, higher resolution, measurements of stenosis, and are methods of choice for measuring IMT and calcification, respectively. However, these methods have shown mixed results in attempts to characterize the entire breadth of plaque features resolved by MRI. The most important imaging advancement on the horizon appears to be the use of targeted imaging agents that highlight the presence and amount of molecular receptors associated with plaque instability.

Applications of these techniques in the near term will continue to be in assessing group characteristics and responses to therapy. Thus, the immediate clinical benefit will be in clinical trials that determine which treatment option offers the most promising outcome to all patients. The challenge for these techniques is to reach a level of accuracy, precision and clinical significance to dictate treatment options for the individual patient. Once outcome trials establish which parameters are meaningful indicators of risk for an individual, these techniques will likely be used to select between options such as CEA, stenting, or aggressive drug therapy. The addition of these evaluations to standard patient assessments can ultimately save cost by eliminating unnecessary surgery or indicating the need for aggressive therapy before a patient presents emergently.

Acknowledgement

The author thanks Chun Yuan, Xingde Li, Jianming Cai, and Marina Ferguson for contributions to this chapter.

References

[1] ACAS: ACAS Endarterectomy for asymptomatic carotid artery stenosis. JAMA 273: 1421–1428 (1995).
[2] Adame IM, van der Geest RJ, Wasserman BA, Mohamed MA, Reiber JH, Lelieveldt BP: Automatic segmentation and plaque characterization in atherosclerotic carotid artery MR images. MAGMA 16: 227–234 (2004).
[3] Adams GJ, Greene J, Vick GW 3rd, Harrist R, Kimball KT, Karmonik C, Ballantyne CM, Insull W Jr, Morrisett JD: Tracking regression and progression of atherosclerosis in human carotid arteries using high-resolution magnetic resonance imaging. Magn Reson Imaging 22: 1249–1258 (2004).
[4] Akopov S, Cohen SN: Preventing stroke: a review of current guidelines. J Am Med Dir Assoc 4: S127–S132 (2003).
[5] American Heart Association. Heart Disease and Stroke Statistics Update (2005).
[6] Barnett HJ, Taylor DW, Eliasziw M, Fox AJ, Ferguson GG, Haynes RB, Rankin RN, Clagett GP, Hachinski VC, Sackett DL, Thorpe KE, Meldrum HE, Spence JD: Benefit of carotid endarterectomy in patients with symptomatic moderate or severe stenosis. North American Symptomatic Carotid Endarterectomy Trial Collaborators. N Engl J Med 339: 1415–1425 (1998).
[7] Bots ML, Hofman A, Grobbee DE: Increased common carotid intima-media thickness. Adaptive response or a reflection of atherosclerosis? Findings from the Rotterdam Study. Stroke 28: 2442–2447 (1997).

[8] Bots ML, Hoes AW, Koudstaal PJ, Hofman A, Grobbee DE: Common carotid intima-media thickness and risk of stroke and myocardial infarction: the Rotterdam Study. Circulation 96: 1432–1437 (1997).

[9] Burke AP, Farb A, Kolodgie FD, Narula J, Virmani R: Atherosclerotic plaque morphology and coronary thrombi. J Nucl Cardiol 9: 95–103 (2002).

[10] Cai JM, Hatsukami TS, Ferguson MS, Small R, Polissar NL, Yuan C: Classification of human carotid atherosclerotic lesions with in vivo multicontrast magnetic resonance imaging. Circulation 106: 1368–1373 (2002).

[11] Carr S, Farb A, Pearce WH, Virmani R, Yao JS. Atherosclerotic plaque rupture in symptomatic carotid artery stenosis. J Vasc Surg 23: 755–765 (1996).

[12] Chu B, Kampschulte A, Ferguson MS, Kerwin WS, Yarnykh VL, O'Brien KD, Polissar NL, Hatsukami TS, Yuan C: Hemorrhage in the atherosclerotic carotid plaque: a high-resolution MRI study. Stroke 35: 1079–1084 (2004).

[13] Clarke SE, Hammond RR, Mitchell JR, Rutt BK: Quantitative assessment of carotid plaque composition using multicontrast MRI and registered histology. Magn Reson Med 50: 1199–1208 (2003).

[14] Corti R, Fuster V, Fayad ZA et al.: Lipid lowering by simvastatin induces regression of human atherosclerotic lesions: two years' follow-up by high-resolution non-invasive magnetic resonance imaging. Circulation 106: 2884–2887 (2002).

[15] Crouse JR 3rd, Grobbee DE, O'Leary DH, Bots ML, Evans GW, Palmer MK, Riley WA, Raichlen JS: Measuring Effects on intima media Thickness: an Evalution of Rosuvastatin study group. Related Measuring Effects on intima media Thickness: an Evaluation of Rosuvastatin in subclinical atherosclerosis – the rationale and methodology of the METEOR study Cardiovasc Drugs Ther 18: 231–238 (2004).

[16] del Sol AI, Moons KG, Hollander M, Hofman A, Koudstaal PJ, Grobbee DE, Breteler MM, Witteman JC, Bots ML: Is carotid intima-media thickness useful in cardiovascular disease risk assessment? The Rotterdam Study. Stroke 32: 1532–1538 (2001).

[17] Devuyst G, Ruchat P, Karapanayiotides T, Jonasson L, Cuisinaire O, Lobrinus JA, Pusztaszeri M, Kalangos A, Despland PA, Thiran JP, Bogousslavsky J: Ultrasound measurement of the fibrous cap in symptomatic and asymptomatic atheromatous carotid plaques. Circulation 111: 2776–2782 (2005).

[18] Espeland MA, O'leary DH, Terry JG, Morgan T, Evans G, Mudra H: Carotid intimal-media thickness as a surrogate for cardiovascular disease events in trials of HMG-CoA reductase inhibitors. Curr Control Trials Cardiovasc Med 6: 3 (2005).

[19] European Carotid Surgery Trialists' Collaborative Group. Randomised trial of endarterectomy for recently symptomatic carotid stenosis: final results of the MRC European carotid surgery trial (ECST). Lancet 351: 1379–1387 (1998).

[20] Fisher M, Paganini-Hill A, Martin A, Cosgrove M, Toole JF, Barnett HJ, Norris J: Carotid plaque pathology: thrombosis, ulceration, and stroke pathogenesis. Stroke 36: 253–257 (2005).

[21] Flacke S, Fischer S, Scott MJ et al.: Novel MRI contrast agent for molecular imaging of fibrin: implications for detecting vulnerable plaques. Circulation 104: 1280–1285 (2001).

[22] Goldstein LB, Adams R, Becker K, Furberg CD, Gorelick PB, Hademenos G, Hill M, Howard G, Howard VJ, Jacobs B, Levine SR, Mosca L, Sacco RL, Sherman DG, Wolf PA, del Zoppo GJ: Primary prevention of ischemic stroke: A statement for healthcare professionals from the Stroke Council of the American Heart Association. Circulation 103: 163–182 (2001).

[23] Geroulakos G, Ramaswami G, Nicolaides A, James K, Labropoulos N, Belcaro G, Holloway M: Characterization of symptomatic and asymptomatic carotid plaques using high-resolution real-time ultrasonography. Br J Surg 80: 1274–1277 (1993).

[24] Gorelick PB: Carotid endarterectomy: where do we draw the line? Stroke 30: 1745–1750 (1999).

[25] Gray-Weale AC, Graham JC, Burnett JR, Byrne K, Lusby RJ: Carotid artery atheroma: comparison of preoperative B-mode ultrasound appearance with carotid endarterectomy specimen pathology. J Cardiovasc Surg (Torino) 29: 676–681 (1988).

[26] Gronholdt ML, Nordestgaard BG, Schroeder TV, Vorstrup S, Sillesen H: Ultrasonic echolucent carotid plaques predict future strokes. Circulation 104: 68–73 (2001).

[27] Halm EA, Chassin MR, Tuhrim S, Hollier LH, Popp AJ, Ascher E, Dardik H, Faust G, Riles TS: Revisiting the appropriateness of carotid endarterectomy. Stroke 34: 1464–1471 (2003).

[28] Han C, Hatsukami TS, Hwang JN, Yuan C: A fast minimal path active contour model. IEEE Trans Med Imaging 10: 865–873 (2001).

[29] Han C, Kerwin WS, Hatsukami TS, Hwang JN, Yuan C: Detecting objects in image sequences using rule-based control in an active contour model. IEEE Trans Biomed Eng 50: 705–710 (2003).

[30] Hatsukami TS, Thackray BD, Primozich JF, Ferguson MS, Burns DH, Beach KW, Detmer PR, Alpers C, Gordon D, Strandness DE Jr: Echolucent regions in carotid plaque: preliminary analysis comparing three-dimensional histologic reconstructions to sonographic findings. Ultrasound Med Biol 20: 743–749 (1994).

[31] Hatsukami TS, Ross R, Polissar NL, Yuan C: Identification of fibrous cap thickness and cap rupture in hu-

man atherosclerotic carotid plaque in-vivo with high resolution magnetic resonance imaging. Circulation 102: 959–964 (2000).
[32] Hedblad B, Wikstrand J, Janzon L, Wedel H, Berglund G: Low-dose metoprolol CR/XL and fluvastatin slow progression of carotid intima-media thickness: Main results from the Beta-Blocker Cholesterol-Lowering Asymptomatic Plaque Study (BCAPS). Circulation 103: 1721–1726 (2001).
[33] Itskovich VV, Samber DD, Mani V, Aguinaldo JG, Fallon JT, Tang CY, Fuster V, Fayad ZA: Quantification of human atherosclerotic plaques using spatially enhanced cluster analysis of multicontrast-weighted magnetic resonance images. Magn Reson Med 52: 515–523 (2004).
[34] Kampschulte A, Ferguson MS, Kerwin WS, Polissar NL, Chu B, Saam T, Hatsukami TS, Yuan C: Differentiation of intraplaque versus juxtaluminal hemorrhage/thrombus in advanced human carotid atherosclerotic lesions by in vivo magnetic resonance imaging. Circulation 110: 3239–3244 (2004).
[35] Kang XJ, Polissar NL, Han C, Lin E, Yuan C: Analysis of the measurement precision of arterial lumen and wall areas using high resolution magnetic resonance imaging. Magn Reson Med 44: 968–972 (2000).
[36] Kang S, Wu Y, Li X: Effects of statin therapy on the progression of carotid atherosclerosis: a systematic review and meta-analysis. Atherosclerosis 177: 433–442 (2004).
[37] Kardoulas DG, Katsamouris AN, Gallis PT, Philippides TP, Anagnostakos NK, Gorgoyannis DS, Gourtsoyannis NC: Ultrasonographic and histologic characteristics of symptom-free and symptomatic carotid plaque. Cardiovasc Surg 4: 580–590 (1996).
[38] Kerwin WS, Yuan C: Active edge maps for medical image registration. Proc SPIE 4322: 516–526 (2001).
[39] Kerwin WS, Cai J, Yuan C: Noise and motion correction in dynamic contrast-enhanced MRI for analysis of atherosclerotic lesions. Magn Reson Med 47: 1211–1217 (2002).
[40] Kerwin W, Hooker A, Spilker M et al.: Quantitative magnetic resonance imaging analysis of neovasculature volume in carotid atherosclerotic plaque. Circulation 107: 851–856 (2003).
[41] Kerwin WS, Ferguson MS, O'Brien KD, Hatsukami TS, Yuan C: Quantitative detection of inflammation in carotid atherosclerosis by dynamic contrast enhanced magnetic resonance imaging. J Amer Coll Cardiol 43: 534A (2004).
[42] Kooi ME, Cappendijk VC, Cleutjens KB et al.: Accumulation of ultrasmall superparamagnetic particles of iron oxide in human atherosclerotic plaques can be detected by in vivo magnetic resonance imaging. Circulation 107: 2453–2458 (2003).
[43] Liu F, Xu D, Yuan C, Kerwin WS: In vivo carotid plaque segmentation using probability maps and multiple active contour competition. J Cardiovasc Magn Resonance 7: 215–217 (2005).
[44] Luo Y, Polissar N, Han C, Yarnykh V, Kerwin WS, Hatsukami TS, Yuan C: Accuracy and uniqueness of three in vivo measurements of atherosclerotic carotid plaque morphology with black blood MRI. Magn Reson Med 50: 75–82 (2003).
[45] Mackay J, Mensah G: Atlas of Heart Disease and Stroke. World Health Organization (2004).
[46] Manca G, Parenti G, Bellina R, Boni G, Grosso M, Bernini W, Palombo C, Paterni M, Pelosi G, Lanza M, Mazzuca N, Bianchi R, De Caterina R: 111 In platelet scintigraphy for the noninvasive detection of carotid plaque thrombosis. Stroke 32: 719–727 (2001).
[47] McCarthy MJ, Loftus IM, Thompson MM et al.: Angiogenesis and the atherosclerotic carotid plaque: an association between symptomatology and plaque morphology. J Vasc Surg 30: 261–268 (1999).
[48] McKinney AM, Casey SO, Teksam M, Lucato LT, Smith M, Truwit CL, Kieffer S: Carotid bifurcation calcium and correlation with percent stenosis of the internal carotid artery on CT angiography. Neuroradiology 47: 1–9 (2005).
[49] Mitsumori LM, Hatsukami TS, Ferguson MS, Kerwin WS, Cai J, Yuan C: In vivo accuracy of multisequence MR imaging for identifying unstable fibrous caps in advanced human carotid plaques. J Magn Reson Imaging 17: 410–420 (2003).
[50] Moody AR, Murphy RE, Morgan PS, Martel AL, Delay GS, Allder S, MacSweeney ST, Tennant WG, Gladman J, Lowe J, Hunt BJ: Characterization of complicated carotid plaque with magnetic resonance direct thrombus imaging in patients with cerebral ischemia. Circulation 107: 3047–3052 (2003).
[51] Murphy RE, Moody AR, Morgan PS, Martel AL, Delay GS, Allder S, MacSweeney ST, Tennant WG, Gladman J, Lowe J, Hunt BJ: Prevalence of complicated carotid atheroma as detected by magnetic resonance direct thrombus imaging in patients with suspected carotid artery stenosis and previous acute cerebral ischemia. Circulation 107: 3053–3058 (2003).
[52] Naghavi M, Libby P, Falk E, Casscells SW, Litovsky S, Rumberger J, Badimon JJ, Stefanadis C, Moreno P, Pasterkamp G, Fayad Z, Stone PH, Waxman S, Raggi P, Madjid M, Zarrabi A, Burke A, Yuan C, Fitzgerald PJ, Siscovick DS, de Korte CL, Aikawa M, Juhani Airaksinen KE, Assmann G, Becker CR, Chesebro JH, Farb A, Galis ZS, Jackson C, Jang IK, Koenig W, Lodder RA, March K, Demirovic J, Navab M, Priori SG, Rekhter MD, Bahr R, Grundy SM, Mehran R, Colombo A, Boerwinkle E, Ballantyne C, Insull W Jr,

Schwartz RS, Vogel R, Serruys PW, Hansson GK, Faxon DP, Kaul S, Drexler H, Greenland P, Muller JE, Virmani R, Ridker PM, Zipes DP, Shah PK, Willerson JT: From vulnerable plaque to vulnerable patient: a call for new definitions and risk assessment strategies: Part I. Circulation 108: 1664–1672 (2003).

[53] North American Symptomatic Carotid Endarterectomy Trial Collaborators. The beneficial effect of carotid endarterectomy in symptomatic patients with high–grade stenosis. N Engl J Med 325: 445–453 (1991).

[54] Oliver TB, Lammie GA, Wright AR, Wardlaw J, Patel SG, Peek R, Ruckley CV, Collie DA: Atherosclerotic plaque at the carotid bifurcation: CT angiographic appearance with histopathologic correlation. AJNR 20: 897–901 (1999).

[55] Picano E, Landini L, Distante A et al: Angle dependence of ultrasonic backscatter in arterial tissues: a study in vitro. Circulation 72: 572–576 (1985).

[56] Pignoli P, Tremoli E, Poli A, Oreste P, Paoletti R: Intimal plus medial thickness of the arterial wall: a direct measurement with ultrasound imaging. Circulation 74: 1399–1406 (1986).

[57] Rothwell PM, Gutnikov SA, Warlow CP: Reanalysis of the final results of the European Carotid Surgery Trial. Stroke 34: 514–523 (2003).

[58] Saam T, Ferguson MS, Yarnykh VL, Takaya N, Xu D, Polissar NL, Hatsukami TS, Yuan C: Quantitative evaluation of carotid plaque composition by in vivo MRI. Arterioscler Thromb Vasc Biol 25: 234–239 (2005).

[59] Saam T, Cai JM, Cai YQ, An NY, Kampschulte A, Xu D, Kerwin WS, Takaya N, Polissar NL, Hatsukami TS, Yuan C: Carotid plaque composition differs between ethno-racial groups: an MRI pilot study comparing mainland Chinese and American Caucasian patients. Arterioscler Thromb Vasc Biol 25: 611–616 (2005).

[60] Schulte-Altedorneburg G, Droste DW, Haas N, Kemeny V, Nabavi DG, Fuzesi L, Ringelstein EB: Preoperative B-mode ultrasound plaque appearance compared with carotid endarterectomy specimen histology. Acta Neurol Scand 101: 188–194 (2000).

[61] Schminke U, Hilker L, Motsch L, Griewing B, Kessler C: Volumetric assessment of plaque progression with 3-dimensional ultrasonography under statin therapy. J Neuroimaging 12: 245–251 (2002).

[62] Shaalan WE, Cheng H, Gewertz B, McKinsey JF, Schwartz LB, Katz D, Cao D, Desai T, Glagov S, Bassiouny HS: Degree of carotid plaque calcification in relation to symptomatic outcome and plaque inflammation. J Vasc Surg 40: 262–269 (2004).

[63] Shinnar M, Fallon JT, Wehrli S et al.: The diagnostic accuracy of ex vivo MRI for human atherosclerotic plaque characterization. Arterioscler Thromb Vasc Biol 19: 2756–2761 (1999).

[64] Tearney GJ, Yabushita H, Houser SL, Aretz HT, Jang IK, Schlendorf KH, Kauffman CR, Shishkov M, Halpern EF, Bouma BE: Quantification of macrophage content in atherosclerotic plaques by optical coherence tomography. Circulation 107: 113–119 (2003).

[65] Tegos TJ, Sohail M, Sabetai MM, Robless P, Akbar N, Pare G, Stansby G, Nicolaides AN: Echomorphologic and histopathologic characteristics of unstable carotid plaques. AJNR Am J Neuroradiol 21: 1937–1944 (2000).

[66] Vallabhajosula S, Fuster V: Atherosclerosis: imaging techniques and the evolving role of nuclear medicine. J Nucl Med 38: 1788–1796 (1997).

[67] Virmani R, Kolodgie FD, Burke AP, Farb A, Schwartz SM: Lessons from sudden coronary death: a comprehensive morphological classification scheme for atherosclerotic lesions. Arterioscler Thromb Vasc Biol 20: 1262–1275 (2000).

[68] Virmani R, Burke AP, Kolodgie FD, Farb A: Vulnerable plaque: the pathology of unstable coronary lesions. J Interv Cardiol 15: 439–446 (2002).

[69] Walker LJ, Ismail A, McMeekin W, Lambert D, Mendelow AD, Birchall D: Computed tomography angiography for the evaluation of carotid atherosclerotic plaque: correlation with histopathology of endarterectomy specimens. Stroke 33: 977–981 (2002).

[70] Wasserman BA, Smith WI, Trout HH 3rd, Cannon RO 3rd, Balaban RS, Arai AE: Carotid artery atherosclerosis: in vivo morphologic characterization with gadolinium-enhanced double-oblique MR imaging initial results. Radiology 223: 566–573 (2002).

[71] Wilhjelm JE, Gronholdt ML, Wiebe B, Jespersen SK, Hansen LK, Sillesen H: Quantitative analysis of ultrasound B-mode images of carotid atherosclerotic plaque: correlation with visual classification and histological examination. IEEE Trans Med Imaging 17: 910–922 (1998).

[72] Winter PM, Caruthers SD, Yu X, Song SK, Chen J, Miller B, Bulte JW, Robertson JD, Gaffney PJ, Wickline SA, Lanza GM: Improved molecular imaging contrast agent for detection of human thrombus. Magn Reson Med 50: 411–416 (2003).

[73] Winter PM, Morawski AM, Caruthers SD, Fuhrhop RW, Zhang H, Williams TA, Allen JS, Lacy EK, Robertson JD, Lanza GM, Wickline SA: Molecular imaging of angiogenesis in early-stage atherosclerosis with alpha(v)beta3-integrin-targeted nanoparticles. Circulation 108: 2270–2274 (2003).

[74] Wong M, Edelstein J, Wollman J, Bond MG: Ultrasonic-pathological comparison of the human arterial wall. Verification of intima-media thickness. Arterioscler Thromb 13: 482–486 (1993).

[75] Xu D, Kerwin WS, Saam T, Ferguson M, Yuan C: CASCADE: Computer aided system for cardiovascular disease evaluation. Proc ISMRM 1922 (2004).

[76] Yabushita H, Bouma BE, Houser SL, Aretz HT, Jang IK, Schlendorf KH, Kauffman CR, Shishkov M, Kang DH, Halpern EF, Tearney GJ: Characterization of human atherosclerosis by optical coherence tomography. Circulation 106: 1640–1645 (2002).

[77] Yadav JS, Wholey MH, Kuntz RE, Fayad P, Katzen BT, Mishkel GJ, Bajwa TK, Whitlow P, Strickman NE, Jaff MR, Popma JJ, Snead DB, Cutlip DE, Firth BG, Ouriel K: Protected carotid-artery stenting versus endarterectomy in high-risk patients. N Engl J Med 351: 1493–1501 (2004).

[78] Yao J, van Sambeek MR, Dall'Agata A et al.: Three-dimensional ultrasound study of carotid arteries before and after endarterectomy; analysis of stenotic lesions and surgical impact on the vessel. Stroke 29: 2026–2031 (1998).

[79] Yuan C, Lin E, Millard J et al.: Closed contour edge detection of blood vessel lumen and outer wall boundaries in black-blood MR images. Magn Reson Imaging 17: 257–266 (1999).

[80] Yuan C, Mitsumori LM, Ferguson MS et al.: In vivo accuracy of multispectral magnetic resonance imaging for identifying lipid-rich necrotic cores and intraplaque hemorrhage in advanced human carotid plaques. Circulation 104: 2051–2056 (2001).

[81] Yuan C, Kerwin WS, Ferguson MS et al.: Contrast-enhanced high resolution MRI for atherosclerotic carotid artery tissue characterization. J Magn Reson Imaging 15: 62–67 (2002).

[82] Yuan C, Zhang SX, Polissar NL et al.: Identification of fibrous cap rupture with magnetic resonance imaging is highly associated with recent TIA or stroke. Circulation 105: 181–185 (2002).

[83] Zhao XQ, Yuan C, Hatsukami TS et al.: Effects of prolonged intensive lipid-lowering therapy on the characteristics of carotid atherosclerotic plaques in vivo, by MRI: a case-control study. Arterioscler Thromb Vasc Biol 21: 1623–1629 (2001).

Chapter 1.3

SONOGRAPHIC EVALUATION IN CAROTID ARTERY STENOSIS

B. K. Lal

Department of Surgery, New Jersey Medical School, University of Medicine and Dentistry of New Jersey, Newark, New Jersey, USA

Introduction

Over three decades ago, Doppler was introduced as the first ultrasonographic method for evaluation of cerebrovascular disease. Since then, the development of new ultrasound techniques has revolutionized the clinical applications for extracranial carotid disease. Interpretation of pulse wave Doppler signals involves an analysis of audio signals and the frequency spectrum. It is based on the Doppler frequency shift resulting from moving red blood cells in the carotid artery. In experienced hands, pulse wave Doppler ultrasound can identify significant luminal narrowing based on increased velocity of blood flow across a stenotic lesion. High-resolution B-mode ultrasound scanning uses linear array transducers (7–12 MHz) to display morphological features of the arterial wall. Duplex ultrasonography (DUS) combines integrated PW Doppler spectrum analysis and B-mode sonography. The B-mode image offers information about morphology in addition to serving as a guide for accurate PW Doppler velocity measurement. Color Doppler flow imaging based on the direction of flow superimposes color-coded blood flow patterns over the B-mode image. Power Doppler imaging color codes blood flow according to the amplitude of the Doppler signal. Both these modalities afford greater sensitivity to blood flow detection allowing improved detection of near-occlusive stenoses, tortuosity, and other morphological abnormalities in the arterial wall. The noninvasive nature of DUS makes this testing modality more attractive than the "gold standard" of cervical angiography. If the diagnosis of significant carotid stenosis can be accurately made with DUS, the risk of stroke inherent in angiography (1.2% in the Asymptomatic Carotid Atherosclerosis Study [9]) can be avoided. Currently, many patients (90% at the authors' institution) undergo carotid revascularization based solely on a duplex examination.

Indications for testing

Symptomatic patients

Prospective randomized trials have documented the efficacy of carotid endarterectomy (CEA) in reducing stroke in symptomatic carotid stenosis. The North American Symptomatic Carotid Endarterectomy Trial (NASCET) confirmed that CEA offered a 65% relative risk reduction compared to best medical therapy in patients with 70-99% carotid stenosis who present with transient ischemic attack (TIA) or non-disabling stroke [23]. Similarly, symptomatic patients with a 50–69% carotid stenosis derived a 29% relative risk reduction at 5 years [4]. Therefore all patients with hemispheric neurological symptoms attributable to the carotid circulation should undergo carotid imaging. This test should be performed even in the absence of a carotid bruit because NASCET data revealed that over one third of patients with high-grade carotid stenosis lacked a carotid bruit [28]. Testing in asymptomatic patients with hemispheric infarcts identified on computed tomographic (CT) or magnetic resonance (MR) is also indicated to rule out carotid disease. Patients with non-lateralizing symptoms such as dizziness or lightheadedness cannot be assumed to be caused by carotid stenosis. Other symptoms such as cranial nerve dysfunction (e.g., dysphasia, double vision, or blurred vision) and drop attacks are more likely to be vertebro-basilar in origin.

Asymptomatic patients with a carotid bruit

The Asymptomatic Carotid Atherosclerosis Study (ACAS) documented a 53% relative risk reduction in ipsilateral stroke and any perioperative stroke or death at 5 years when comparing CEA with medical therapy for asymptomatic $\geq$ 60% carotid stenosis [9]. Controversy continues regarding who best to screen since widespread imaging of all asymptomatic patients is unlikely to be cost-effective. Most physicians have adopted a selective approach; however, it is clear that additional studies are necessary to clarify this issue.

The most commonly used selection criteria include the presence of a carotid bruit. Carotid bruits, expected to be found in up to 8.2% of patients $\geq$ 75 years of age [14] have been associated with a three-times increased risk of stroke in a population-based prospective cohort study [33]. One third of patients with an asymptomatic carotid bruit can be expected to harbor a carotid stenosis $\geq$ 50% when studied with DUS [27]. Of note, 21% of patients with a bruit ultimately progressed to 50–79% stenosis; while 27% of patients with 50–79% stenosis progressed to $\geq$ 80% stenosis at 7 years [17]. It is clear that the presence of a carotid bruit should prompt a carotid duplex ultrasound to screen for carotid stenosis and the patients must be followed regularly for possible disease progression in case their disease is not severe enough to warrant revascularization.

Asymptomatic patients without a bruit

Significant carotid stenosis can exist in the absence of cervical bruit. For this reason, recommendations for carotid duplex scanning have been made based on specific risk factors such as age, hypertension, smoking, coronary artery disease (CAD), and peripheral arterial occlusive disease (PAD). Significant carotid stenosis was present in 17.5% of patients aged $\geq$ 50 years with CAD, tobacco abuse, and PAD [12]. Claudication and decreased ankle-brachial index have both been found to be predictive of carotid stenosis [21]. In a prospective evaluation of 1087 patients undergoing coronary artery bypasses, 17% had carotid stenoses $\geq$ 50% and 5% had stenoses $\geq$ 80%. Age $>$ 60 years, hypertension, diabetes mellitus, and smoking, increase the risk of significant carotid stenosis in patients undergoing cardiac surgery [3]. Based on these data, duplex scanning can be recommended selectively based on the presence of several risk factors.

Post-carotid revascularization surveillance

Carotid duplex scanning has been used as a surveillance tool for carotid restenosis. Widely varying protocols exist for the follow-up of patients after carotid revascularization. In addition, despite the absence of conclusive cost-effectiveness data, it is likely that carotid duplex scanning for surveillance in this setting will continue to be a common indication, given the restenosis rates associated with CEA [8] and carotid artery stenting [20]. Data supporting surveillance of the contralateral carotid artery after ipsilateral revascularization is more forthcoming since a substantial number of contralateral arteries have been observed to progress to high-grade stenoses on follow-up [29]. The optimal frequency of this surveillance has not been defined but the author follows patients with $<$ 50% stenoses once a year; and those with $\geq$ 50% disease twice a year.

Quantifying the degree of carotid stenosis

Arteriography is the standard against which all non-invasive assessments of carotid luminal narrowing are commonly compared. While several methodologies have been proposed for the angiographic quantification of stenosis, the Committee on Standards for Noninvasive Vascular Testing of the Joint Council of the Vascular Societies recommended that percent diameter reduction should be determined relative to the distal uninvolved internal carotid artery (ICA) [30]. Doppler measures that have been correlated with angiographic stenosis include ICA peak systolic velocity (PSV), and end-diastolic velocity (EDV), as well as ratios of ICA PSV and CCA PSV [1].

Initially, ICA PSV and the relative distribution of velocities within the spectral profile based on PW Doppler measurements, were used to define the degree of narrowing of the ICA [5]. The University of Washington criteria were subsequently refined with the addition of EDV [28]. Accordingly, stenoses were classified as mild (1–15%), moderate (16–49%), severe (50–99%) and occluded. These criteria remained useful until the publication of the results of the North American Symptomatic Carotid Endarterectomy Trial (NASCET) [23], [4], and the Asymptomatic Carotid Atherosclerosis Study (ACAS) [9]. The NASCET demonstrated an early and significant benefit associated with carotid endarterectomy (CEA) in symptomatic patients with an ipsilateral ICA stenosis ≥ 70%, and a significant benefit over a longer follow-up in symptomatic patients with ICA stenosis of 50–69%. Additionally, the ACAS concluded that asymptomatic patients with an ICA stenosis ≥ 60% could also benefit from CEA. These new criteria did not correspond to the categories previously defined by researchers at the University of Washington. Using receiver operator characteristic (ROC) curves to compare sensitivity, specificity, positive predictive value (PPV) and negative predictive value (NPV) for new criteria to define degrees of stenosis relevant to clinical management, Faught et al. [10] concluded that the combination of a PSV > 130 cm/s and an EDV > 100 cm/s defined a stenosis of 70–99%. Using a similar approach, Moneta et al. [22] concluded that an ICA PSV/common carotid artery PSV ratio > 4.0 provided optimal accuracy for the diagnosis of a stenosis of 70–99%. Yet a third set of criteria for the same degree of stenosis were proposed by Carpenter et al. [7] such that a combination of PSV > 210 cm/s, EDV > 70 cm/s, ICA PSV/CC PSV > 3.0, and ICA EDV/CCA EDV > 3.3 was most accurate. It is clear that DUS results are more accurate when a single cutoff point for stenosis is used (e.g., ≥ 50% or ≥ 60%), or when a broad category is used rather than a small range of stenosis (e.g., 50–99% vs. 60–69%).

Recent studies demonstrate that Doppler criteria are influenced by equipment used [11], laboratories [2] and the technologist performing the test [24]. Additionally, contralateral disease has been associated with increased carotid volume flow resulting in an overestimation of the severity of disease [31]. Most diagnostic laboratories simply use the well-established criteria of others to diagnose severe carotid stenosis. However, for the reasons cited above, it is recommended that each laboratory validate its own Doppler criteria for clinically relevant stenoses [18]. One such methodology is to subject the vascular laboratory to certification by an independent auditing organization such as the Intersocietal Commission for Accreditation of Vascular Laboratories (ICAVL) [6], [16]. Studies comparing the accuracy of duplex ultrasound examinations have noted consistently superior results from accredited versus non-accredited laboratories [6].

A group of experts from different medical specialties met in October 2002 to arrive at a consensus document with regard to the use of DUS in the diagnosis of ICA [13]. Table 1 illustrates their recommendations when using grayscale imaging and Doppler ultrasound. Technical considerations, diagnostic stratification, imaging and Doppler parameters, Doppler diagnostic thresholds, structure and content of the final report, and quality assessment issues were all discussed and suggestions were made. Recommendations were also made for follow-up of patients at high risk or with asymptomatic carotid stenosis, and research topics were suggested for the future. Ideally, each center should perform its own validation; however, in the absence of such validation, the criteria suggested in Table 1 may serve as a useful guideline.

Ultrasound and carotid artery stenting

Carotid artery stenting (CAS) has emerged as an alternative to CEA in the management of carotid stenosis under specific high-risk circumstances [32]. The ultimate value of CAS when compared with CEA will be based upon ongoing prospective randomized clinical trials [15]. In the interim, however, the number of patients undergoing CAS is increasing rapidly and these patients require intensive follow-up to monitor for instent restenosis [20]. US velocity criteria have not been well established for patients undergoing CAS. We have

Table 1. Representative Doppler ultrasound velocity criteria for the diagnosis of internal carotid artery stenosis

Primary parameters		Additional parameters	
Degree of stenosis (%)	ICA PSV (cm/sec)	ICA/CCA PSV ratio	ICA EDV (cm/sec)
Normal	< 125	< 2.0	< 40
< 50	< 125	< 2.0	< 40
50–69	125–230	2.0–4.0	40–100
70–99	> 230	> 4.0	> 100
Near occlusion	High/low/undetectable	Variable	Variable
Occlusion	Undetectable	Not applicable	Undetectable

Adapted from: Grant EG et al.: Carotid artery stenosis: Gray-scale and Doppler ultrasound diagnosis. Society of Radiologists in Ultrasound consensus conference. Radiology 229: 340–346 (2003).

reported that the introduction of a stent into the ICA alters arterial biomechanical properties such that the resultant stent-arterial complex has decreased compliance [19]. Additional studies have demonstrated that when velocity criteria for non-stented ICAs were used in stented ICAs, several normal diameters were diagnosed as having in-stent stenosis [25], [26]. We have also reported that normal luminal diameters in recently stented ICAs were most accurately defined by revised velocity criteria: PSV < 150 cm/sec with ICA PSV/CCA PSV ratio < 2.16 [19]. Correlation studies with evolving in-stent restenosis (ISR) and angiographic diameter reduction will help define velocity criteria for increasing grades of stenosis in the stented ICA. Meanwhile, the author's laboratory routinely registers baseline velocities immediately post-CAS, and utilizes a combination of planimetric measurements on B-mode imaging and rising intra or peri-stent velocities as indicators of evolving ISR during follow-up.

Testing procedure

The DUS examination must include a blood pressure measurement in both arms. A blood pressure differential of ≥ 20 mmHg is indicative of possible brachiocephalic, subclavian or axillary artery stenosis. Testing proceeds with the patient in the supine position with the head turned away from the side being examined. The carotid sheath travels along the anterior border of the sternocleidomastoid muscle and this is where imaging can commence. The common carotid artery is identified at its origin in the base of the neck just above the clavicle and followed to the carotid bifurcation usually located below the mandible. Abnormal locations of the bifurcation must be reported since they impact on the extent of surgical exposure (mandibular subluxation during CEA for high bifurcations) or decision regarding the type of revascularization to be offered (CAS for extremely high bifurcations).

The transducer may be placed anterior, medial, or posterior to the sternocleidomastoid muscle to optimize flow visualization. Any luminal or wall abnormalities should be reported. Velocity measurements are recorded with an angle of insonation of 60°. Commonly, velocity measurements are obtained at the proximal and distal common carotid artery (CCA), external carotid artery (ECA); ICA (proximal, middle, and distal); and vertebral. Every effort should be made to follow the ICA as far cephalad as possible. The location of the distal extent of the plaque should be reported since this again impacts on the revascularization procedure. If the plaque continues cephalad into the distal ICA it entails extensive surgical dissection in the distal carotid triangle.

The vertebral arteries can be found posterior to the CCA between the vertebral bodies. While the tortuous course of these arteries makes diagnosis of a stenosis difficult; every effort must be made to report antegrade versus retrograde (i.e., reverse) flow.

Validation

The standard technique of validating DUS is through comparison to angiography. The goal for a definitive examination would be a high positive predictive value (PPV) to minimize the number of patients who would undergo an unnecessary operation. A high PPV is achieved by missing the diagnosis in some patients with a stenosis (decreased sensitivity). The laboratory at the authors' institution has a high PPV, and thus diagnostic angiography may be avoided before recommending revascularization. In elderly, asymptomatic patients, the few patients under-diagnosed would be at a low risk for stroke which is why such an approach is utilized by all participating centers in large multicenter trials for carotid revascularization (e.g., NASCET). A younger, otherwise healthy patients with a bruit, TIA, or an atherosclerotic carotid artery on a B-mode scan, who does not meet the flow criteria of a significant stenosis, should have additional diagnostic studies (e.g., contrast angiography, MRA, or CTA). The patient's physician needs to ensure that a potential stroke-prone lesion is not left untreated.

Other diagnostic laboratories may use DUS as a screening test only. They wish to have a high negative predictive value (NPV) so that few patients with a stenosis are under-diagnosed. A high NPV is achievable by decreasing the specificity. Many patients will be over-diagnosed so that few are missed. Thus all patients in this setting will need an additional study before proceeding to revascularization.

Planimetric evaluation

As the discussion above indicates, velocity criteria for equivalent degrees of stenosis may vary between different centers. Conversely diameter and percent area stenosis measurements do not have this disadvantage. In addition, unlike ipsilateral velocity measurements, area and diameter measurements remain unaffected by contralateral stenosis/occlusion, ipsilateral proximal or distal stenosis/occlusion, or low cardiac output/cardiac arrhythmia. However, planimetry has not gained universal popularity since the measurements are hindered by heavy arterial calcification or tortuosity leading to inadequate B-mode imaging of the stenosis. This may occur in as high as 10–15% of all arteries imaged. These issues affect velocity recordings much less because the highest velocities are seen at the exit of the stenosis. Planimetry, however, complements velocity measurements and these methods should be used together. It is an especially important adjunct in the follow-up of stented carotid arteries.

Conclusions

Carotid DUS is the established method for diagnosing a cervical carotid artery stenosis. In medical centers with a vascular laboratory that has established an excellent PPV, angiography may be avoided before embarking on carotid revascularization. Other laboratories may emphasize the screening aspect of their testing and will have a higher NPV. Patients diagnosed in this setting must undergo a confirmatory study prior to undergoing revascularization. The criteria used for diagnosing specific categories of stenoses vary between laboratories. The hallmark of a good laboratory is one that establishes its own criteria and continually validates them in an ongoing quality assurance program.

References

[1] Alexandrov AV, Brodie DS, McLean A et al.: Correlation of peak systolic velocity and angiographic measurement of carotid stenosis revisited. Stroke 28: 339–342 (1997).
[2] Alexandrov AV, Vital D, Brodie DS et al.: Grading carotid stenosis with ultrasound. An interlaboratory comparison. Stroke 28: 1208–1210 (1997).
[3] Ascher E, Hingorani A, Yorkovich W et al.: Routine preoperative carotid duplex scanning in patients undergoing open heart surgery: is it worthwhile? Ann Vasc Surg 15: 669–678 (2001).
[4] Barnett HJ, Taylor DW, Eliasziw M et al.: North American Symptomatic Carotid Endarterectomy Trial Collaborators. Benefit of carotid endarterectomy in patients with symptomatic moderate or severe stenosis. N Engl J Med 339: 1415–1425 (1998).
[5] Blackshear WM Jr, Phillips DJ, Thiele BL et al.: Detection of carotid occlusive disease by ultrasonic imaging and pulsed Doppler spectrum analysis. Surgery 86: 698–706 (1979).
[6] Brown OW, Bendick PJ, Bove PG et al.: Reliability of extracranial carotid artery duplex ultrasound scanning: value of vascular laboratory accreditation. J Vasc Surg 39: 366–371; discussion 371 (2004).

[7] Carpenter JP, Lexa FJ, Davis JT: Determination of duplex Doppler ultrasound criteria appropriate to the North American Symptomatic Carotid Endarterectomy Trial. Stroke 27: 695–699 (1996).

[8] DeGroote RD, Lynch TG, Jamil Z et al.: Carotid restenosis: long-term noninvasive follow-up after carotid endarterectomy. Stroke 18: 1031–1036 (1987).

[9] Executive Committee for the Asymptomatic Carotid Atherosclerosis Study: Endarterectomy for asymptomatic carotid artery stenosis. JAMA 273: 1421–1428 (1995).

[10] Faught WE, Mattos MA, van Bemmelen PS et al.: Color-flow duplex scanning of carotid arteries: new velocity criteria based on receiver operator characteristic analysis for threshold stenoses used in the symptomatic and asymptomatic carotid trials. J Vasc Surg 19: 818–827; discussion 827–818 (1994).

[11] Fillinger MF, Baker RJ Jr, Zwolak RM et al.: Carotid duplex criteria for a 60% or greater angiographic stenosis: variation according to equipment. J Vasc Surg 24: 856–864 (1996).

[12] Fowl RJ, Marsch JG, Love M et al.: Prevalence of hemodynamically significant stenosis of the carotid artery in an asymptomatic veteran population. Surg Gynecol Obstet 172: 13–16 (1991).

[13] Grant EG, Benson CB, Moneta GL et al.: Carotid artery stenosis: gray-scale and Doppler US diagnosis—Society of Radiologists in Ultrasound Consensus Conference. Radiology 229: 340–346 (2003).

[14] Heyman A, Wilkinson WE, Heyden S et al.: Risk of stroke in asymptomatic persons with cervical arterial bruits: a population study in Evans County, Georgia. N Engl J Med 302: 838–841 (1980).

[15] Hobson RW 2nd: Rationale and status of randomized controlled clinical trials in carotid artery stenting. Semin Vasc Surg 16: 311–316 (2003).

[16] ICAVL: The Intersocietal Commission for the Accreditation of Vascular Laboratories: Standards for Accreditation in Noninvasive Vascular Testing. Columbia, MD: ICAVL (2005).

[17] Johnson BF, Verlato F, Bergelin RO et al.: Clinical outcome in patients with mild and moderate carotid artery stenosis. J Vasc Surg 21: 120–126 (1995).

[18] Kuntz KM, Polak JF, Whittemore AD et al.: Duplex ultrasound criteria for the identification of carotid stenosis should be laboratory specific. Stroke 28: 597–602 (1997).

[19] Lal BK, Hobson RW 2nd, Goldstein J et al.: Carotid artery stenting: is there a need to revise ultrasound velocity criteria? J Vasc Surg 39: 58–66 (2004).

[20] Lal BK, Hobson RW 2nd, Goldstein J et al.: In-stent recurrent stenosis after carotid artery stenting: life table analysis and clinical relevance. J Vasc Surg 38: 1162–1168; discussion 1169 (2003).

[21] Marek J, Mills JL, Harvich J et al.: Utility of routine carotid duplex screening in patients who have claudication. J Vasc Surg 24: 572–577; discussion 577–579 (1996).

[22] Moneta GL, Edwards JM, Chitwood RW et al.: Correlation of North American Symptomatic Carotid Endarterectomy Trial (NASCET) angiographic definition of 70% to 99% internal carotid artery stenosis with duplex scanning. J Vasc Surg 17: 152–157; discussion 157–159 (1993).

[23] North American Symptomatic Carotid Endarterectomy Trial Collaborators: Beneficial effect of carotid endarterectomy in symptomatic patients with high-grade carotid stenosis. N Engl J Med 325: 445–453 (1991).

[24] Ranke C, Trappe HJ: Blood flow velocity measurements for carotid stenosis estimation: interobserver variation and interequipment variability. Vasa 26: 210–214 (1997).

[25] Ringer AJ, German JW, Guterman LR et al.: Follow-up of stented carotid arteries by Doppler ultrasound. Neurosurgery 51: 639–643; discussion 643 (2002).

[26] Robbin ML, Lockhart ME, Weber TM et al.: Carotid artery stents: early and intermediate follow-up with Doppler US. Radiology 205: 749–756 (1997).

[27] Roederer GO, Langlois YE, Jager KA et al.: The natural history of carotid arterial disease in asymptomatic patients with cervical bruits. Stroke 15: 605–613 (1984).

[28] Sauve JS, Laupacis A, Ostbye T et al.: Does this patient have a clinically important carotid bruit? The rational clinical examination. Jama 270: 2843–2845 (1993).

[29] Strandness DE Jr: Screening for carotid disease and surveillance for carotid restenosis. Semin Vasc Surg 14: 200–205 (2001).

[30] Thiele BL, Jones AM, Hobson RW et al.: Report from the Committee on Standards for Noninvasive Vascular Testing of the Joint Council of the Society for Vascular Surgery and the North American Chapter of the International Society for Cardiovascular Surgery. Standards in noninvasive cerebrovascular testing. J Vasc Surg 15: 495–503 (1992).

[31] van Everdingen KJ, van der Grond J, Kappelle LJ: Overestimation of a stenosis in the internal carotid artery by duplex sonography caused by an increase in volume flow. J Vasc Surg 27: 479–485 (1998).

[32] Veith FJ, Amor M, Ohki T et al.: Current status of carotid bifurcation angioplasty and stenting based on a consensus of opinion leaders. J Vasc Surg 33: S111–S116 (2001).

[33] Wiebers DO, Whisnant JP, Sandok BA et al.: Prospective comparison of a cohort with asymptomatic carotid bruit and a population-based cohort without carotid bruit. Stroke 21: 984–988 (1990).

Chapter 1.4

DIGITAL SUBTRACTION ANGIOGRAPHY IN CAROTID ARTERY STENOSIS

A. Srinivasan and M. Goyal

Department of Diagnostic Imaging, University of Ottawa, Ottawa, Canada

Introduction

Atherosclerotic disease of the craniocervical vessels is the underlying basis for cerebral thromboembolic stroke in more than 90% of cases in industrialized nations [19]. Craniocervical atherosclerotic vascular disease most commonly and severely affects the internal carotid artery (ICA) origin and the distal basilar artery [19]. The clinical symptoms and morbidity that result from carotid artery disease, the primary cause of stroke, are mainly due to plaque ulceration, thrombosis, intraplaque hemorrhage, and thinned fibrous caps [24]. Clinical benefit of treating symptomatic, severe carotid stenosis has been demonstrated in a number of trials [18], [10]. Therefore the goals of imaging in atherosclerotic craniocervical disease are to determine the degree of carotid stenosis, identify 'tandem' lesions in the carotid siphon or intracranial circulation and to evaluate the existing and potential collateral circulation [27]. Conventional catheter angiography remains the standard technique against which other non-invasive modalities (CT, MR) are assessed.

Experimental and clinical knowledge

Measuring carotid stenosis

Both the North American Symptomatic Endarterectomy Trial (NASCET) and European Carotid Surgery Trial (ECST) demonstrated definite benefit of carotid endarterectomy (CEA) in symptomatic patients with severe stenosis (70–99%) of the ICA [18], [10]. The Asymptomatic Carotid Atherosclerosis Study (ACAS) also showed benefit of surgery for asymptomatic stenosis greater than 60% [10]. In an analysis published in 1998 by the NASCET collaborators, they showed that CEA yielded only a moderate reduction in the risk of stroke in patients with symptomatic moderate (50–69%) carotid stenosis whereas patients with severe stenosis ($\geq$ 70 percent) had a durable benefit from CEA at eight years of follow-up [2]. They suggested that decisions about treatment for patients in the moderate stenosis category must take into account recognized risk factors, and that exceptional surgical skill was obligatory if CEA was to be performed. As a result, it is essential to determine accurately the degree of stenosis in an individual patient since this has an impact on management decisions.

In both the NASCET and ECST trials, the degree of stenosis was determined using digital subtraction angiography (DSA), which has since become the reference standard. In the NASCET trial, the stenosis was calculated from the ratio of the linear luminal diameter of the narrowest segment of the diseased portion of the artery to the diameter of the artery beyond any poststenotic dilatation (% stenosis = [1 − minimum residual lumen/normal distal cervical internal carotid artery diameter] $\times$ 100) [18] (Fig. 1). The ECST trial measured the percentage diameter stenosis on the best angiographic view of the point of maximum narrowing, using as the denominator an estimate of the original width of the artery at this narrowest point and bearing in mind the slight widening of the normal ICA origin, which is where most of the stenoses were found [10]. The reproducibility of these measurements was also internally validated in both the studies. Gagne et al. prospectively studied the reliability of carotid stenosis measurements performed by practicing physicians of different specialties and different levels of clinical experience and concluded that physicians could easily

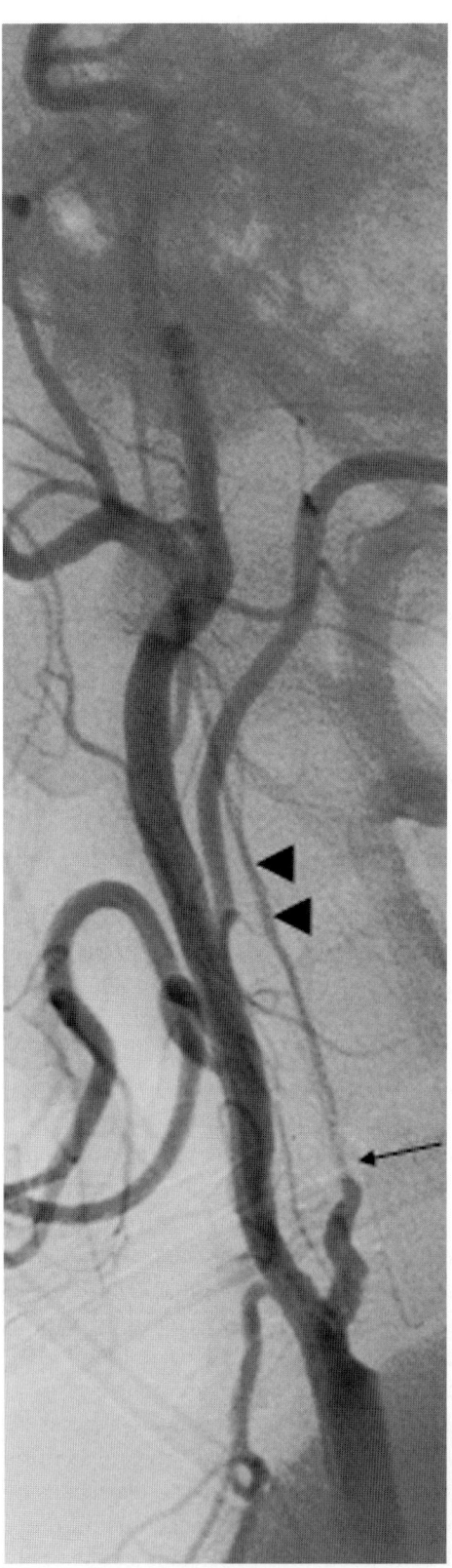

Fig. 1. Lateral common carotid angiogram in a 50-year-old male patient reveals severe stenosis involving the internal carotid artery bulb (arrow) with a 'string-sign' (arrowheads) noted distal to the stenosis. DSA still remains the best modality for distinguishing complete ICA occlusion from the 'string-sign' due to 99% stenosis.

learn the NASCET technique for quantification of carotid stenosis and reliably implement it for appropriate identification of candidates for CEA [12].

Limitations of measurement techniques

There are, however, limitations with both the NASCET and ECST angiographic methods [1], [5], [11]. With the NASCET method, the distal ICA may be obscured by overlying vessels or inadequate contrast enhancement. It is often difficult to decide the appropriate segment of distal ICA on which to base a measurement. With severe stenosis, there is the risk of underestimation of stenosis since the ICA beyond the stenosis may be significantly narrowed. Furthermore, minor degrees of stenosis (<50% bulb diameter reduction) may result in a "negative stenosis" because the carotid bulb is larger than the distal ICA [1]. For ECST measurements, variations in anatomy or irregular stenoses can make it difficult, even for the experienced observer, to predict the normal position of the carotid bulb.

Also, significant discrepancies between the NASCET and the ECST angiographic methods may arise such that a 50% stenosis by NASCET is equivalent to approximately 70% by ECST [3], [23]. For a clinician considering CEA in an individual symptomatic patient, this could cause management dilemmas. This is due to the fact that CEA has a proven benefit in severe stenosis and may only be moderately beneficial in moderate stenosis [2]. The principal difficulty, therefore, with both methods is establishing the diameter of the normal ICA. An alternative approach is to use the well-established physiological and anatomic relationship between the common carotid artery (CCA) and proximal ICA, so that the normal ICA diameter can be derived from measurement of the CCA. For example, duplex ultrasound studies have consistently shown normal ICA/CCA peak blood flow velocity ratios of 0.7 [3], [23], and studies of normal angiograms [25] have shown the ICA/CCA diameter ratio is 1:1.19 (±0.09).

Alternate methods of quantifying stenosis

Thus there are different methods for estimating the stenosis of the ICA proposed in the literature. The use of various methods, which produce different values on the same angiograms, has caused confusion and reduced the generalizability of the results of research. If the results of future studies are to be properly applied to clinical practice, and if noninvasive methods of imaging are to be properly validated against angiography, a single, standard method of measurement of stenosis on angiograms should be adopted. This standard method should be selected on the bases of its ability to predict risk of ipsilateral carotid distribution ischemic stroke and its reproducibility.

Bladin et al. compared stenosis measurements using the NASCET and ECST methods and, two new techniques, the Common Carotid (CC) and Carotid Stenosis Index (CSI) [4]. The CC method was based on a direct comparison of the residual lumen to the distal CCA diameter adjacent to the bulb. The CSI was based on the known relationship between the proximal CCA and ICA (1.2 × CCA diameter = proximal ICA diameter). Of the different angiographic techniques, CSI was found to be the most reliable validated method of measuring carotid stenosis. Hence the authors proposed CSI as a bridge between results of carotid surgery trials, and to validate noninvasive modalities against angiography [4].

Staikov et al. compared three angiographic methods for grading of carotid stenosis (ECST, NASCET, and CC methods) and also examined the correlation between angiographic and ultrasound findings [21]. They concluded that measurements using the CC method were the most reproducible and those using the NASCET method the least. Also, interobserver reproducibility was found to be best for the CC and ECST methods and least for the NASCET method. Ultrasound provided an accuracy of 94% compared to ECST and CC methods and 84% compared to the NASCET method in this study [21].

In another study, Rothwell et al. [20] concluded that there was little difference in the ability of the three angiographic methods (NASCET, ECST and CC) to predict ipsilateral carotid distribution ischemic stroke but found the CC method to be consistently the most reproducible of the three, particularly for stenosis in the clinically important range of 50–90%. Hence, they recommended that the CC method of measurement should be adopted as the standard method of measuring the degree of carotid stenosis on angiograms [20].

However, other authors have felt that CC method is neither superior nor easier to calculate than the NACSET method [8]. They also point out that benefits of CEA have been established in patients with 70–99% carotid stenosis using the NASCET criteria in a clinical trial (unlike the CC method which has not figured in any major clinical trial) and hence did not recommend conversion from the NASCET method to the CC method [8].

Role of rotational angiography

DSA measurement techniques used traditionally involve the anterior-posterior, lateral and oblique views of the carotid bifurcation. However, these projections may not always be optimal for demonstrating the maximum stenosis. Three-dimensional reformations of CT angiogram and MR angiogram can provide visualization from any angle desired and may be as or more accurate than DSA for determining the degree of stenosis. Newer techniques like 3D computed rotational angiography (CRA) can provide a larger number of views than DSA, which may influence the estimated degree of stenosis. CRA provides stenosis grades equivalent to DSA, as well as absolute measurements, providing a comparison for newer 3D techniques [16].

In a study comparing depiction of ICA stenosis on rotational angiography and DSA and its impact on patient treatment, both rotational angiography and DSA were performed in 47 stenotic ICAs. In three ICAs, rotational angiography was non-diagnostic. In 28 of the remaining 44 ICAs, the degree of stenosis was categorized similarly with DSA and rotational angiography, whereas with rotational angiography, 15 ICAs were classified one category higher and one ICA was classified two categories higher, owing to the increased number of projections available. Seventy percent to 99% stenosis was demonstrated in 18 ICAs with DSA and in 25 ICAs with rotational angiography. The authors concluded that rotational angiography frequently depicts more severe ICA stenosis and that rotational angiography could have facilitated a change in the optimal treatment (from non-surgical treatment to CEA) in seven ICAs [7].

Interobserver variability

Interobserver variability in the measurement of carotid stenoses from DSA displayed in different ways (non-magnified or magnified, white or black arteries) was studied by Chow et al., who also compared human readers with computer-generated densitometric measurements of vessel stenosis [6]. The most reliable measurements of stenosis were obtained from the non-magnified black and white artery images. The interobserver variability in the measurement of internal carotid stenoses using non-magnified images was small and increased with magnified images. Also, the computer-generated stenosis measurements were consistently much higher than those of the radiologists. The authors concluded that readers of digital angiographic images must determine the most reliable, reproducible images generated by their equipment, as these measurements significantly affect treatment of patients with symptomatic ICA stenosis [6].

Another study evaluating the interobserver variability for carotid artery stenosis measurements resulted in good overall interrater agreement using the NASCET/ACAS and ECST criteria [22]. However, the authors found that the agreement for therapeutic decisions on carotid surgery was less strong and concluded that accurate stenosis measurement alone may not suffice for reliable treatment decisions in patients with high grade carotid artery stenosis [22].

Young et al. evaluated the reporting of carotid stenosis using four different techniques (three techniques with caliper measurements and the fourth was visual assessment) on both DSA and MRA [28]. The variability in reporting and the number of clinically significant differences arising as a result were similar for each of the four techniques using DSA. While the typical measurement errors for each of the techniques studied were on the order of ± 5%, each technique produced some sizable individual differences for the same angiogram, with resultant wide 95% limits of agreement. Also, the observer variability for reporting MRA was generally a little greater than for DSA. Compared with the caliper techniques, the visual impression of stenosis technique performed well, particularly for MRA. The authors concluded that although observer variability in reporting can be considerable, no important differences were found among the different techniques widely used for measuring carotid stenosis [28].

Advantages of DSA

Distinction between near-occlusion and occlusion of the ICA is crucial because patients can benefit from a surgical treatment in the former scenario [27]. DSA is the best neuroimaging technique for this distinction since other non-invasive modalities may fail to show antegrade flow in severely stenotic vessels [27]. An example of 'string sign' is depicted in Fig. 1.

Detection of tandem lesions (or distal stenosis) is important since some patients may be included from CEA or endovascular therapy depending on the severity of the individual lesions. DSA is probably the best test to reliably demonstrate tandem lesions compared to other non-invasive modalities [27] (Fig. 2).

DSA also provides information about accessibility from the femoral route, demonstrates any aortic pathology (e.g., dissection, aneurysm) that may preclude endovascular therapy or make it difficult and assesses feasibility of using present day angiographic equipment to access tortuous vessels.

Complications of angiography

Hankey et al. prospectively evaluated 382 patients with symptomatically mild carotid ischemia who had cerebral angiography to visualize a potentially resectable lesion at the carotid bifurcation [13]. They encountered complications in 14 angiograms done in 13

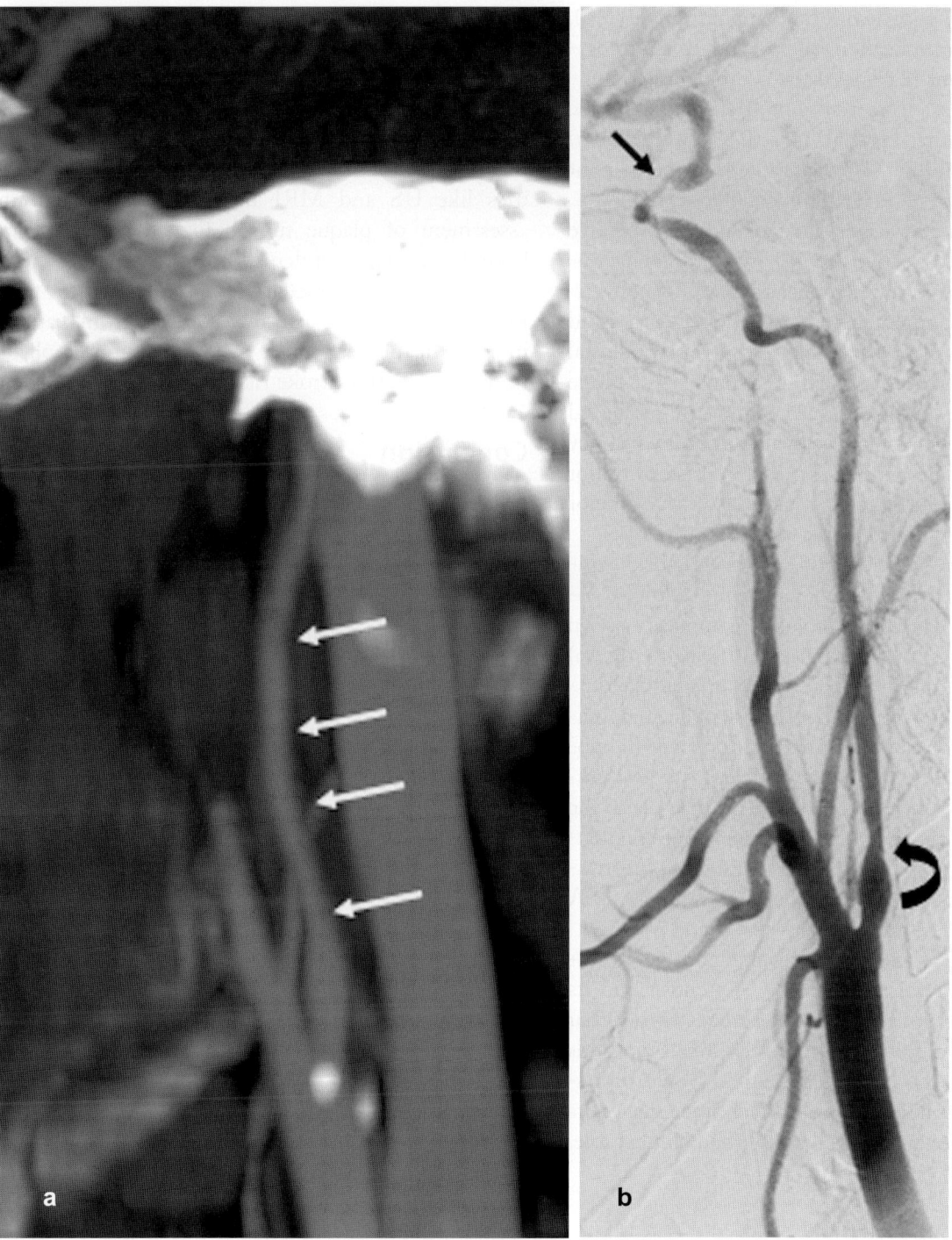

Fig. 2. A 47-year-old female patient presented with right middle cerebral artery territory stroke. CT angiogram (**a**) revealed focal stenosis at the right ICA bulb and a long segment narrowing involving the cervical ICA starting from the bulb upwards (arrows). Carotid angioplasty and stenting was planned. However, on the common carotid angiogram (**b**), there was tandem stenosis detected with a proximal internal carotid stenosis (curved arrow) and a significant distal intracranial stenosis in the supraclinoid segment (arrow), which was difficult to appreciate even retrospectively on the CTA due to adjacent bone.

patients (3.4%) with two local complications (0.5%), two systemic complications (0.5%) and 10 neurological complications (2.6%). Of the neurological complications 2 (0.5%) were transient (transient ischemic attack 1, generalized seizure 1), 3 (0.8%) were reversible strokes and 5 (1.3%) resulted in permanent strokes. There were no deaths encountered [13].

Hankey et al. also evaluated eight prospective and seven retrospective studies from which it was possible to derive the complication rate of conventional cerebral angiography for patients with mild ischemic cerebrovascular disease, who were potential candidates for carotid endarterectomy [14]. Three studies of intravenous and one of intra-arterial digital subtraction angiography were also examined. They reported that angiography carries a 4% risk of minor stroke or transient ischemic attacks, 1% risk of major stroke and a less than 1% risk of even death [14].

In another study evaluating the neurological complications in cerebral angiography, the authors encountered 39 (1.3%) neurologic complications in 2,899 procedures; 20 were transient (0.7%), five (0.2%) were reversible, and 14 (0.5%) were permanent [26].

These studies suggest that the risk of an angiographic procedure is not negligible and therefore the potential benefit to symptomatic patients may be diminished by the invasive nature of DSA. There is also the additional risk of contrast reactions and contrast induced nephropathy with DSA. Amongst the non-invasive modalities, CTA shares the same risks as DSA whereas these risks are avoided with US and MRA.

Thus there is still ongoing work about determining the best way of measuring ICA stenosis and its clinical application. However, it suffices to say that till a proper trial with the other mentioned methods are performed, the NASCET method would probably be the most commonly used technique due to its simplicity of use and its well established clinical role.

Aspects to the future

Carotid plaque instability is considered an important determinant of stroke risk [17]. There are now various imaging techniques that can provide information on carotid plaque morphology. Some characteristics that may reflect a high risk of vulnerability are outward, abluminal plaque remodelling, the presence of intra-plaque haemorrhage, inflammation, severe flow disturbances around the encroaching lesion, plaque cap thinning and ulceration, and abnormal plaque motion [15]. While non-invasive modalities like US and MRI have shown potential in assessment of plaque morphology, DSA may not have the capability of demonstrating the above mentioned plaque characteristics. Non-invasive tests may, therefore, play an increasing role in carotid imaging in the near future due to potential implications in predicting stroke risk.

Conclusion

DSA has long since been established as the gold standard for assessment of vascular disease. Clinical trials using DSA for measurement of carotid artery stenosis have been found DSA to be reasonably reproducible and reliable. But ultrasound Doppler, CTA and MRA are replacing DSA in most centers as the initial tool for assessment of vascular disease in the neck and intracranial circulation. Not only do these modalities have the obvious advantage of being non-invasive unlike DSA, they also have demonstrated good sensitivity in detecting and grading carotid artery stenosis in multiple studies. Also demonstration of plaque morphology may be better with MRI and US and this may play a key role in predicting stroke risks. However, DSA is still the modality of choice for distinguishing between near occlusion and occlusion and will continue to be used for problem solving purposes.

References

[1] Alexandrov AV, Bladin CF, Maggisano R, Norris JW: Measuring carotid stenosis: time for a reappraisal. Stroke 24: 1292–1296 (1993).
[2] Barnett HJ, Taylor DW, Eliasziw M, Fox AJ, Ferguson GG, Haynes RB, Rankin RN, Clagett GP, Hachinski VC, Sackett DL, Thorpe KE, Meldrum HE, Spence JD: Benefit of carotid endarterectomy in patients with symptomatic moderate or severe stenosis. North American Symptomatic Carotid Endarterectomy Trial Collaborators. N Engl J Med 339: 1415–1425 (1998).

[3] Blackshear WM, Phillips DJ, Chikos PM, Harley JD, Thiele BL, Strandness DE: Carotid artery velocity patterns in normal and stenotic vessels. Stroke 11: 67–71 (1980).

[4] Bladin CF, Alexandrova NA, Murphy J, Alexandrov AV, Maggisano R, Norris JW: The clinical value of methods to measure carotid stenosis. Int Angiol 15: 295–299 (1996).

[5] Bousser MG: Benefits from carotid surgery? Yes, but ... Cerebrovasc Dis 2: 122–126 (1992).

[6] Chow V, Burbridge B, Friedland R, Kudel B, Chappell B, Tan L: Interobserver variability in the measurement of internal carotid stenosis. Can Assoc Radiol J 50: 37–40 (1999).

[7] Elgersma OE, Buijs PC, Wust AF, van der Graaf Y, Eikelboom BC, Mali WP: Maximum internal carotid arterial stenosis: assessment with rotational angiography versus conventional intraarterial digital subtraction angiography. Radiology 213: 777–783 (1999).

[8] Eliasziw M, Smith RF, Singh N, Holdsworth DW, Fox AJ, Barnett HJ: Further comments on the measurement of carotid stenosis from angiograms. North American Symptomatic Carotid Endarterectomy Trial (NASCET) Group. Stroke 25: 2445–2449 (1994).

[9] Endarterectomy for asymptomatic carotid artery stenosis. Executive Committee for the Asymptomatic Carotid Atherosclerosis Study. JAMA 273: 1421–1428 (1995).

[10] European Carotid Surgery Trialists' Collaborative Group. Randomised trial of endarterectomy for recently symptomatic carotid stenosis: final results of the MRC European Carotid Surgery Trial (ECST). Lancet 351: 1379–1387 (1998).

[11] Fox AJ: How to measure carotid stenosis. Radiology 186: 316–318 (1993).

[12] Gagne PJ, Matchett J, MacFarland D, Hauer-Jensen M, Barone GW, Eidt JF, Barnes RW: Can the NASCET technique for measuring carotid stenosis be reliably applied outside the trial? J Vasc Surg 24: 449–456 (1996).

[13] Hankey GJ, Warlow CP, Molyneux AJ: Complications of cerebral angiography for patients with mild carotid territory ischaemia being considered for carotid endarterectomy. J Neurol Neurosurg Psychiatry 53: 542–548 (1990).

[14] Hankey GJ, Warlow CP, Sellar RJ: Cerebral angiographic risk in mild cerebrovascular disease. Stroke 21: 209–222 (1990).

[15] Hennerici MG: The unstable plaque. Cerebrovasc Dis; 17 Suppl 3: 17–22 (2004).

[16] Hyde DE, Fox AJ, Gulka I, Kalapos P, Lee DH, Pelz DM, Holdsworth DW: Internal carotid artery stenosis measurement: comparison of 3D computed rotational angiography and conventional digital subtraction angiography. Stroke 35: 2776–2781 (2004).

[17] Lovett JK, Redgrave JN, Rothwell PM: A Critical Appraisal of the Performance, Reporting, and Interpretation of Studies Comparing Carotid Plaque Imaging With Histology. Stroke [Epub ahead of print] (2005).

[18] NASCET Collaborators. Beneficial effect of carotid endarterectomy in symptomatic patients with high-grade carotid stenosis. N Engl J Med 325: 445–453 (1991).

[19] Okazaki H: Fundamentals of Neuropathology, 2nd ed., pp. 27–70. Tokyo: Igaku-Shoin (1989).

[20] Rothwell PM, Gibson RJ, Slattery J, Warlow CP: Prognostic value and reproducibility of measurements of carotid stenosis. A comparison of three methods on 1001 angiograms. European Carotid Surgery Trialists' Collaborative Group. Stroke 25: 2440–2444 (1994).

[21] Staikov IN, Arnold M, Mattle HP, Remonda L, Sturzenegger M, Baumgartner RW, Schroth G: Comparison of the ECST, CC, and NASCET grading methods and ultrasound for assessing carotid stenosis. European Carotid Surgery Trial. North American Symptomatic Carotid Endarterectomy Trial J Neurol 247: 681–686 (2000).

[22] Stapf C, Hofmeister C, Hartmann A, Seyfert S, Koch HC, Mohr JP, Marx P, Mast H: Interrater agreement for high grade carotid artery stenosis measurement and treatment decision. Eur J Med Res 5: 26–31 (2000).

[23] Vaisman U, Wojciechowski M: Carotid artery disease: new criteria for evaluation by sonographic duplex scanning. Radiology 158: 253–255 (1986).

[24] von Ingersleben G, Schmiedl UP, Hatsukami TS, Nelson JA, Subramaniam DS, Ferguson MS, Yuan C: Characterization of atherosclerotic plaques at the carotid bifurcation: correlation of high-resolution MR imaging with histologic analysis-preliminary study. Radiographics 17: 1417–1423 (1997).

[25] Williams MA, Nicolaides AN: Predicting the normal dimensions of the internal and external carotid arteries from the diameter of the common carotid. Eur J Vasc Surg 1: 91–96 (1986).

[26] Willinsky RA, Taylor SM, TerBrugge K, Farb RI, Tomlinson G, Montanera W: Neurologic complications of cerebral angiography: prospective analysis of 2,899 procedures and review of the literature. Radiology 227: 522–528 (2003).

[27] Wolpert SM, Caplan LR: Current role of cerebral angiography in the diagnosis of cerebrovascular diseases. Am J Roentgenol 159: 191–197 (1992).

[28] Young GR, Humphrey PR, Nixon TE, Smith ET: Variability in measurement of extracranial internal carotid artery stenosis as displayed by both digital subtraction and magnetic resonance angiography: an assessment of three caliper techniques and visual impression of stenosis. Stroke 27: 467–473 (1996).

Chapter 1.5

COMPUTED TOMOGRAPHY IMAGING IN CAROTID ARTERY STENOSIS

M. Berg, R. Vanninen, and H. Manninen

Department of Clinical Radiology, Kuopio University Hospital, Kuopio, Finland

Technical evolution of CT-angiography

Volumetric imaging with single and multidetector-row detector spiral scanners

Since the advent of computed tomography (CT) equipment for clinical imaging, the development of spiral (or helical) CT with a slip ring scanner was the main step towards the evolution of CT angiography. Continuous CT spiral scanning with breath-holding of the patient and simultaneous patient transport through the gantry allowed volumetric imaging of whole organs without discontinuities [29], [17]. This rapid spiral volumetric CT scanning permitted imaging of the organs optimally in the arterial or venous phase during the first pass of an intravenously injected bolus of contrast media. Soon after spiral CT scanning was introduced in 1990, several of the first reports on the clinical applications of spiral CT concentrated on CT angiography [16], [47], [68], [25]. With a singledetector spiral CT scanner (SDCT), rapid volumetric scanning increased image noise slightly and induced a minor decrease in the z-axis resolution compared to previous sequential technique, but did not decrease the diagnostic quality of the study [11]. Methods for three-dimensional (3D) display were generated before the introduction of CT angiography. The 3D display with 'angiographic-like' images was quickly adopted for demonstration of CT angiography studies [47], [63], [69], [70], [66]. With overlapping axial source images the z-axis resolution was improved, upgrading also the quality of reconstructed images [30].

In the first series the scanning volume in SDCT angiography was relatively short, depending on the imaging parameters such as collimation and table feed. The introduction of 180 linear and higher-order interpolation algorithms showed that table feed could be increased over the length of slice collimation (pitch values over 1), with a slight increase in image noise, but longer scanning volumes [51], [62]. In the early days of CT angiography the total examination time, including the time for scanning, postprocessing of the images and the image display, was up to 1.5 hours. Gradually, the overall duration of CT angiography has decreased. The capacity and heat-resistance of X-ray tubes increased, also allowing longer scan times. Furthermore, data acquisition time has decreased with subsecond scanning, which also improves the imaging of small arteries [58]. Computers have become more powerful, resulting in faster reconstruction of raw data. With effective computers the real time interactive volume rendering (VR) method for 3D display has become available for clinical use [34].

Because individual circulation time sometimes led to suboptimal arterial contrast enhancement, a method for the detection of optimal scan delay time was developed, replacing partly the use of fixed delay time [62]. Later manufacturers produced special programs for automatic detection of contrast material arrival into target vessels, i.e., bolus triggering methods. Within five years, CT angiography has been used to image almost all arteries from head to toe [69], [70], [36], [31], and also venous structures [69], [70], [13].

CT angiography examination using a single slice device must be planned with caution due to the limited coverage of imaging volume obtained with the SDCT device. The scanning time also extends up to 30–40 seconds with the larger imaging volumes, which may exceed the breath-holding capability of the patient. This problem has been solved with the multidetector-row CT (MDCT) scanners allowing both the increase of the scanning volume and the faster scanning using a narrow collimation. With a 16-row MDCT the entire carotid circulation with the arteries of circle of Willis can be scanned with a sufficient image quality in nine seconds.

Carotid imaging with a SDCT scanner

In general, with a SDCT device a thin collimation should be chosen to optimise longitudinal (z-axis) resolution. A slow table feed and a small reconstruction interval are preferable to image small vessels, especially those running in the axial plane [10]. Naturally, minimising those parameters will decrease the length of the scanning volume. To meet the need for good resolution and sufficient scan volume, it is preferable to increase the pitch (P) (=table increment per gantry rotation/collimation) rather than to increase the width of collimation. Then the pitch value increases to over 1, but it should not exceed the value of 2 [51]. In addition, with SDCT the radiation dose is consequently reduced with the greater pitch, if the other imaging parameters remain constant. Most clinical applications of CT angiography can be performed with 3–5 mm collimation using an SDCT device, but for carotid arteries, a thin collimation of 1–2 mm is preferable. The reconstruction increment for axial source images should be chosen so that axial slices overlap at least 50%. The noise is related to other imaging parameters such as collimation and X-ray tube output (kilovoltage, tube current) and to reconstruction kernel, but not to the pitch value [78]. Table 1 shows the designs of SDCT studies used for carotid imaging.

Towards multiple-row detector scanners

CT equipment with multiple-row detectors (MDCT) opened a new era for CT angiography, eliminating many disadvantages such as limited scan volume coverage, long scanning times, some artifacts and large doses of contrast media [6], [61]. MDCT using thin section width for standard protocols with increased longitudinal resolution has enabled multiplanar reformats (MPR) and 3D reconstructions of excellent quality for CT angiography in various anatomic areas including carotid circulation. Nowadays, this 'multislice' CT angiography with rapid interactive modes for image display has achieved a firm standing in the repertoire of noninvasive methods for carotid imaging.

Actually, the earliest prototypes of CT scanner were dual scanners in the early seventies, but single detector CT devices went to production. In 1993 a dual section scanner was introduced again. Advanced MDCT devices with two different detector array designs (matrix detectors and adaptive array detectors) were introduced in 1998. Those detector array designs are used for four- and eight-row detector devices. The MDCT technology allowed larger anatomic coverage, for example imaging of the entire aortoilac system and lower extremity inflow and run-off [61], [64]. Also with MDCT the table speed and the tube rotation time of the scanner influence the scanning volume coverage. The limited scan coverage of four detector row MDCT devices is evident with a high-resolution protocol [55].

At present, MDCT devices with subsecond tube rotation are available with up to 32 rows of detectors for 64 slices. However, MDCT technology using 16-row adaptive array detector has already allowed faster scanning, excellent spatial resolution with near-isotropic imaging for routine scanning protocols, multiphase studies and convenience for the patient because the breath-holding time is shortened. Also new applications, i.e., cardiac and coronary artery imaging, have been introduced. All these advancements can contribute to the increase of diagnostic utility also for carotid imaging. The newest MDCT technonology with 32 detector rows for 64 slices has better spatial resolution than other MDCT scanners but the sufficient volume coverage and speed for routine clinical use has already been obtained with 16-row detector CT device. Faster scanning with 16- and 32-row detector CT devices permits CT angiography of carotid arteries without venous enhancement.

One of the advantages of MDCT imaging is flexibility. For the MDCT scanners with z filter approach such as produced by Siemens, spiral raw data can retrospectively be reconstructed at different slice thickness values and increment values, but the section width (slice thickness) should not be less than the thickness of the collimation [23]. Both the axial images with thin section width (1 mm or less) of high resolution and with wide section width of less noise can be reconstructed from the same study. One disadvantage of modern MDCT technology is the overwhelming number of axial images, and therefore image reconstruction with wide section thickness for archiving axial source images with additional 2D reformats and 3D reconstructions are needed. Detailed descriptions about the MDCT technology have been published [23], [53], [54].

There have been two definitions for the pitch value of MDCT [55], but after recommendations given by International Electrotechnical Commission only the definition equal to SDCT pitch definition is preferable to use [23]. Then pitch is defined as in SDCT: P = Table feed (mm) per gantry rotation/ beam collimation (mm). Pitch value in spiral CT examinations reveals the intersection cap (P > 1) or overlapping of the sections (P < 1). The main principle of cervicocranial imaging with fast MDCT scanners is to use thin collimation at pitch < 1. Axial image overlap is recommended to be 20–50%. Thus the good quality of 2D and 3D reconstructions is ensured.

The challenge for CT imaging is the dose reduction. CT imaging is highly responsible for the radiation dose produced by medical X-ray imaging. Using SDCT devices the increase in pitch value enabled dose reduction. Also with faster MDCT the reduction of dose is possible but the requirements for larger anatomic coverage and better spatial resolution increases the radiation dose subsequently. It is important to adapt the tube current and the imaging parameters to the size of the patient (the body diameter) for reducing the dose and maintaining constant noise. It must be noted that the dose is unrelated to the pitch with MDCT using z-filter approach [23]. CT equipments nowadays registry the dose, which is calculated to the weighted CT dose index (CTDIvol) and dose length product (DLP) available for the radiologist and the technologist at each study.

Clinical knowledge

Cerebrovascular disease with disabling stroke is still the leading cause of long-lasting morbidity. Atherosclerotic plaques in the carotid arteries may cause life-threatening or strongly disabling disorders. Atherosclerosis in the artery wall supplying the brain is a risk factor for stroke and other cerebrovascular disorders, i.e. amaurosis fugax, transient ischaemic attacks and dizziness. Stenosis, wall thickness, the lipid or necrotic core of the plaque, plaque ulceration and intraplaque haemorrhage are supposed to be related to the risk of stroke and other cerebrovascular disorders, but the data concerning the relationship between plaque morphology and clinical outcome are still conflicting [18], [27], [44]. However, both haemodynamic and embolic mechanism are supposed to produce disorders [18]. The degree of stenosis has been reliably verified to be related with stroke risk. The European Carotid Surgery Trial (ECST) and the North American Symptomatic Carotid Endarterectomy Trial (NASCET) have shown that carotid endarterectomy is beneficial in the secondary prevention of stroke in symptomatic patients with high-grade stenosis [48], [43], [20]. An ongoing randomised study includes the plaque characterisation for the observation of subgroups at stroke risk [49]. Obstructing arterial stenosis due to either a large plaque or sudden intraplaque haemorrhage of a plaque and plaque rupture with thrombosis are the main causes of symptomatic disease. Before the choice of the treatment, the extent of the atherosclerotic disease and the need for interventions are verified by imaging.

Despite some disadvantages of CT angiography imaging, such as radiation and use of potentially nephrotoxic contrast media, CT angiography is feasible for the imaging of atherosclerotic carotid arteries when the patient selection and preparation before the scanning are well done. Over the last decade, the development of CT devices has widened the scope of this nowadays rapid and easy imaging method for carotid circulation. Furthermore, CT angiography is more convenient and less time consuming for the patient than catheter angiography.

The advantages of CT angiography are the possibility to evaluate extracranial arteries simultaneously with delineation of soft tissues, including the plaque, and to achieve good spatial resolution in any direction with the three-dimensional display [67]. The anatomic orientation of carotid arteries running perpendicular to the imaging plane is favourable for CT angiography [33]. The designs and results of various studies of the use of SDCT angiography in the evaluation of carotid arteries are shown in Tables 1 and 2.

The diversity of various elements in CT angiography, including variability in the CT devices, contrast agent infusion implementation techniques, scanning parameters and variable image display for diagnosis, complicates the comparison of various studies. In addition, the studies had different scales for stenosis grading. However, these studies have proved that CT angiography is a promising tool for the assessment of carotid arteries and the detection of stenoses. The study by Moll et al. [45] has in a large study population shown that CT angiography had higher sensitivity than CD-US for the detection of severe (70–99%) stenosis in the carotid artery. In that study the results of various imaging methods were compared with the findings of subsequent surgical operation as a reference. CT angiography was as sensitive and specific as DSA [45].

The MDCT technique facilitates rapid scanning of the head and neck, thus allowing either smaller volume high-resolution imaging with isotropic voxel size or imaging of a larger coverage of anatomic areas, i.e. the whole cerebrovascular circulation from aortic arch to intracranial arteries [61] (Fig. 1). MDCT has a high resolution in z-direction, facilitating good quality 2D reformats or 3D reconstructions and accurate measurements. In a preliminary study with five patients using MDCT for carotid CT angiography excellent image quality and good demonstration of carotid plaques was reported [39].

Preparing of the patient for CT angiography

Preparing the patient for CT angiography is simple. To perform CT angiography, it is mandatory that the patient can co-operate. Before the study all phases of the examination should be explained to the patient to obtain good quality images without moving artefacts. A history of previous hypersensibility reactions of the patient should be asked, especially if caused by iodinated contrast agents. Because the contrast media may be nephrotoxic, before CT angiography renal function should be evaluated to avoid use of contrast media for patients at risk for contrast-induced renal failure [72]. The screening of renal function with laboratory tests, most often serum creatinine, from patients without risk factors has been questioned based on a study with 2034 outpatients, because renal function impairment is very seldom among patients without known risk factors [73]. Recently, the European Society of Urogenital Radiology has produced a simple guideline on serum creatinine measurements before iodinated contrast medium administration [72]. If needed, sufficient hydration for the patient should be arranged. For the contrast media infusion, an 18-gauge cannula is placed in the antecubital vein. Unenhanced images from the target area for localising anatomical structures are obtained, if necessary.

Imaging protocols for carotid CT angiography

Different protocols are available for carotid circulation in different multidetector-row CT devices [59], [24], [53]. For patients with overweight it is possible to change imaging parameters and the interpolation algorithm to improve the quality of images [64]. A noteworthy point for the improvement of the CT angiography quality is appropriate scanning technique, because low kVp enhances the attenuation of radiation in vascular studies increasing the ratio of resolution to noise and visualisation of vascular structures [79]. Furthermore, with the use of low kVp the dose of radiation decreases concurrently. Our protocol for carotid imaging for scientific purposes including carotid circulation and aortic arch with a 16-row CT device (Siemens Somatotom Sensation 16) is described in the Table 1.

Table 1. CT angiography protocol for the cervicocranial arteries at the authors' institution

slice collimation	16 × 0.75mm
table feed	12mm
tube rotation time	0.5 s
pitch	0.5
kV	100
mAs(eff)	120–160
reconstruction increment for axial slices	0.8 mm
section width	1mm
medium smooth reconstruction kernel	(B30f)
contrast media infusion volume	100 ml with a flow rate of 5 ml/s
contrast media concentration	300 mgI/ml
saline chaser bolus	30 ml with a flow rate of 5 ml/s
bolus triggering ROI	in the aortic arch

Another section width of 2–3mm is also used for the multiplanar reformats and 3D reconstructions. The 2 mm thick miniMIP reconstructions are routinely made in sagittal and coronal planes at the level of the carotid bifurcations and (double)oblique sagittal planes are applied when necessary. In addition to the carotid bifurcations and common carotid arteries, the distal internal carotid arteries and the M1 segments should also be evaluated as well as the vertebrobasilar arteries for the presence of tandem lesions and hemodynamically significant lesions in the collateral circulation. For the optimal enhancement in aorta and carotid arteries during scanning, the bolus triggering is used placing the ROI circle in the aortic arch, and the delay-time of 6s is used for the monitoring scans. A thorough review about the scanning protocols with various MDCT scanners has been published [53].

Contrast media application

It is desirable to perform the contrast media injection with a double-syringe power injector for the contrast media injection and subsequent saline flush. The saline flush pushes the contrast media to central circulatory and flushes the veins free from high concentration of contrast media related to strike artifacts. Artifacts from contrast-filled veins also can be avoided by changing the scanning direction (i.e., caudocranial for the imaging of carotid arteries). With recently introduced three-syringe power injector it is possible to infuse a dilution of contrast media between the contrast media and saline for decreasing strike artifacts properly.

The circulation time of the patient should be determined if there is doubt about decreased cardiac output increasing the time between the start of the contrast media infusion and the arrival of contrast media in the target vessel. The determination of circulation time can be carried out with a test bolus or with specific programs, i.e., bolus triggering methods, which are nowadays widely available in CT devices [74], [28]. These bolus triggering methods monitor the inflow of contrast media to the target vessel with continuous low-dose scanning. The use of bolus triggering during CT angiography ensures sufficient contrast density in target vessels. In addition, the use of high-concentration contrast media for CT angiography studies has been recommended [21].

Enhancement in the target vessels is affected by patient-related and injection-related factors. Body weight is the most important patient-related factor; an increase in body weight decreases the arterial enhancement [8]. Low cardiac output delays the peak enhancement, but increases the enhancement magnitude. In vascular imaging, the enhancement is directly related to the iodine concentration in target vessels [8], [3]. A high concentration in target vessels can be reached with an increase in flow rate of commonly used contrast media (300 mgI/ml) or with the use of high-concentration contrast media (370 or 400 mgI/ml). Additional benefit can be achieved with the use of high-concentration contrast media with early enhancement [3], especially with very short scanning times of MDCT devices.

Because the resolution to noise relationship is proportionally affected by the contrast media concentration in target vessel, the contrast media infusion should be planned carefully. The duration of the scanning is critical for the planning of contrast media application. Using SDCT the scanning duration time is almost always long, up to 40 seconds. Some special

MDCT imaging protocols with a long scanning time for example ECG-gated cardiac imaging, require extended contrast media infusion. With the use of extended contrast media infusion, the total amount of iodine given to the patient should be controlled.

A basic understanding of the contrast media kinetics after intravenous bolus infusion is essential to perform CT angiography studies [21]. In general, the iodine administration rate has to be increased for angiography examinations with MDCT to obtain satisfactory enhancement in the target vessels. The iodine administration rate could be increased using a higher flow rate of the infusion or alternatively using high-concentration contrast media. However, due to faster scanning of MDCT the total volume of contrast media infusion is substantially lower than using SDCT for CT angiography. The critical point for contrast media infusion for MDCT angiography examinations is the very short time window for the data acquisition, because in most general applications for vascular imaging the scanning lasts only 5–10 seconds [21]. The exact time delay from the beginning of the intravenous infusion to the arrival of the contrast media in the target vessel is crucial due to the short data acquisition time, because if timing fails, the enhancement in target vessels could be totally missed. Therefore, the use of bolus triggering technique is essential for the MDCT angiography studies. Specific contrast infusion protocols for different duration of data acquisitions are published and it is also recommended to use biphasic protocols to achieve uniform enhancement in CT angiography [21], [22].

Reformations and 3D reconstructions of carotid CT angiography

The axial data of CT angiography can be demonstrated with reformations (two-dimensional display) or with 3D reconstructions. The reformation techniques, multiplanar reformation (MPR) and curved planar reformation (CPR), retain the original image data of axial source images including high attenuation structures such as enhanced vessels and mural calcifications and low attenuation structures such as intimal plaques and trombi. Two-dimensional MPR is a widely used postprocessing technique and with arbitrary chosen views, it is very useful in CT angiography [59], [32], [75]. Thin MPR with good resolution for vessel display shows usually only restricted views of the tortuous vessels demanding serial of thin MPRs over the region of interest or MPR with a thickness covering the entire artery diameter. In eccentric stenoses two perpendicular MPRs are needed to display the lesion in the artery wall. With CPR it is possible to follow the entire course of the vessel (Fig. 1). In general, CPR is operator dependent and not suitable for measurement of diameters

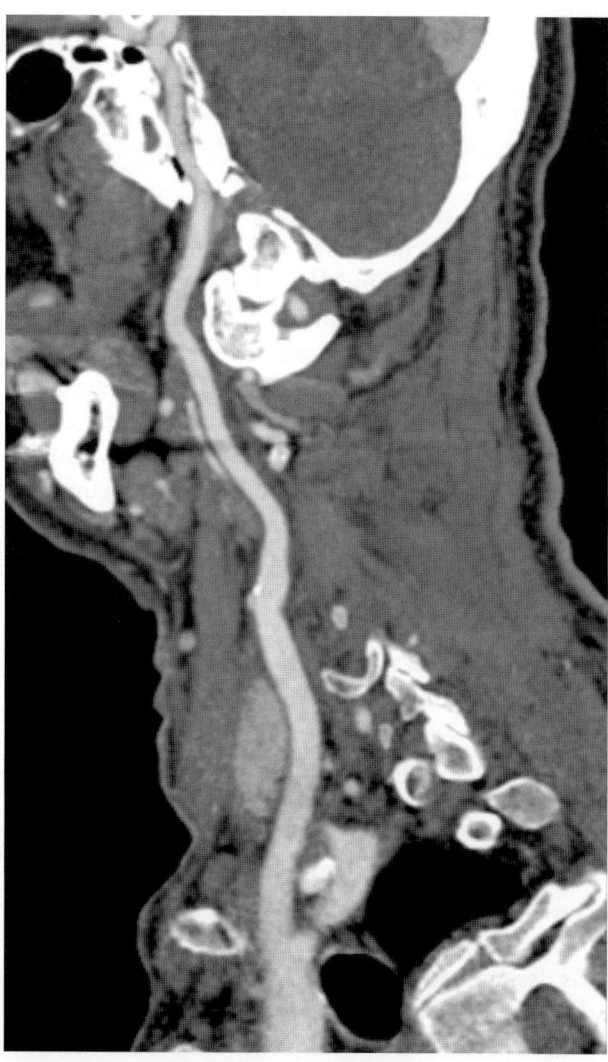

Fig. 1. Curved planar reformation of the left carotid artery with no hemodynamically significant stenosis.

while the operator may not accurately point the centre of the vessel leading to distortions of anatomic structures. However, there is commercially available software with automatic assessment of the vessel using CPR, where the automatic assessment of the center of the lumen facilitates automatic measurements of vessel cross-sectional dimensions in diameters and in area value [81].

For the 3D display using maximum intensity projection (MIP) or shaded surface display (SSD) the editing of unnecessary structures, such as bones and enhancing veins and organs, is essential [59]. MIP retains the voxel with the maximum intensity in each line, in CT angiography mainly the voxels containing enhanced vascular structures [56]. MIP misses the visualisation of depth, leading sometimes to misinterpretation of the anatomical relationships. In MIPs, differences in attenuation can be detected, thus plaque mural calcifications are distinguishable but especially an extensive mural calcification hampers the demonstration of vessel lumen. Intraluminal pathology may be obscured if it is surrounded by enhanced blood flow; hence the detection of intravascular trombi, emboli or dissection is limited in MIP [56]. Sliding thin-slab MIPs are also useful for the demonstration of the complex vascular structures [46]. Targeted MIP is useful to avoid artefacts from overlying structures.

For SSD images, one or two user-defined thresholds are chosen, and only those high attenuation voxels inside chosen two thresholds or over one chosen threshold are displayed [9]. The impression of depth is computed with a virtual light source. SSD images in CT angiography are feasible for visualising complex vascular anatomy, but this method suffers from the inability to show structures separately, i.e., in CT angiography this method fuses vascular structures and plaque calcifications [63].

With the aid of powerful computers the volume rendering (VR) technique has developed into one of the most fascinating technique for 3D image display. The primary principle of the VR technique is to maintain the original data of CT examination without cumbersome and obsolete editing of the axial data. VR technique uses data from all imaged voxels through volume data management. VR image formation for display consists of algorithms for transfer functions [12]. In VR the voxels are assigned with an opacity value and this value can be chosen between total transparency and opacity. The VR images are lighted similarly as the SSDs. Maintainance of the data from all voxels in VR allows the editing of 3D display with a clip plane in real time. Coloring of the structures having different opacity value for each anatomic structure is possible. VR technique can also be used for the purpose of virtual endoscopy in addition to the SSD technique [60].

Table 2 presents the advantages and limitations of each reformation and 3D reconstruction method.

Carotid CT angiography interpretation

For the purpose of CT angiography image display several methods are available as described above. However, the radiologist must be aware of the technical principles underlying those 3D reconstruction methods to avoid pitfalls in the evaluation of vascular lesions [59], [53], [32]. The editing of axial slices must be done with caution to avoid removal of valid data. MIP lacks impression of depth, leading to overprojection of structures. While only those voxels containing the highest intensity are displayed, other valid data of the same ray with lower attenuation might be obscured. The selection of threshold is of greater significance for SSD. Incorrect threshold selection can falsely imply or exclude lesions, i.e., stenosis, in arteries. Although the VR technique for 3D image display consists more of the original data than MIP or SSD, all the pathology detected in VR must be confirmed from the source images. This also applies to other 3D display techniques [32].

Instead of immediate use of the 3D display methods, it is preferable first to interpret a CT angiography study using original data without data editing or conversion [56]. Axial source images as a secondary raw data and additional MPRs contain all the information of the entire imaged volume, such as enhanced vascular structures, plaques in the arterial wall with or without mural calcifications and extravascular tissues. The quality of MPR images has improved since the advent of MDCT, which has al-

Table 2. Advantages and pitfalls of different carotid CT angiography reformations and 3D reconstruction techniques

Technique	Advantage	Pitfalls
Original axial source images	Excellent for the use of interactive interpretation, all information from the study available	Interpretation operator dependent. Not useful for the demonstration of the findings
MPR	Excellent for the use of interactive interpretation. All information from the study available in arbitrary planes	Interpretation operator dependent. Not very useful for the demonstration of the findings
CPR	Useful for the demonstration of the findings needing two perpendicular views	Operator dependent. Not useful for the measurements, with the exception of specific automated methods for the stenosis assessment
MIP	Useful for the demonstration of the findings	Needs editing of the original data. Especially volume MIP time consuming and lacks depth information
Thin slab MIP	2 mm slices excellent for the evaluation of bifurcation area. Visualization of the mural calcifications	Thicker slices may loose information of thin structures such as intimal flap
SSD	Useful for the demonstration of complex vascular anatomy with depth information	Fusion of mural calcifications with enhanced vascular lumen. Prone for operator dependent (thresholding) artefacts
VR	Useful for the demonstration of complex vascular anatomy with some density information and with depth information. Interactive 3D display method for CT angiography findings	Needs good hardware capacity of the computer. Still somewhat operator dependent

lowed the routine use of thin collimation, leading to high spatial resolution and nearly isotropic or isotropic voxel size [55]. In addition, MPR images, thin-slicing MIPs and targeted MIP image are easy to reconstruct without time-consuming editing of source images or removal of mural calcifications. MPR does not suffer from the overprojection of the other enhanced vessels. However, a single axial image or thin MPR view displays only a substructure of an arterial tree. The interpretation of the complex vascular system necessitates viewing of several contiguous axial images or MPRs. Therefore the interpretation has to be done on a workstation using a cine mode. This is called interactive interpretation [53]. The interactive interpretation of CT angiography in our daily practice includes scrolling of axial source images together with two MPR views in orthogonal directions (sagittal and coronal) to analyse vascular anatomy and pathology. If necessary, additional MPR views angled by the direction of the viewed vessel or curved reformats are done. CT angiography with this interactive volumetric interpretation is an advisable and beneficial tool for the radiologist to analyse vascular anatomy and pathology. The 3D display methods are an additional tool for the overview of the anatomy, for the search of possible sites of pathology, and for the demonstration of the diagnosis to the referring physician [32]. In addition, the 3D images can display complex arterial anatomy in a single view, as shown in Fig. 2 displaying 3D reconstruction images of the epiaortic and entire carotid circulation imaged with a 16-row multidetector device.

Diagnostic performance of CT angiography for carotid stenosis assessment

Based on the results of a carotid SDCT angiography study where intravascular ultrasound (IVUS) was

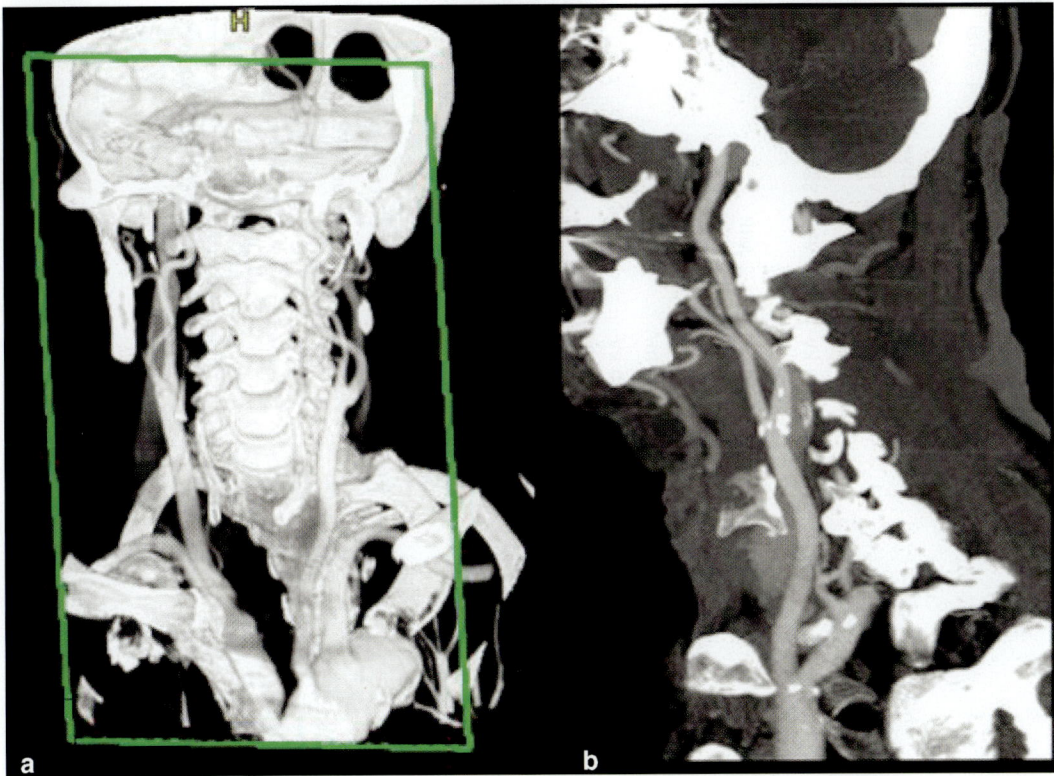

Fig. 2. Carotid artery anatomy of two different patients shown with 3D reconstructions. VR image (**a**) shows the entire course of both carotid arteries. Thin slab MIP (**b**) shows the entire course of the extracranial right carotid artery with mural calcifications at the bifurcation.

used as the reference method, the repeatability of CT angiography for the measurements of lumen diameter, plaque thickness and diameter stenosis from the axial source images is excellent [5]. Even for subtle stenoses, the sensitivity of SDCT angiography was excellent (96–100%) when IVUS was used as a standard of reference. Intraplaque calcifications and anatomic vascular structures facilitate the precise localisation and identification of atherosclerotic plaque as a target for measurements, even between successive studies. CT angiography seems to be an adequate follow-up imaging method for the aims of prospective studies.

In the same study, CT angiography depicted all stenotic lesions of the carotid arteries evident in contrast angiography. Moreover, CT angiography also detected concentric stenoses not detectable in contrast angiography [4]. Contrast angiography with only luminal display fails to detect atherosclerotic lesions, which are concentric. The difference between contrast angiography and CT angiography diameter stenosis measurements may be even greater because of the inability of contrast angiography to detect the compensatory arterial enlargement during the development of the atherosclerotic process [26]. Complex vascular anatomy does not hamper the quality of CT angiography, and the reconstructions can be created in any projection without artefacts from surrounding structures [55].

CT angiography with MDCT technique has excellent spatial resolution also for smaller structures, but artefacts sometimes still hamper the visualisation of short stenoses [53]. The capacity of newer MDCT devices with up to 64 slices per rotation is superior to the older devices used in the reviewed literature shown in Table 2. The 16-row multidetector

Table 3. The design of SDCT angiography studies on carotid arteries

Study	Contrast media				Imaging parameters					Reformat or reconstruction used for the diagnosis
	Volume ml	Concentration mg I/ml	Flow rate ml/s	Bolus triggering* (s)	Collimation mm	Feed mm	pitch	Incr. mm	Tube Current	
Papp, 1997	100	(30 g iodine)	1.5	−(30)	3	3	1	2	120 kV 250 mA	SSD, interactive SSD + axial
Magarelli, 1998	80	350	3	+(15–22)	3	3	1	NA	120 kV 160 mAs	Interactive MIP + axial
Cinat, 1998	125	370	2.5–3	−(12)	2	NA	1.25	2	NA	Interactive MIP + axial
Leclerc, 1999	120	350	3	−(20)	2	2	1	1	120 kV 220 mA	Axial, VR, MIP
Marcus, 1999	140	300	3.5	NA(15–26)	3	3	1	1.5	120 kV 210 mAs	VRT, SSD
Sameshima, 1999	90	300	3–4	−(15–25)	3	3–4	1–1.5	1	120 kV 210 mA	MIP
Verhoek, 1999	100	350	3	−	2	3	1.5	1	120 kV 240 mA	MIP, VR, t-CT
Anderson, 2000	120	300	3	−	3 with 1mm section width	NA	1.5	NA	120 kV 200–320 mA	Axial, MIP, SSD
Binaghi, 2001	100	300	NA	−(13–15)	3	3	1	1	120 kV 200 mA	Interactive axial + MPR + MIP
Moll, 2001	120	300	2.5–3.0	±(15,18,20)	2	3	1.5	1 or 2	140 kV 140 mA	Interactive axial + SSD + VR + MIP
Randoux, 2001	140	250	2.5	+	3 with 1mm section width	3	NA	1	NA	Interactive axial + oblique MPR
Alvarez-Linera, 2003	150	NA	3	+	2	2	1	NA	120 kV 210 mA	Interactive MIP + SSD +axial[†] + multiplanar rendering reconstructions[†]

Note — NA, not available; HU, Hounsfield unit; MIP, maximum intensity projection; SSD, shaded surface display; VR(T), volume rendering (technique); MPR, multiplanar reformation; t-CT, transverse 2D-CT.
* The fixed delay time in parenthesis.
[†] Those images used only for calcified stenoses.

Table 4. Diagnostic performance of carotid SDCT angiography in comparison to conventional angiography: A review of the literature

Study	n vessels (patients)	Evaluation method for the degree of stenosis	Scales for grading	Criteria for the significant finding	Results Sensitivity %	Specificity %	Overall accuracy %	Agreement	Other result
Papp, 1997	96 (48)	"Evaluation of the degree of stenosis"	5	>70%	SSD 65–66* SSD + axial 76–80*	NA	NA	NA	Mean error: SSD f[1.93] = 5.98 SSD + axial images f[1.93] = 0.00
Magarelli, 1998	40 (20)	Measurement of the DSD	5	>70%	81.4	96.4	91.3	NA	
Cinat, 1998	106 (53)	Measurement of area reduction	5	>80%	87	90	89	NA	PPV 89%, NPV 88%
Leclerc, 1999	44 (22)	Measurement of the DSD	5	>70%	Axial 67 MIP 86 VR 100	Axial 96 MIP 91 VR 92	NA	NA	Axial κ = 0.90 MIP κ = 0.87 VR κ = 0.85
Marcus, 1999	46 (23)	Measurement of the DSD	4	≥70%	VRT 89–94† SSD 88–94†	VRT 96–97† SSD 93†	NA	NA	Interobserver agreement (κ): VRT 0.90 – 0.97 SSD 0.95 – 0.97
Sameshima, 1999	128 (64)	Estimation of the DSD	5		NA	NA	NA	NA	r = 0.987
Verhoek, 1999	38 (19)	Measurement of the DSD	4		NA	NA	NA	VR 76 MIP 71 t-CT 89	VR κ = 0.67 MIP κ = 0.62 t-CT κ = 0.85
Anderson, 2000	80 (40)	Measurement of the DSD	5	> 50%	Axial 89 MIP 90 SSD 85	Axial 91 MIP 82 SSD 86	Axial 90 MIP 86 SSD 86	NA	PPV NPV Axial 86% Axial 93% MIP 78% MIP 93% SSD 75% SSD 90%
Binaghi, 2001	49 (25)	Measurement of the DSD	4	≥70%	89	100	NA	NA	PPV 100%, NPV 94% κ = 0.94
Moll, 2001	356 (178)	Measurement of DSD and area stenosis with reference to surgery	3	≥50%	98.3	100	NA	NA	
Randoux, 2001	44 (22)	Measurement of the DSD	6	>70%	100	100	NA	NA	r = 0.93 Interobserver κ = 0.92
Alvarez-Linera, 2003	80 (40)	Measurement of the DSD	5	≥70%	74.3	97.6	NA	NA	κ = 0.72 Pearson correlation=0.86

Note – NA, not available; κ, statistic kappa; r, Spearman's correlation; DSD, diameter stenosis degree; MIP, maximum intensity projection; SSD, shaded surface display; VR(T), volume rendering (technique); PPV, positive predictive value; NPV, negative predictive value.
* The approximation of values from the bar chart done by the author (MB).
† Minimum and maximum values for three different observers.

CT device nowadays available for carotid imaging in our department produces images with fewer artifacts (Fig. 2) with considerably shorter acquisition time. The advent of the CT with 64 slices does not provide anymore advance in scanning time but better spatial resolution acquired with very thin slices, which may provide additional benefit for the carotid imaging. In addition, the use of ECG-gated imaging significantly reduces the movement artifacts in CT angiography, and also can be used for carotid arteries in cases with suspicion of tight stenoses. Alternatively, in ambiguous cases the use of conventional angiography is advisable. Arguments for the use of conventional angiography for the confirmation of high-grade stenosis in symptomatic patients have also been proposed earlier to ensure appropriate treatment decisions [19].

Although measurements of the absolute diameter by CT angiography were inaccurate compared with rotational angiography especially in cases of high-grade stenosis, the diagnostic performance of CT angiography performed with a four-channel CT device using DSA as a standard of reference proved to be good in a study of 35 patients with carotid artery stenosis [4]. In this study, in addition to the interpretation based on absolute diameter measurements, a third radiologists visually interpreted CT angiography using interactive interpretation of axial slices and MPR views for the diagnosis and simply estimated the degree of stenosis. Visual estimation proved to be the most sensitive method for identification of carotid stenosis of 50% or more, but specificity was only modest. Simple visual estimation of the degree of stenosis in four-detector row CTA has been reported to yield sensitivity of 100%, specificity of 73% and overall accuracy of 86% for the detection of carotid stenosis ≥ 50%, when using DSA as the standard of reference [4]. When using the highly sensitive visual estimation as the first line screening step for the detection of a significant stenosis (50%), the measurement of the degree of stenosis can be used as the second step only for the positive cases selected by visual estimation. The combination of interactive interpretation of CT angiography with subsequent MPR measurements for selected cases achieved the best diagnostic accuracy; CT angiography for the symptomatic side showed a sensitivity of 95%, specificity of 93% and overall accuracy of 94% [4]. In another study by Anderson et al. [2], SDCT angiography with the interpretation of axial source images proved to be 89% sensitive, 91% specific and 90% accurate in the detection of carotid stenosis over 50%.

In the study of Josephson et al. MDCT showed high sensitivity (100%) for the assessment of carotid stenosis with measurement using 70% cutoff for stenosis degree [35]. Most of the major overestimations of diameter stenosis degree with CT angiography seem to occurr because of the enlargement of intraplaque calcifications by the partial volume effect. This phenomenon is a disadvantage of CT angiography when precisely assessing the diameter stenosis, but it is not particularly problematic in follow-up.

Irregular eccentric stenoses with a noncircular lumen as well as mural calcifications are common in carotid arteries. Good experience of the radiologist interpreting CT angiography studies is essential. There are several possible reasons for the inaccurate determination of the diameter in the carotid artery with a high-grade stenosis using electronic caliper for measuring the diameters of the stenosed artery manually. One reason may be the inability of the observer to place the digital calipers accurately in a stenosed artery with very small diameter, where the caliper almost hides the vessel. When magnifying the displayed image, some blurring of the structures occurs. Wide window and level settings in CT angiography interpretation can be used in order to visualise mural calcifications properly. The study by Liu et al. [40] with a vessel phantom showed that the application of optimised window and level settings on CT angiography can reduce the measurement variability, because suboptimal window and level settings are the reason for edge blurring of the enhanced vessel. The smaller the actual luminal diameter, the greater the potential measurement error. This phenomenon may partly explain the possible failing of CT angiography measurement to assess accurately the diameter in cases of high-grade stenoses.

In another phantom study, the reconstruction kernel for axial slices and insufficient contrast density has been proposed to be possible sources of errors for the contrast column diameter assessment with automated software [71]. The movement of pulsating carotid artery during CT angiography may also cause blurring of the vessel edges and even obscure high-grade stenosis in CT angiography. It is sometimes obvious that the measured stenosis degree is not reasonably precise, and it is not reasonable to base the diagnosis only on a single measurement of the degree of carotid stenosis, but rather on multiple measurements and interactive viewing of original images. Perhaps further studies will give information on the optimal display of CT angiography to accurately measure the degree of carotid stenosis.

Automated vessel analysis program

An automated 3D CTA analysis program can be used to assess the degree of stenosis of carotid arteries. The program assesses the cross-section area of the artery lumen based on density and reconstructed a three-dimensional image. After selection of the level of reference and the lower and upper margins of the stenosis on the lumen image, the workstation automatically assesses the level of maximal stenosis. However, several misregistrations of the enhanced carotid artery lumen can occur when using 3D CTA automated analysis method. Intramural calcifications have been found to be the most common interfering factors leading to the misregistration of the borders of contrast enhanced lumen in the carotid bifurcations [81]. The other interfering factors include bifurcating vessels, adjacent bypassing vessels, partial-volume effects from short segment stenosis, and intraluminal low contrast media density. Most of those interfering factors causing misregistrations by the automated 3D CTA analysis program are quite easy to recognise and correct. Mural calcifications are common in atherosclerotic carotid stenoses. Mural calcifications are problematic for the assessment of the degree of stenosis with CT angiography due to beam hardening and partial volume effect enlarging the size of the mural calcification. Mural calcification obscures the arterial lumen, leading to inaccuracies in the assessment of stenoses. After manual corrections of the misregistrations of the 3D CTA analysis system, the reproducibility of this method is good, and the intra- and interobserver correlations are better than those of MPR measurements measured manually with electronic caliper [81]. However, the diagnostic performance of the 3D CTA analysis method still lacks robustness.

CT angiography as a true cross-sectional imaging method

The amount of flow in a tubular structure (vessel) is directly related to the cross-sectional area, and the measurements based on two-dimensional diameter values are inevitably only an approximation of the actual flow. Therefore, evaluation of stenosis degree with true lumen area measurements is theoretically a more accurate method in the optimal evaluation of real flow restriction through a stenosed carotid segment often with irregular lesion morphology. CT-angiography non-invasively provides the three-dimensional information of the vessel morphology, and new automated analysis software programmes provide quantitative information on cross-sectional lumea area values. The stenosis degree based on lumen area values can be obtained by the following equation:

$$100 \times (\text{area}^{\text{reference level}} - \text{area}^{\text{maximal stenosis level}})/\text{area}^{\text{reference level}}.$$

Theoretically, when carotid lumen is circular in shape (L/S-ratio = 1.0) as in cases of concentric stenoses, the diameter stenosis degrees of 70%, 50% and 30% correspond to area stenosis degrees of 91%, 75% and 51%, respectively. Zhang et al. [80] compared diameter and area stenosis degrees in carotid CTA in a clinical population with complex lesion morphology. In those carotids with L/S-ratio of >1.5, i.e. in vessels with obvious eccentric and complex lesions, stenosis degree poorly correlated with the lumen area at the maximal stenosis [80]. This finding indicates that the calculated stenosis degree based on diameter measurements may not be optimal for the assessment of carotid stenosis with eccentric or complex plaques. In this study, calculated with regression analysis from the actual area stenosis values of the study material, the threshold of 74% area stenosis corresponded to the clinically important threshold of 70% diameter stenosis. The threshold of 56% area stenosis corresponded to the threshold of 50% diameter stenosis, and the threshold of 36% area stenosis corresponded to 30% diameter stenosis in this study, respectively. Correspondingly, the thresholds of 5 mm^2, 8 mm^2, and 12 mm^2 for the lumen area at the level of maximal stenosis corresponded to the thresholds of 70%, 50%, and 30% diameter stenosis. In eccentric lesions with noncircular lumen area stenosis often seemed to provide a less severe estimate of the hemodynamic significance of the carotid stenosis than the conventional diameter stenosis [80]. The value of the assessment of area stenosis easily provided by CT angiography needs to be further evaluated in large clinical trials with comparison to the better established lumen diameter measurement techniques.

The role of CT angiography for complete evaluation of the carotid circulation

The detection of calcification is valuable for the estimation of the thromboembolic predisposition of the carotid atherosclerotic lesion, since plaque calcifications are thought to be associated with more stable plaques. With CT angiography more calcifications in the carotid arteries can be detected than with other imaging studies. However, without histopathologic verification the diagnostic accuracy of CT angiography for the detection of punctate calcifications remains unknown.

Ulcerative plaques in carotid arteries may be the source of thromboembolism into the cerebral circulation [42]. Moderate agreement between the modalities for the detection of ulceration has been reported [4]. Without proper verification of the plaque (pathoanatomical diagnosis), the true accuracy of each modality remains unknown. The accuracy of CT angiography for detecting carotid artery occlusion is high [2], [4], [38], [15] (Fig. 3). The sensitivity of CT angiography seems to be excellent for the detection of distal lesions in the ICA [4]. Other clinically relevant findings may also be revealed, such as intracranial aneurysms [77].

Aspects to the future

CT angiography of supra aortic arteries is still under a rapid technical development. It is probable that algorithms for decreasing the harmful effect of artifacts from bony skull base and inaccuracies in the assessment of the degree of stenosis in carotid arteries with heavy plaque calcifications will be diminished with newer visualisation techniques and MDCT devices. Moreover, the scanning time has become amazingly short compared to the first experiences with SDCT, and at the same time the anatomic coverage has increased dramatically. Improved temporal and spatial resolution may facilitate fully diagnostic imaging in a single session from the heart to intracranial vessels in a neurological patient for search of, e.g., source of embolism. Thus, CT may replace transthoracic/esophacial US and catheter angiography as a primary imaging modality for these patients. Similarly, cerebral CT can be combined with CT perfusion study for the brain and CT angiography for supra-aortic arteries as a proper evaluation set for stroke patients. In addition, a scanner located next to the emergency room seems to provide the quickest and most secure diagnostic algoritm for selection of stroke patients to arterial or venous thrombolysis therapy.

Take home message

Regardless of slight underestimation of near-occlusion stenoses or overestimation of the calcified stenoses in MDCT angiography, the diagnostic performance of CT angiography with interactive interpretation has been shown to be good when using DSA as a standard of reference. MDCT angiography seems to be highly sensitive for the detection of carotid artery stenosis, suggesting the suitability of CT angiography as a screening method for symptomatic patients. The specifity of this highly sensititive method can be increased with the aid of measuring the degree of stenosis. The radiation dose of CT angiography study is a challenge, and the technical solutions for the reduction of the radiation dose (i.e., CAREdose etc.) should be used.

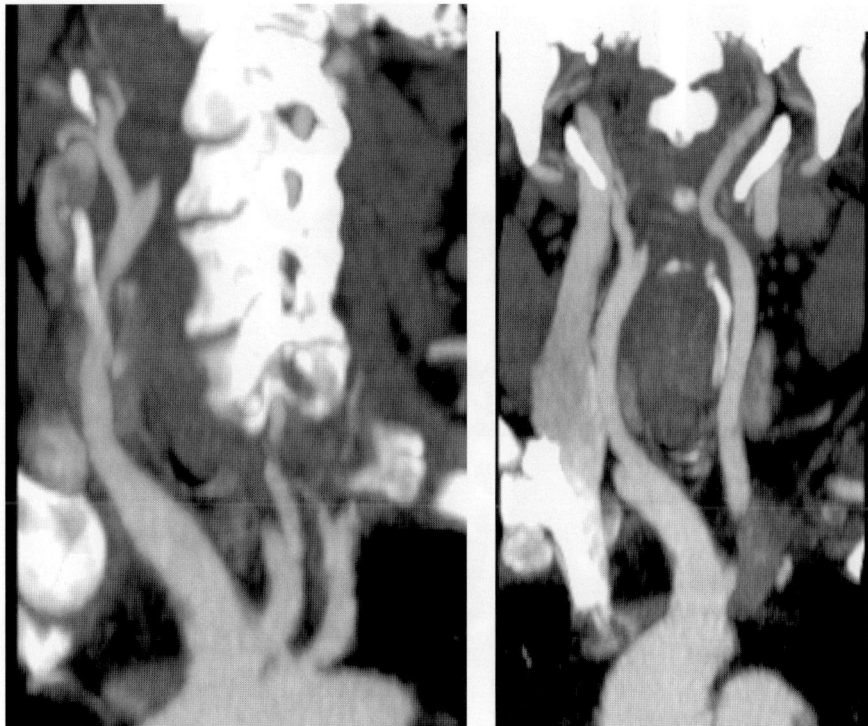

Fig. 3. A flame-like total occlusion of the right internal carotid artery, typical of dissection, detected on CT angiography (2 mm thin-slice MIP reconstructions, sagittal plane left, coronal plane right).

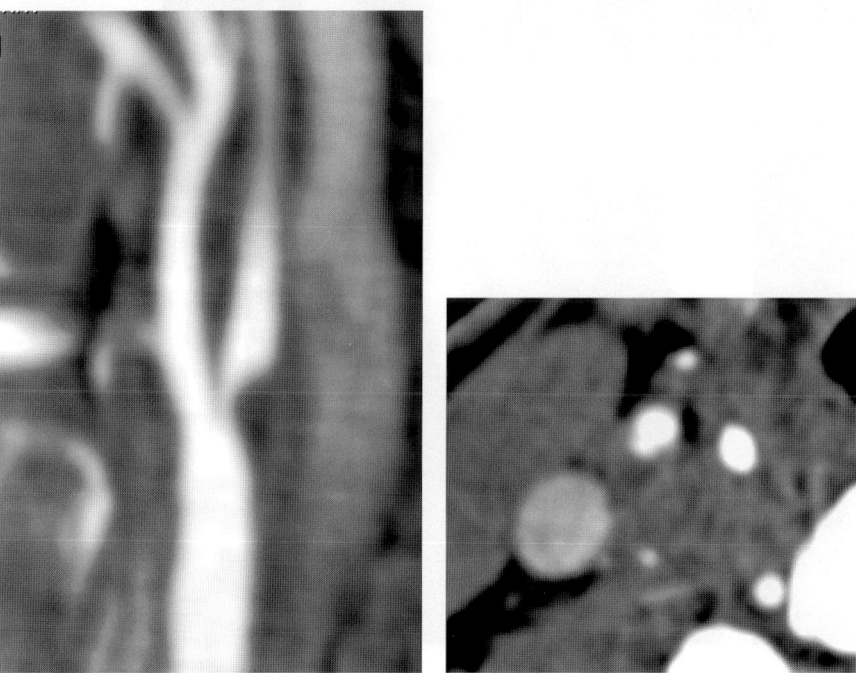

Fig. 4. CT angiography shows a smooth, soft, lipid-rich (HU 21) plaque at the origin of the right internal carotid artery (sagittal and axial planes).

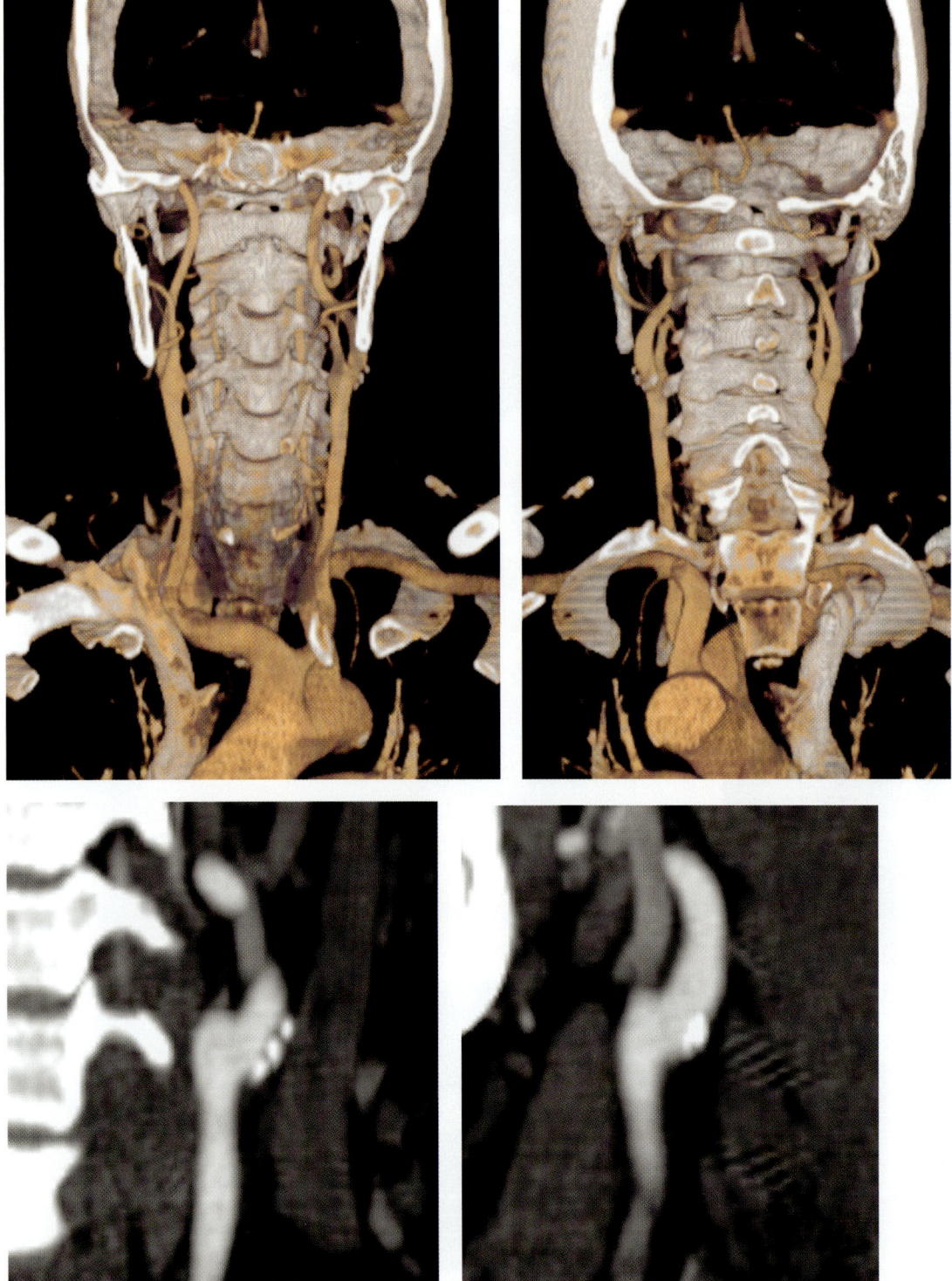

Fig. 5. A small mixed plaque with multiple small calcifications but no hemodynamically significant stenosis in the left carotid bifurcation. VR reconstructions with the anterior and posterior view (top row) and 2 mm thin-slice MIP reconstructions, coronal and sagittal plane (bottom row).

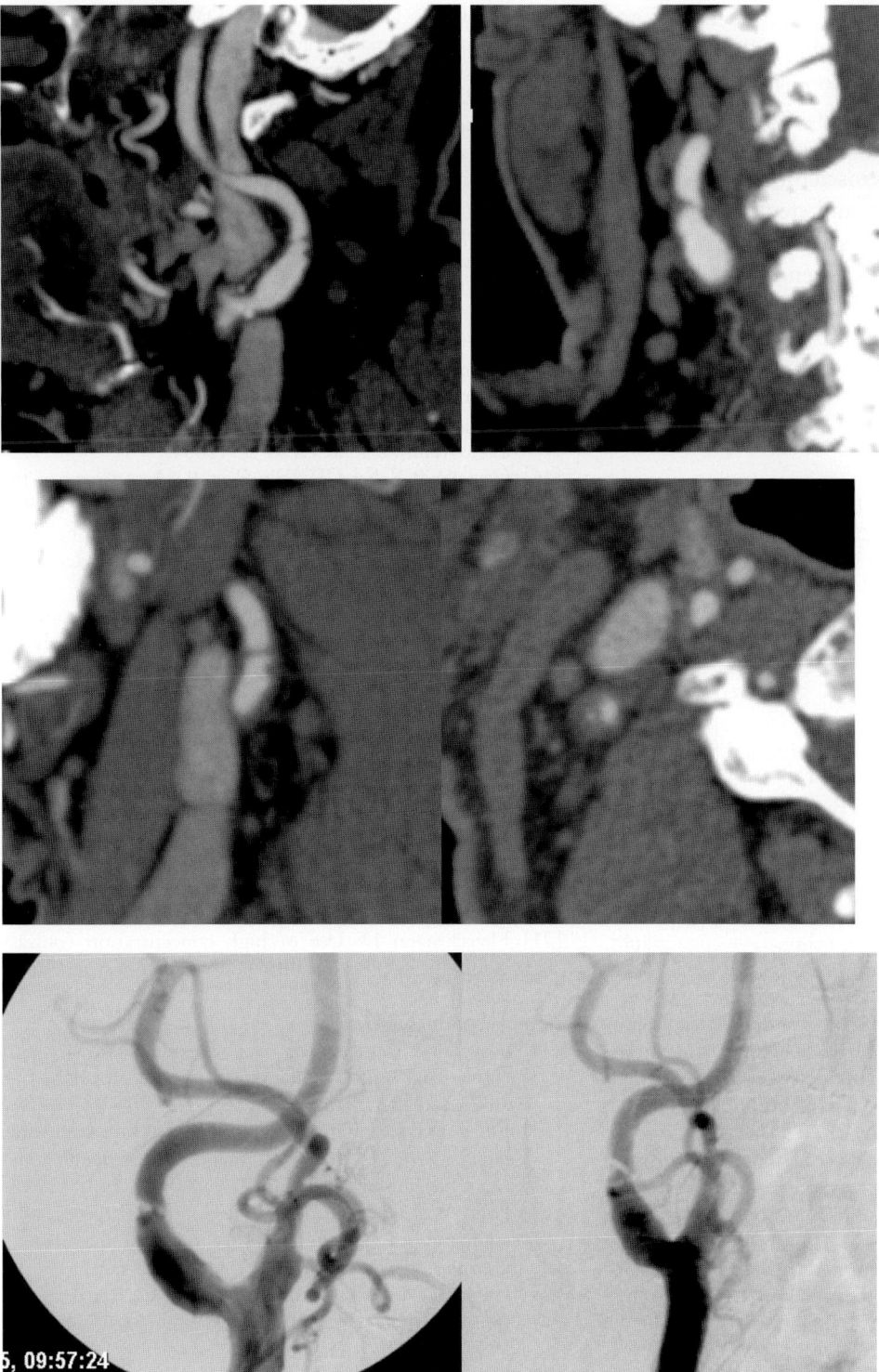

Fig. 6. A thin, web-like stenosis in the right internal carotid artery distal to the bulb. The 2 mm thin-slice MIP reconstructions in different planes (top and middle row) show the horizontally oriented thin margin of the plaque with an ulcerative pouch. DSA angiography confirms the hemodynamical significance of the lesion (bottom row).

Proper verification of the reproducibility and accuracy of MDCT angiography with the newest technology in large patient population studies are needed to define the actual indications in which CT angiography should be used in clinical practice, in selecting patients with atherosclerotic stenosis to carotid artery endarterectomy and stenting and in the differential diagnostics of less frequent types of carotid artery lesions. Good experience of the radiologist interpreting carotid CT angiography studies is essential.

References

[1] Alvarez-Linera J, Benito-Leon J, Escribano J et al.: Prospective evaluation of carotid artery stenosis: elliptic centric contrast-enhanced MR angiography and spiral CT angiography compared with digital subtraction angiography. AJNR 24: 1012–1019 (2003).

[2] Anderson GB, Ashforth R, Steinke DE et al.: CT angiography for the detection and characterization of carotid artery bifurcation disease. Stroke 31: 2168–2174 (2000).

[3] Bae KT, Heiken JP, Brink JA: Aortic and hepatic contrast medium enhancement at CT. Part I. Prediction with a computer model. Radiology 207: 647–655 (1998).

[4] Berg M, Zhang Z, Ikonen A et al.: Multi-detector row CT angiography in the assessment of carotid artery disease in symptomatic patients: comparison with rotational angiography and digital subtraction angiography. AJNR 26: 1022–1034 (2005).

[5] Berg MH, Manninen HI, Rasanen HT et al.: CT angiography in the assessment of carotid artery atherosclerosis. Acta Radiol 43: 116–124 (2002).

[6] Berland LL, Smith JK: Multidetector-array CT: once again, technology creates new opportunities [editorial; comment]. Radiology 209: 327–329 (1998).

[7] Binaghi S, Maeder P, Uske A et al.: Three-dimensional computed tomography angiography and magnetic resonance angiography of carotid bifurcation stenosis. Eur Neurol 46: 25–34 (2001).

[8] Brink JA: Contrast optimization and scan timing for single and multidetector-row computed tomography. J Comput Assist Tomogr 27: S3–S8 (2003).

[9] Brink JA: Technical aspects of helical (spiral) CT. Radiol Clin North Am 33: 825–841 (1995).

[10] Brink JA, Lim JT, Wang G et al.: Technical optimization of spiral CT for depiction of renal artery stenosis: in vitro analysis. Radiology 194: 157–163 (1995).

[11] Brink JA, Heiken JP, Balfe DM et al.: Spiral CT: decreased spatial resolution in vivo due to broadening of section-sensitivity profile. Radiology 185: 469–474 (1992).

[12] Calhoun PS, Kuszyk BS, Heath DG et al.: Three-dimensional volume rendering of spiral CT data: theory and method. Radiographics 19: 745–764 (1999).

[13] Casey SO, Alberico RA, Patel M et al.: Cerebral CT venography. Radiology 198: 163–170 (1996).

[14] Cinat M, Lane CT, Pham H, Lee A, Wilson SE, Gordon I: Helical CT angiography in the preoperative evaluation of carotid artery stenosis. J Vasc Surg 28: 290–300 (1998).

[15] Chen CJ, Lee TH, Hsu HL et al.: Multi-Slice CT angiography in diagnosing total versus near occlusions of the internal carotid artery: comparison with catheter angiography. Stroke 35: 83–85 (2004).

[16] Costello P, Ecker CP, Tello R et al.: Assessment of the thoracic aorta by spiral CT. AJR 158: 1127–1130 (1992).

[17] Crawford CR, King KF: Computed tomography scanning with simultaneous patient translation. Med Phys 17: 967–982 (1990).

[18] Davis SM: Extracranial and intracranial atheroma as causes of stroke. In: Cerebrovascular disease: (Myron D, Ginsberg JB, eds.). Pathophysiology, diagnosis, and management. pp 1373–1391. Malden: Blackwell Science (1998).

[19] Derdeyn CP: Catheter angiography is still necessary for the measurement of carotid stenosis. AJNR 24: 1737–1738 (2003).

[20] ECST: Randomised trial of endarterectomy for recently symptomatic carotid stenosis: final results of the MRC European Carotid Surgery Trial (ECST). Lancet 351: 1379–1387 (1998).

[21] Fleischmann D: Use of high concentration contrast media: principles and rationale-vascular district. Eur J Radiol 2003 45: S88–S93.

[22] Fleischmann D, Rubin GD, Bankier AA et al.: Improved uniformity of aortic enhancement with customized contrast medium injection protocols at CT angiography. Radiology 214: 363–371 (2000).

[23] Flohr TG, Schaller S, Stierstorfer K et al.: Multi-detector row CT systems and image-reconstruction techniques. Radiology 235: 756-773 (2005).

[24] Foley WD, Karcaaltincaba M: Computed tomography angiography: principles and clinical applications. J Comput Assist Tomogr 27: S23–S30 2(2003).

[25] Galanski M, Prokop M, Chavan A et al.: Renal arterial stenoses: spiral CT angiography. Radiology 189: 185–192 (1993).

[26] Glagov S, Weisenberg E, Zarins CK, Stankunavicius R, Kolettis GJ: Compensatory enlargement of human atherosclerotic coronary arteries. N Engl J Med 316: 1371–1375 (1987).

[27] Hatsukami TS, Ferguson MS, Beach KW et al.: Carotid plaque morphology and clinical events. Stroke 28: 95–100 (1997).

[28] Kalender WA, Prokop M: 3D CT angiography. Crit Rev Diagn Imaging 42: 1–28 (2001).

[29] Kalender WA, Seissler W, Klotz E et al.: Spiral volumetric CT with single-breath-hold technique, continuous transport, and continuous scanner rotation. Radiology 176: 181–183 (1990).

[30] Kasales CJ, Hopper KD, Ariola DN et al.: Reconstructed helical CT scans: improvement in z-axis resolution compared with overlapped and nonoverlapped conventional CT scans. AJR 164: 1281–1284 (1995).

[31] Katz DA, Marks MP, Napel SA et al.: Circle of Willis: evaluation with spiral CT angiography, MR angiography, and conventional angiography. Radiology 195: 445–449 (1995).

[32] Kirchgeorg MA, Prokop M: Increasing spiral CT benefits with postprocessing applications. Eur J Radiol 28: 39–54 (1998).

[33] Kuszyk BS, Fishman EK: Technical aspects of CT angiography. Semin Ultrasound CT MR 19: 383–393 (1998).

[34] Johnson PT, Heath DG, Bliss DF et al.: Three-dimensional CT: real-time interactive volume rendering. AJR 167: 581–583 (1996).

[35] Josephson SA, Bryant SO, Mak HK et al.: Evaluation of carotid stenosis using CT angiography in the initial evaluation of stroke and TIA. Neurology 63: 457–460 (2004).

[36] Lawrence JA, Kim D, Kent KC et al.: Lower extremity spiral CT angiography versus catheter angiography. Radiology 194: 903–908 (1995).

[37] Leclerc X, Godefroy O, Lucas C et al.: Internal carotid arterial stenosis: CT angiography with volume rendering. Radiology 210: 673–682 (1999).

[38] Leclerc X, Godefroy O, Pruvo JP et al.: Computed tomographic angiography for the evaluation of carotid artery stenosis. Stroke 26: 1577–1581 (1995).

[39] Lell M, Wildberger JE, Heuschmid M, Flohr T, Stierstorfer K, Fellner FA et al.: CT-angiography of the carotid artery: First results with a novel 16-slice-spiral-CT scanner. Rofo Fortschr Geb Rontgenstr Neuen Bildgeb Verfahr 174: 1165–1169 (2002).

[40] Liu Y, Hopper KD, Mauger DT et al.: CT angiographic measurement of the carotid artery: optimizing visualization by manipulating window and level settings and contrast material attenuation. Radiology 217: 494–500 (2000).

[41] Magarelli N, Scarabino T, Simeone AL et al.: Carotid stenosis: a comparison between MR and spiral CT angiography. Neuroradiology 40: 367–373 (1998).

[42] McCarthy MJ, Loftus IM, Thompson MM et al.: Angiogenesis and the atherosclerotic carotid plaque: an association between symptomatology and plaque morphology. J Vasc Surg 30: 261–268 (1999).

[43] Mayberg MR, Wilson SE, Yatsu F et al.: Carotid endarterectomy and prevention of cerebral ischemia in symptomatic carotid stenosis. Veterans Affairs Cooperative Studies Program 309 Trialist Group. JAMA 266: 3289–3294 (1991).

[44] Milei J, Parodi JC, Ferreira M et al.: Atherosclerotic plaque rupture and intraplaque hemorrhage do not correlate with symptoms in carotid artery stenosis. J Vasc Surg 38: 1241–1247 (2003).

[45] Moll R, Dinkel HP: Value of the CT angiography in the diagnosis of common carotid artery bifurcation disease: CT angiography versus digital subtraction angiography and color flow Doppler. Eur J Radiol 39: 155–162 (2001).

[46] Napel S, Rubin GD, Jeffrey RB Jr.: STS-MIP: a new reconstruction technique for CT of the chest. J Comput Assist Tomogr 17: 832–838 (1993).

[47] Napel S, Marks MP, Rubin GD et al.: CT angiography with spiral CT and maximum intensity projection. Radiology 185: 607–610 (1992).

[48] NASCET: Beneficial effect of carotid endarterectomy in symptomatic patients with high-grade carotid stenosis. North American Symptomatic Carotid Endarterectomy Trial Collaborators. N Engl J Med 325: 445–453 (1991).

[49] Nicolaides A, Sabetai M, Kakkos SK et al.: The Asymptomatic Carotid Stenosis and Risk of Stroke (ACSRS) study. Aims and results of quality control. Int Angiol 22: 263–272 (2003).

[50] Papp Z, Patel M, Ashtari M, Takahashi M, Goldstein J, Maguire W et al.: Carotid artery stenosis: optimization of CT angiography with a combination of shaded surface display and source images. AJNR 18: 759–763 (1997).

[51] Polacin A, Kalender WA, Marchal G: Evaluation of section sensitivity profiles and image noise in spiral CT. Radiology 185: 29–35 (1992).

[52] Prokop M: General principles of MDCT. Eur J Radiol 45: S4–S10 (2003).

[53] Prokop M, Galanski M: Spiral and multislice: computed tomography of the body. Stuttgart New York: Thieme (2003).

[54] Prokop M, Engelke C: Vascular System: In: Spiral and Multislice Computed Tomography of the Body. (Prokop M, Galanski M, eds.) pp 844–851. Stuttgart, New York: Thieme (2003)

[55] Prokop M: Multislice CT angiography. Eur J Radiol 36: 86–96 (2000).

[56] Prokop M, Shin HO, Schanz A: Schaefer-Prokop CM. Use of maximum intensity projections in CT angiography: a basic review. Radiographics 17: 433–451 (1997).

[57] Randoux B, Marro B, Koskas F et al.: Carotid artery stenosis: prospective comparison of CT, three-dimensional gadolinium-enhanced MR, and conventional angiography. Radiology 220: 179–185 (2001).

[58] Remy-Jardin M, Remy J, Artaud D et al.: Peripheral pulmonary arteries: optimization of the spiral CT acquisition protocol. Radiology 204: 157–163 (1997).

[59] Rubin GD: Techniques for performing multidetector-row computed tomographic angiography. Tech Vasc Interv Radiol 4: 2–14 (2001).

[60] Rubin GD, Beaulieu CF, Argiro V, Ringl H, Norbash AM, Feller JF et al.: Perspective volume rendering of CT and MR images: applications for endoscopic imaging. Radiology 199: 321–330 (1996).

[61] Rubin GD, Shiau MC, Schmidt AJ, Fleischmann D, Logan L, Leung AN et al.: Computed tomographic angiography: historical perspective and new state-of-the-art using multi detector-row helical computed tomography. J Comput Assist Tomogr 23: S83–S90 (1999).

[62] Rubin GD, Dake MD, Napel S et al.: Spiral CT of renal artery stenosis: comparison of three-dimensional rendering techniques. Radiology 190: 181–189 (1994).

[63] Rubin GD, Dake MD, Napel SA et al.: Three-dimensional spiral CT angiography of the abdomen: initial clinical experience. Radiology 186: 147–152 (1993).

[64] Rydberg J, Buckwalter KA, Caldemeyer KS et al.: Multisection CT: scanning techniques and clinical applications. Radiographics 20: 1787–1806 (2000).

[65] Sameshima T, Futami S, Morita Y et al.: Clinical usefulness of and problems with three-dimensional CT angiography for the evaluation of arteriosclerotic stenosis of the carotid artery: comparison with conventional angiography, MRA, and ultrasound sonography. Surg Neurol 51: 301–308; discussion 308–309 (1999).

[66] Sato Y, Shiraga N, Nakajima S et al.: Local maximum intensity projection (LMIP): a new rendering method for vascular visualization. J Comput Assist Tomogr 22: 912–917 (1998).

[67] Schwartz RB: Helical (spiral) CT in neuroradiologic diagnosis. Radiol Clin North Am 33: 981–995 (1995).

[68] Schwartz RB, Jones KM, Chernoff DM et al.: Common carotid artery bifurcation: evaluation with spiral CT. Work in progress. Radiology 185: 513–519 (1992).

[69] Stehling MK, Rosen MP, Weintraub J et al.: Spiral CT venography of the lower extremity. AJR 163: 451–453 (1994).

[70] Stehling MK, Lawrence JA, Weintraub JL et al.: CT angiography: expanded clinical applications. AJR 163: 947–955 (1994).

[71] Suzuki S, Furui S, Kaminaga T et al.: Measurement of vascular diameter in vitro by automated software for CT angiography: effects of inner diameter, density of contrast medium, and convolution kernel. AJR 182: 1313–1317 (2004).

[72] Thomsen HS, Morcos SK: In which patients should serum creatinine be measured before iodinated contrast medium administration? Eur Radiol 15: 749–754 Epub 2004 Dec 31 (2005).

[73] Tippins RB, Torres WE, Baumgartner BR et al.: Are screening serum creatinine levels necessary prior to outpatient CT examinations? Radiology 216: 481–484 43(2000).

[74] van Hoe L, Marchal G, Baert AL et al.: Determination of scan delay time in spiral CT-angiography: utility of a test bolus injection. J Comput Assist Tomogr 19: 216–220 (1995).

[75] Van Ooijen PM, Ho KY, Dorgelo J et al.: Coronary Artery Imaging with Multidetector CT: Visualization Issues. Radiographics 7: 7 (2003).

[76] Verhoek G, Costello P, Khoo EW, Wu R, Kat E, Fitridge RA: Carotid bifurcation CT angiography: assessment of interactive volume rendering. J Comput Assist Tomogr 23: 590–596 (1999).

[77] Villablanca JP, Jahan R, Hooshi P et al.: Detection and characterization of very small cerebral aneurysms by using 2D and 3D helical CT angiography. AJNR 23: 1187–1198 (2002).

[78] Wang G, Vannier MW: Maximum volume coverage in spiral computed tomography scanning. Acad Radiol 3: 423–428 (1996).

[79] Weidekamm C: Low kVp settings improve contrast enhancement and reduce radiation exposure in spiral CT of pulmonary emboli. In: Baert AL (ed.) ECR; p. 149. Wien Austria: Springer (2002).

[80] Zhang Z, Berg M, Ikonen A et al.: Carotid stenosis degree in CT angiography: assessment based on luminal area versus luminal diameter measurements. Eur Radiol 14 (2005).

[81] Zhang Z, Berg MH, Ikonen AE et al.: Carotid artery stenosis: reproducibility of automated 3D CT angiography analysis method. Eur Radiol 14: 665–672 (2003).

Chapter 1.6

INTRACEREBRAL IMAGING AND CAROTID ARTERY STENOSIS

K.-O. Lövblad

Radiology Department, HUG Geneva University Hospital, Geneva, Switzerland

Introduction

Cerebrovascular disease is the third cause of death in industrialized countries. Carotid stenosis is associated with an increased risk of acute and chronic infarction. Patients with 80–99% lesions had a 20.6% annual event rate. The main factor that appears to predict increased risk for future stroke is progression of stenosis. A significant carotid stenosis can be found in approximatively one third of patients with cerebral ischemia. Overall carotid atherosclerosis is responsible for approximately 20% of all cerebral ischemic strokes. At 2 years of follow-up, the risk of a repeat stroke is 28 and 13% for symptomatic stenoses of 70–99% and 50–69%. Carotid endarterectomy is now well established as a way to prevent infarction in the presence of carotid stenosis either symptomatic and of a higher grade than 50%, or symptomatic or asymptomatic of a higher grade than 70%. This was proven by two randomized clinical trials, the European Carotid Surgery Trial [3] and the North American Symptomatic Carotid Endarterectomy Trial [1]. The implications of these trials were that beyond surgery treatment of carotid stenosis should be undertaken. For asymptomatic stenosis the same recommendations have been made [2]. Carotid stenting is becoming an accepted alternative approach to carotid revascularization. Stenting has become an established alternative treatment for coronary and peripheral vascular disease and has the advantage of avoiding general anesthesia and neck incision, therefore being associated with lower mortality and morbidity rates. The CAVATAS study (Carotid and Vertebral Artery Transluminal Angioplasty Study) found that endovascular treatment had similar major risks and effectiveness at prevention of stroke during 3 years compared with carotid surgery. A recent randomized trial in 344 patients showed that among patients with severe carotid-artery stenosis and coexisting conditions, carotid stenting with the use of an emboli-protection device is not inferior to carotid endarterectomy [67]. Endovascular treatment with cerebral protection had the advantage of avoiding minor complications.

This chapter studies the impact of carotid artery stenosis on the brain as seen with neuroimaging studies. The aims of neuroimaging studies before stenting are to show or exclude damage as well as to provide information regarding the perfusion of the tissue. We will discuss modalities such as Computed tomography (CT) and Magnetic Resonance Imaging (MRI).

Computer tomography studies

Computed tomography of the brain traditionally can demonstrate the state of ischemia. Newer techniques such as perfusion CT have been shown to provide with maps of Cerebral Blood Flow in cerebrovascular diseases. While CT of the brain is still used it is more and more replaced by MR derived techniques since these can better demonstrate for example watershed lesions observed in carotid stenosis (Fig. 1).

Magnetic Resonance studies

Magnetic Resonance of the brain can now provide many new parameters. In addition to the classic information provided by T1 and T2–weighted imag-

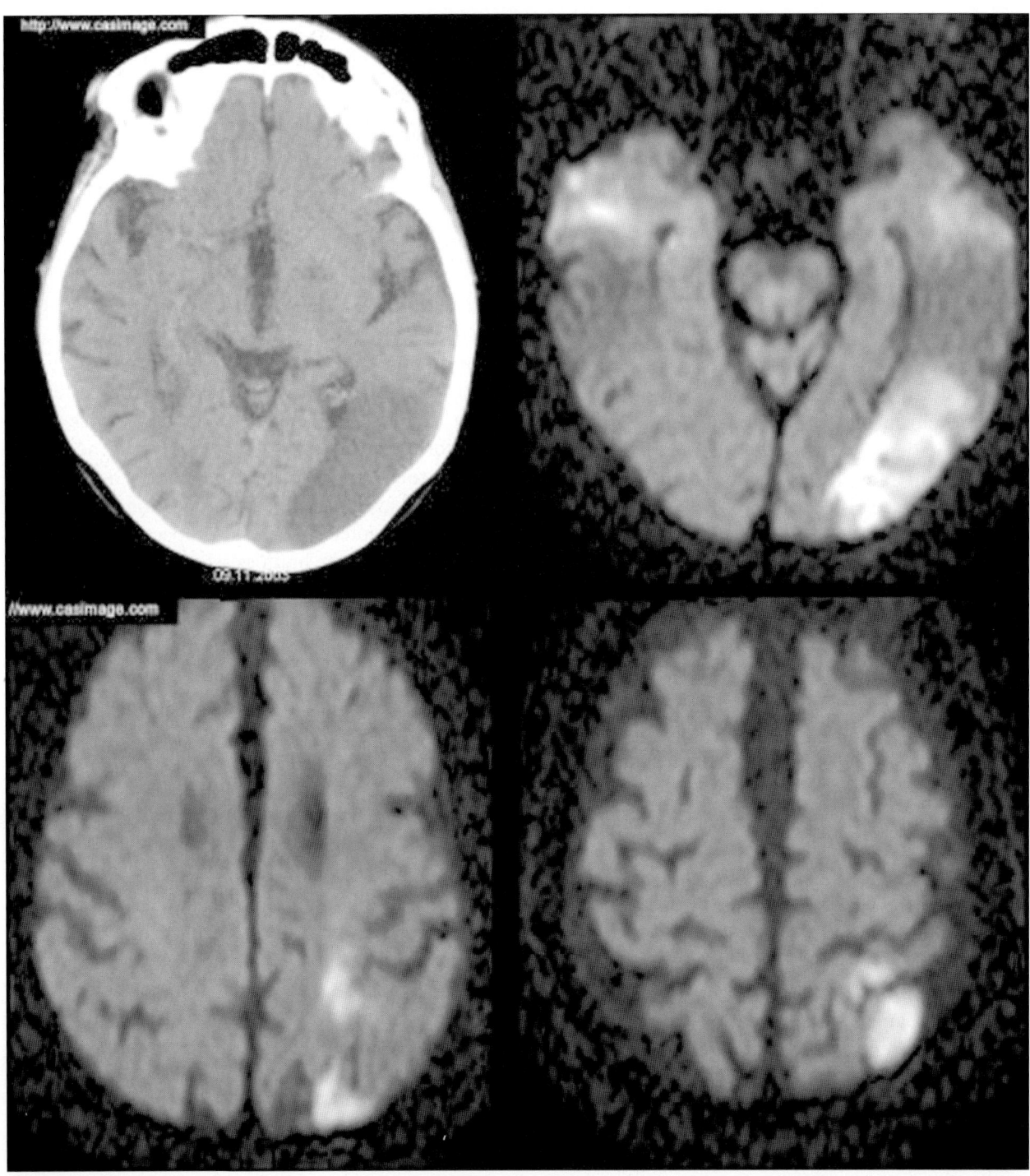

Fig. 1. Patient with watershed infarction due to stenosis: The CT (upper left) shows posterior left-hemispheric hypodensity). The Diffusion-weighted MR images show multiple lesions located in the watershed area.

ing, new information can be provided by techniques such as diffusion imaging, diffusion tensor imaging and perfusion imaging that can all be performed now with MR.

Conventional MR methods

Preinterventionally, MRI can demonstrate the presence or absence of cerebral lesions due to carotid stenosis.

The effect of cerebral hypoperfusion can be seen on many MR sequences. On the Two-dimensional time-of-flight (TOF) sequences that re done at the same time there may be a signal asymmetry between the two internal carotids: due to diminished flow there is less hyperintensity in the affected vessel (Fig. 2). In case of an occluded vessel, one may observe the absence of the normal flow void in the affected vessel with hypersignal in its place which would sign vessel occlusion or slow flow at least (Figs. 3 and 4).

Diffusion and diffusion tensor studies

Diffusion-weighted MR imaging

Diffusion-weighted MR corresponds to a modification of a spin-echo technique. However for any application, MR imaging was initially very slow and examination times for single sequences would run up to ten minutes. Echo-planar imaging changed all this, allowing ultra-fast imaging [61], [14].

Le Bihan developed diffusion-weighted imaging almost 20 years ago [25]. Two diffusion-sensitizing gradients are placed in a sequence, corresponding to

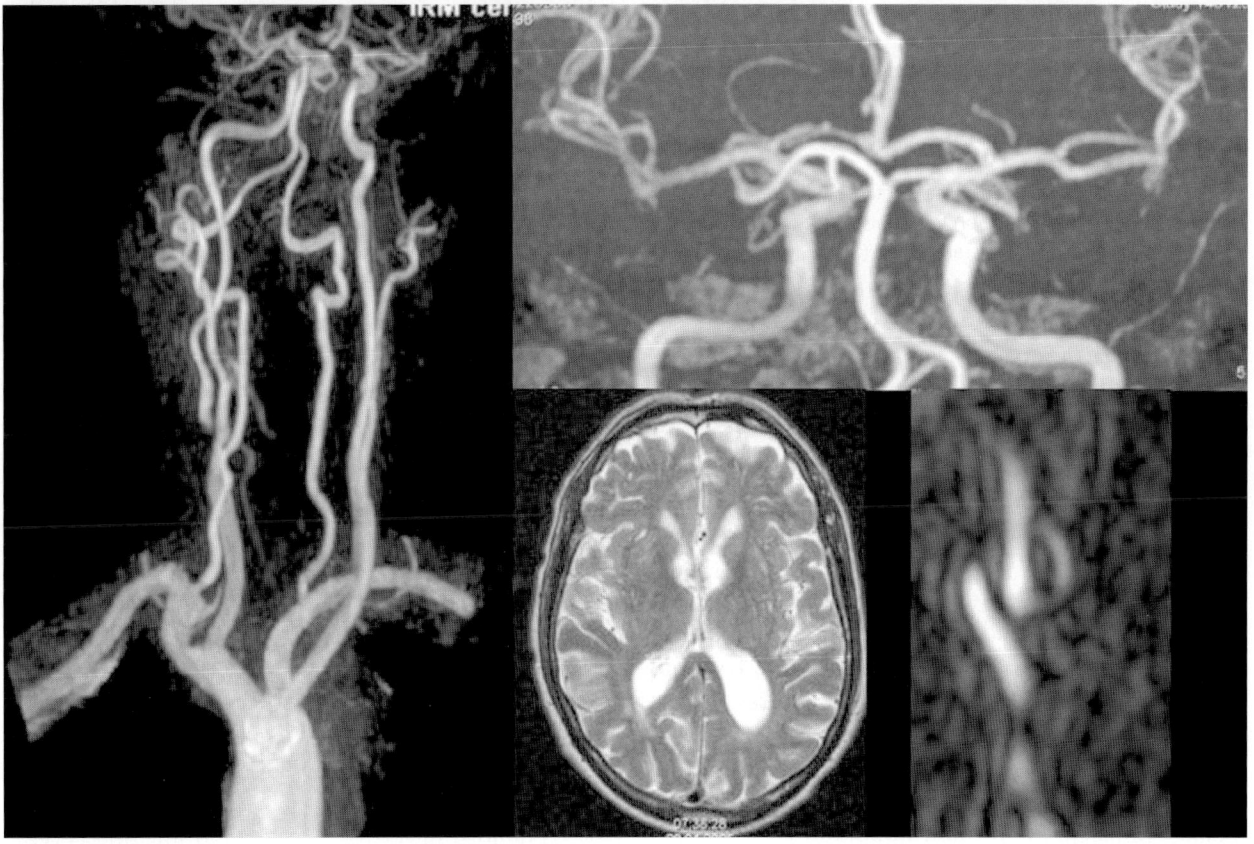

Fig. 2. Patient with right-sided carotid stenosis seen on neck MRA. There is also a slight less bright signal in the internal portion of the carotid system seen on the intracranial time-of-flight MRA due to diminished flow.

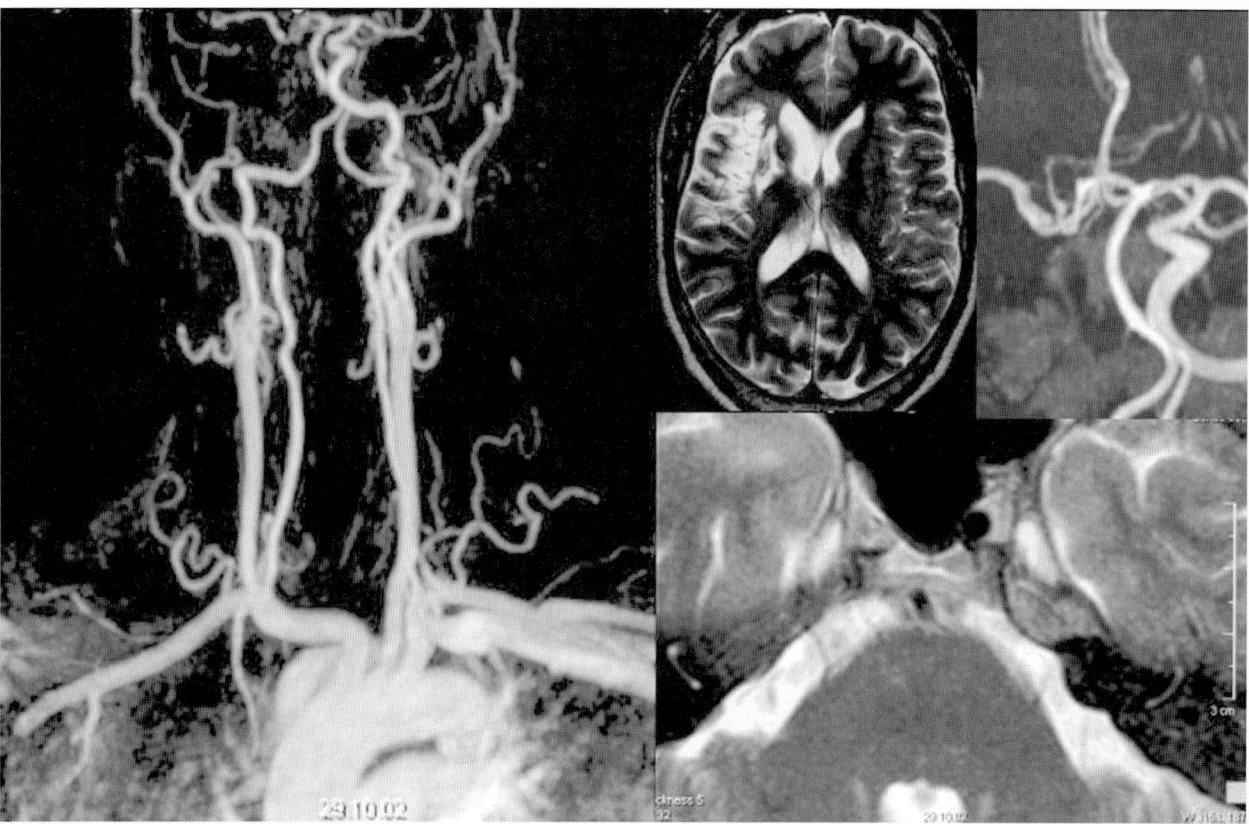

Fig. 3. Patient with occlusion of the right internal carotid artery (image to the left). There is no signal in the intracranial portion of the carotid on the TOF MRA (image on the right). There is chronic lenticular stroke on the right. Note the hyperintensity of the right carotid on the axial T2 image at the intracranial level (lower right).

a Stejskal-Tanner modification [58], giving the sequence a sensitivity to water or tissular motion. Then, M Moseley demonstrated the use of DWI in animal models of stroke, where ischemia was followed by hyperintensity in the DWI images and a decrease in the apparent diffusion coefficient (ADC) [38], further more these changes were found to be reversible on recanalization [10], [37], [18], [56].

The diffusion gradients are usually applied with many b values, at least two (usually 0 and 1000) in order to obtain ADC maps. The b0 image corresponds to a T2 image and the b 1000 image is the b max image and corresponds to what we consider the diffusion-weighted image. On diffusion-weighted images, molecules with high mobility (e.g., cerebrospinal fluid (CSF)) provide little or no signal whereas protons that have not or little moved provide with a hyperintense signal. Therefore on DWI we see CSF as black, brain tissue as grey and tissues with restriction of motion as white [66]. In ischemia there is a shift of intra and extra-cellular water corresponding to cytotoxic edema (Fig. 5). The tissue contrast achieved is high so that even small lesions can be seen.

Previously the images would be acquired at the maximum b value in at least three orthogonal directions in order to rule out the effects of anisotropy, i.e. the presence of natural borders: the presence of the white matter structures such as the internal capsule would induce reduced water motion and therefore hypersignal. Nowadays directly isotropic images are acquired.

The idea of diffusion-weighted imaging (DWI) had been developed early on by Le Bihan; however since it is inherently sensitive to motion, DWI was

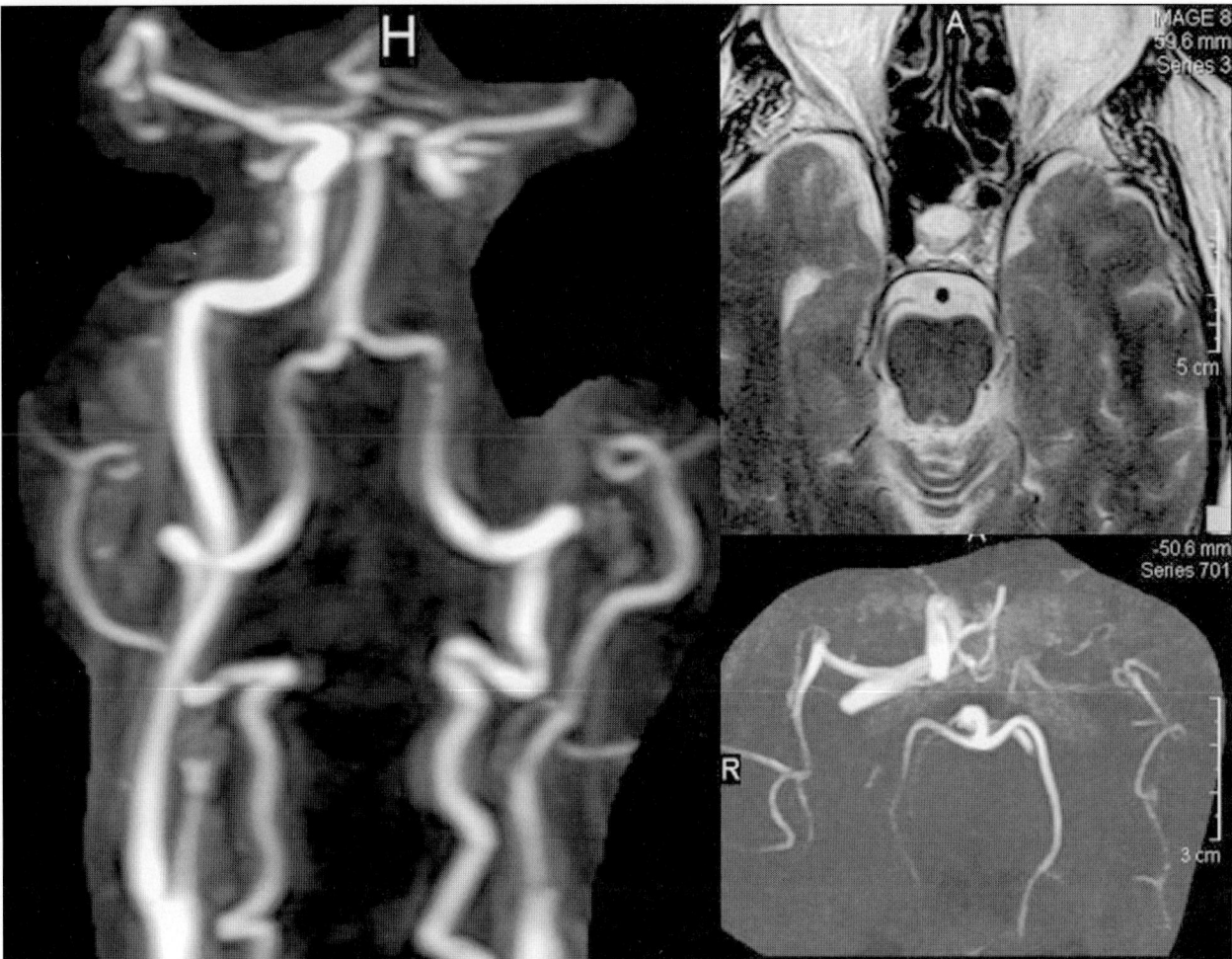

Fig. 4. Left sided carotid occlusion: the T2 image shows hyperintensity of the carotid siphon on the left (left upper image).

difficult to implement clinically. This was due to the presence of patient motion, very often increased in the incooperative stroke patient, as well as important artifacts from pulsations deriving from CSF and blood flow. These problems were partially overcome by the use of stimulated echo acquisition mode (STEAM) sequences and other sequences [62], however these were gain slow and allowed only the acquisition of one slice at a time. All this was changed when echo-planar imaging was rendered available on clinical scanners: indeed these units allow images to be acquired in a few milliseconds; therefore permitting whole-brain scans in less than a minute. This allowed a revolution in neuroimaging that was waiting to occur to arrive. The first papers were by Warach and Chen in 1992 and reported the successful use of DWI in human stroke [62], [9]. Warach followed-up these studies with multi-slice whole brain echo-planar imaging that allowed acquiring lesion volumes [63], [65]. Further studies showed diffusion imaging to be highly sensitive to changes in acute stroke and to correlate with eventual outcomes [33], [29], [4]–[6], [31], [35]. At the same time echo-planer techniques allow to perform fast repetition of perfusion sequences (Figs. 3 and 4), which allows demonstrating the presence of a so-called mismatch and penumbra [47], [15], [32]. Diffusion imaging has been used to demonstrate silent ischemic changes occurring after carotid endarterectomy (CEA) and carotid artery stenting (CAS) [7], [34],

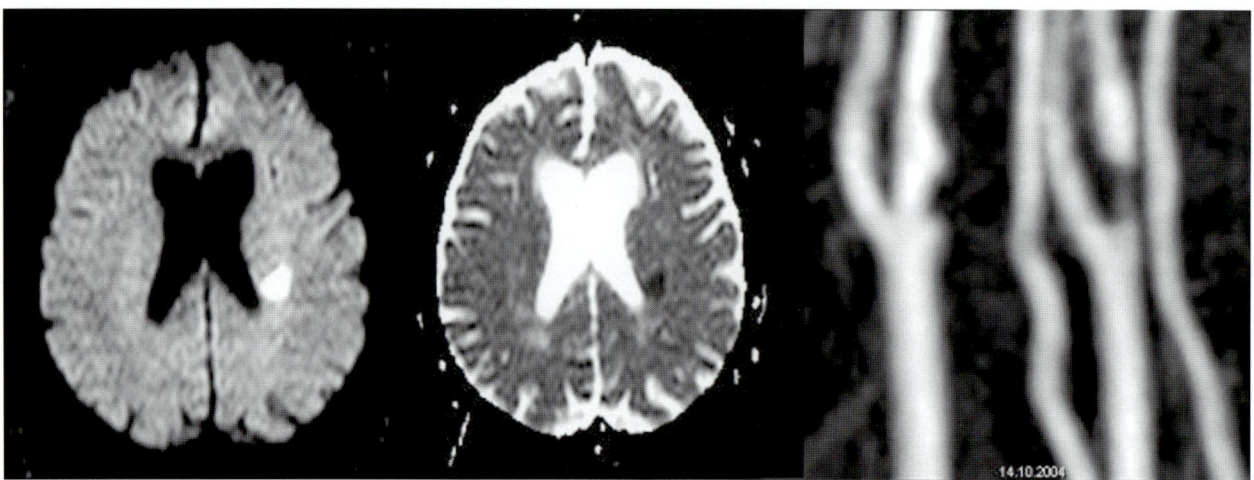

Fig. 5. Ischemic lesion in the left-sided internal capsule, seen as a bright lesion on the diffusion. Weighted image with h b value (left image) and as a hypointensity on the ADC map (middle), due to a carotid stenosis (right image).

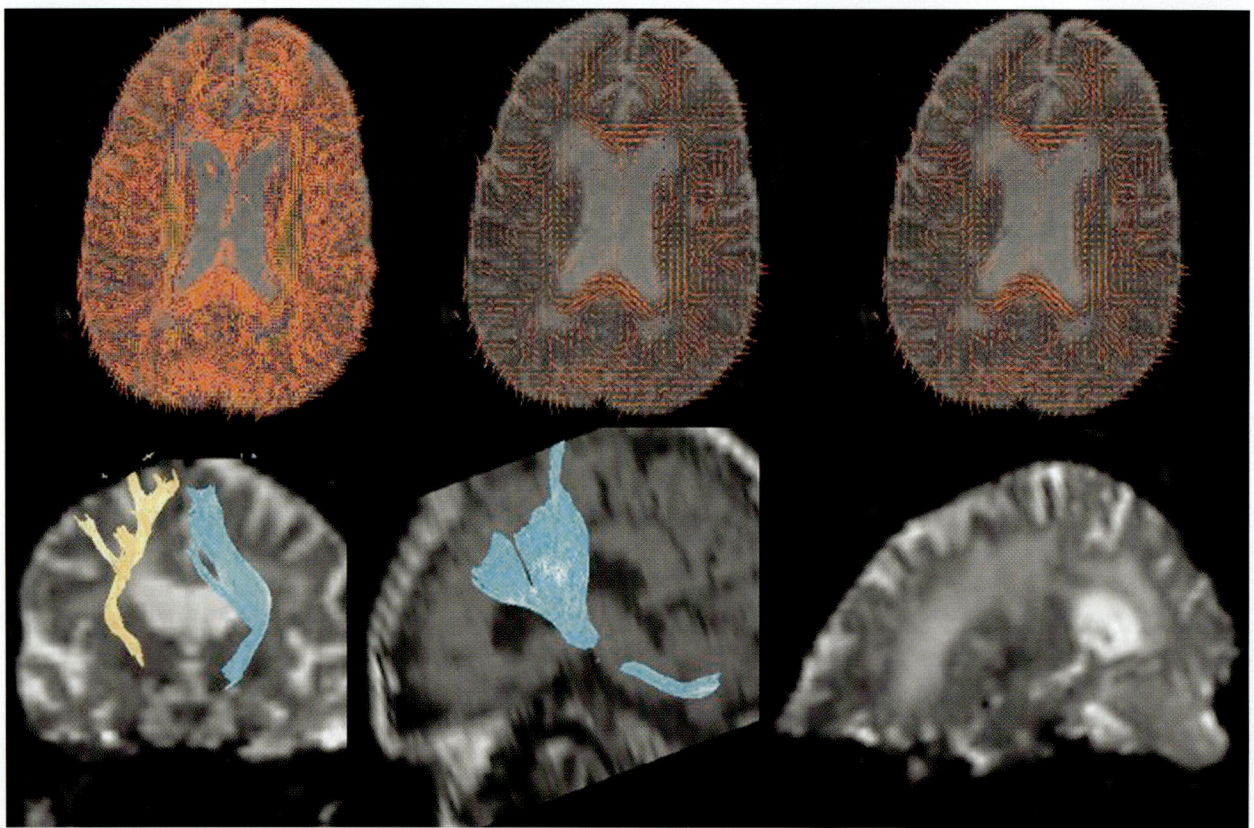

Fig. 6. Alterations in the diffusion tensor due to leucoaraiosis: the disorientation of the tensors (upper row) and the tracts are disorganized on the corresponding reconstructions (lower row).

therefore being of importance in the post-therapeutic assessment of patients undergoing surgical or interventional treatment.

ADC mapping

The early diffusion abnormality is accompanied by changes in the so-called apparent diffusion coefficient [48]. This diffusion coefficient allows measuring and quantifying the changes that are purely observed on the DWI images. In the early phase of stroke, there is a diminished signal on ADC maps that correspond to the diminished diffusion associated with the high DWI signal. After a few days there is a tendency for this ADC signal to increase. Since we often compare the affected area to the contralateral side and report on relative ADCs (affected side/ unaffected side) we observe a so-called pseudo-normalization of the signal after 7 to 10 days approximately: the r ADC is around 1 and there is no signal change observable on the raw ADC map. However as cell lysis continues and there is installation of vasogenic edema, we observe a progressive increase in the ADC with a hypersignal on the ADC maps. Thus ADC measurements provide us with further information: we can assess then age of a diffusion-positive lesion.

Also, when one considers the animal literature, one can see that there is reversibility of these lesions following acute treatment.

Tensor imaging

Diffusion tensor imaging is a further refinement of DWI [26]. In order to acquire tensor images the images must be acquired with the gradients applied in at least 6 directions. This provides with images that can be fusioned to either obtain anisotropy images or even images of tractography [59], [22], [52], [16] (Figs. 6 and 7).

Diffusion MRI can thus demonstrate acute lesions such as brain infarction. In acute stroke there is

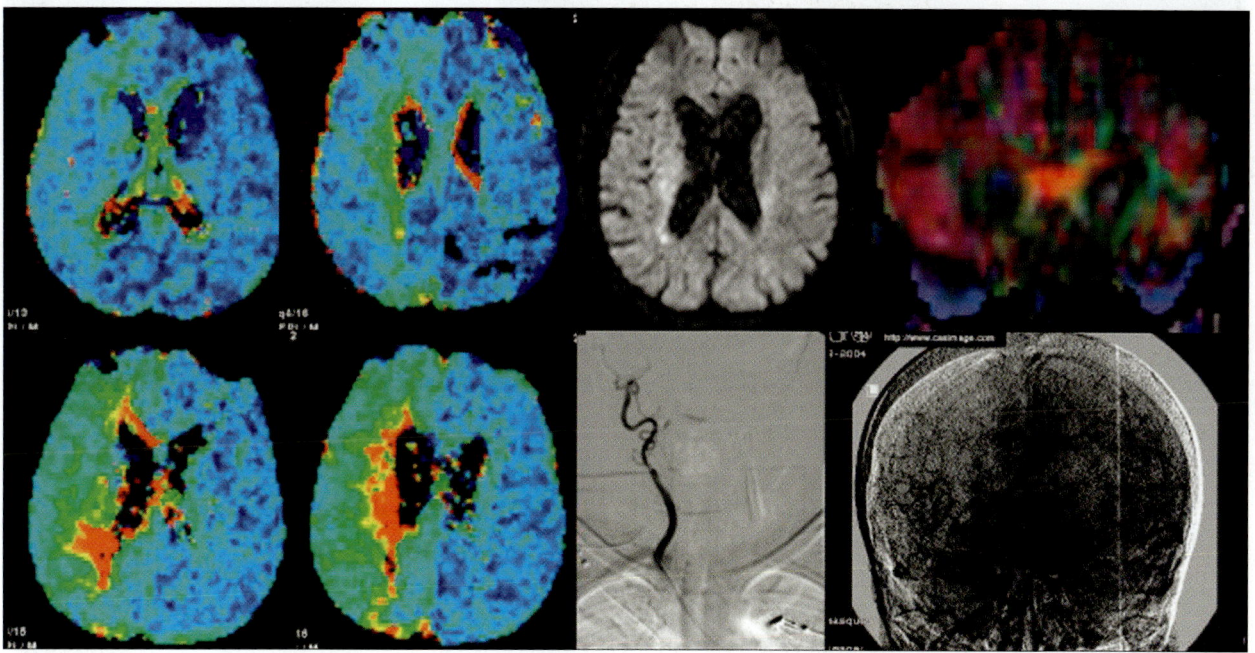

Fig. 7. Hypoperfusion seen on perfusion MR images with alterations on DTI: the perfusion images show a large area of hypoperfusion in the right MCA territory (left images) while there are slight changes on the DWI only. The coronally reconstructed FA shows alterations in the anisotropy in the left frontal lobe. This corresponds to the hypoperfusion seen on the parenchymogramm (lower right) and which is due to carotid occlusion.

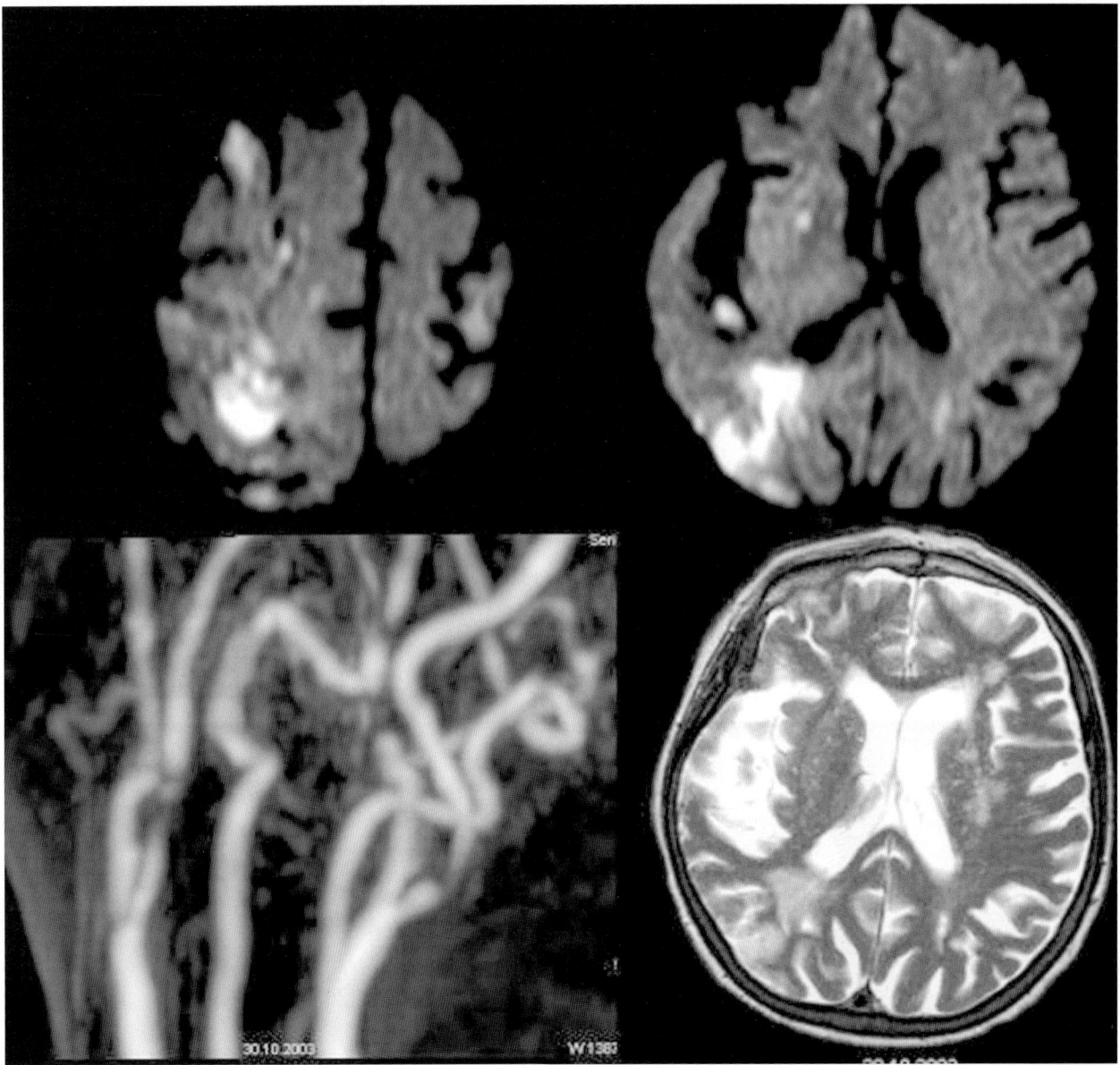

Fig. 8. Severe right-sided carotis stenosis wiith multiple lesions seen on DWI due to hemodynamic insufficiency.

a restriction in motion in the affected tissue with a subsequent hypersignal on diffusion images and a corresponding decrease in the ADC sequences (Fig. 3). These diffusion studies can help elucidate if the lesion is of a hemodynamic type if there is a "string of pearls" disposition of multiple lesions in the watershed areas (Figs. 8 and 9) whereas if there is one lesion located deeply it may be an embolic occurrence (Fig. 10).

Leucoaraiosis and diffusion tensor studies

Hachinski coined the term leucoaraiosis as the hyperintensity found on T2-weighted MR images found in the periventricular cerebral white matter [17]. While its exact pathogenesis is not fully understood it does increase with aging, and the fact that hypodensity is present on CT and hyperintensity on

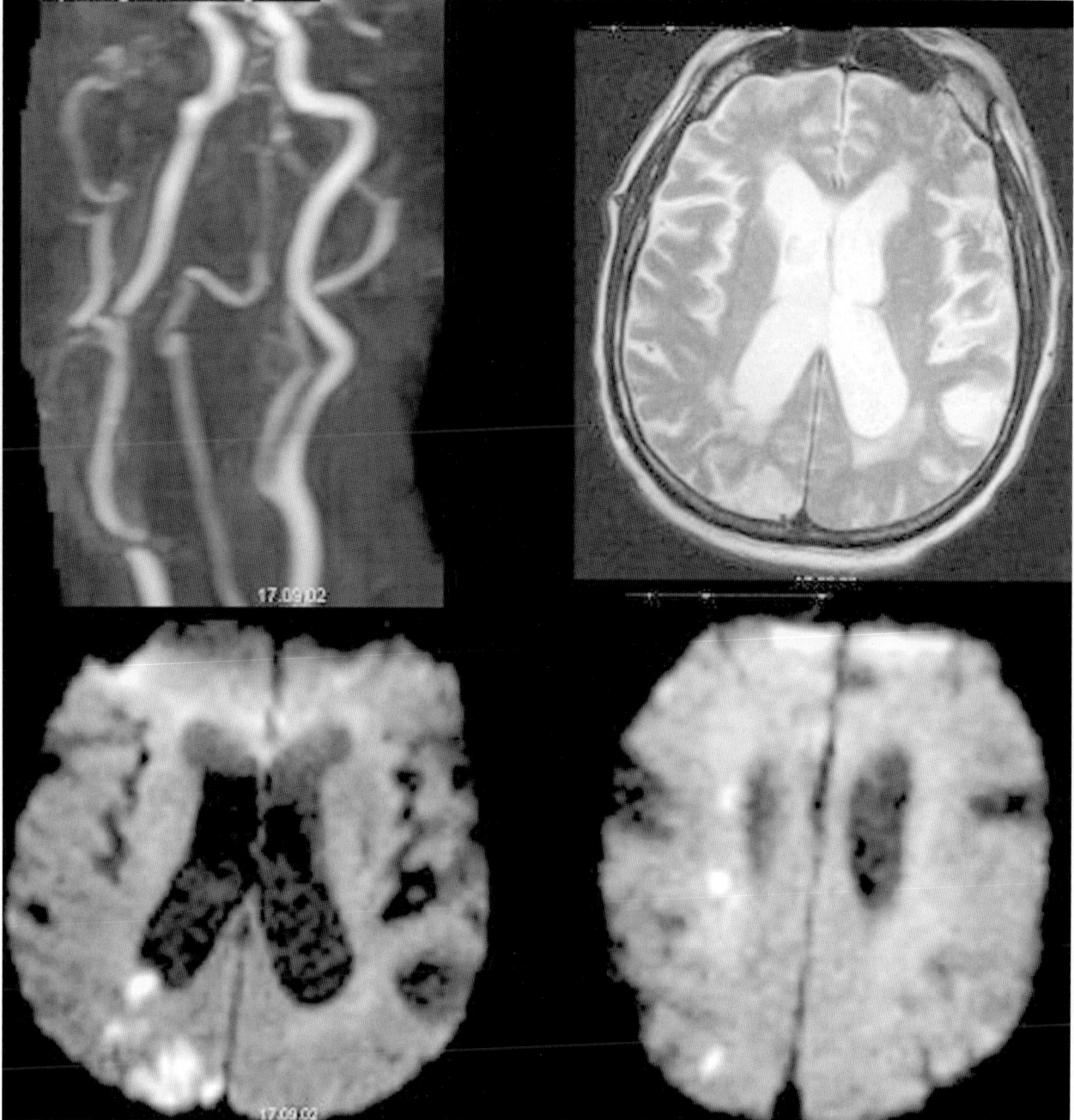

Fig. 9. Severe stenosis of the right carotid with alterations on the DWI.

T2-MRI points towards a probable vascular origin, due to ischemia [45]. White matter hyperintensities on MRI are found frequently [11] with a prevalence increasing with age: de Leeuwa found that only 8% of patients in their study were completely free of lesions. The risk factors most often associated with white matter lesions are high age, diabetes, arterial hypertension atherosclerosis and impairments of cerebral blood flow. Clinically the spectrum is wide with age-related syndromes such as troubles of gait,

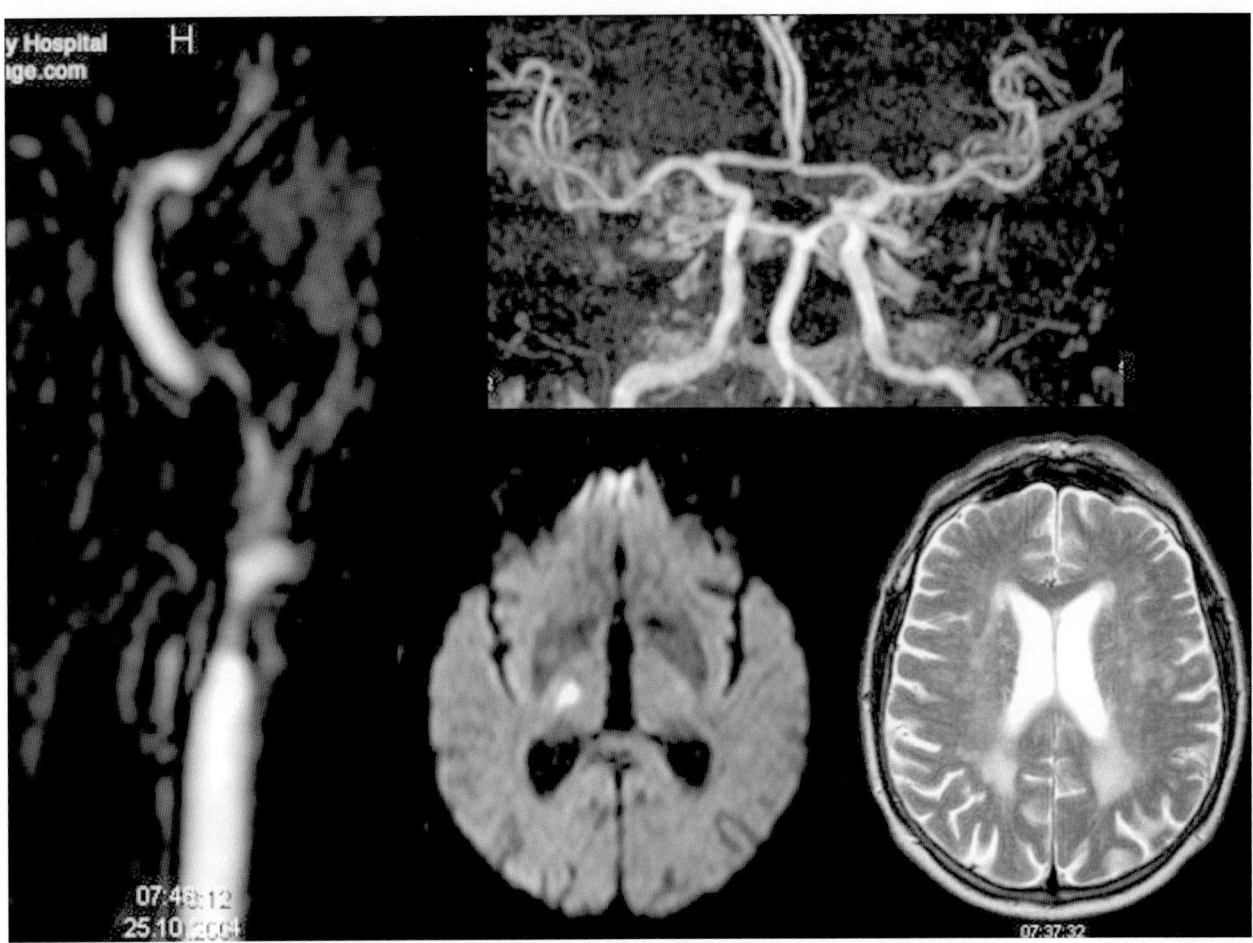

Fig. 10. Severe short stenosis of the right MCA with small embolic infarction in the right internal capsule.

incontinence, cognitive impairment and depression being most often associated with these lesions. When assessing the data from the cardiovascular health study, Yue et al. found that egression models of the entire imaged cohort showed higher grades of all variables with increasing age, and higher ventricular and sulcal grades in men and in nonblack individuals [69]. White matter grade was greater in women and in black individuals. Regression models of the healthier subgroup showed similar associations, except for a lack of association of sulcal and ventricular size with race. They concluded that sulcal width, ventricular size, and white matter signal intensity change with age, sex, and race. Tullberg et al. found that White Matter Hyperintensities in all brain regions were associated with low executive scores in nondemented subjects. They found that these were more frequently found in the frontal white matter [60]. De Carli et al. performing white matter segmentation on fluid-attenuated inversion recovery (FLAIR) images in a series of 55 patients, found that all White Matter Hyperintensities revealed smooth expansion from around central cerebrospinal fluid spaces into more distal cerebral white matter with increasing WMH volume [12]. They based their study on the hypothetical existence of two types of white matter hyperintensities, periventricular and deep white matter hyperintensities; their study failed to rediscover this pattern based on the segmentation techniques they employed. This was in favour of the existence of one underlying vascular watershed area, which is compromised [12]. WT. Longstreth, et al. found that worsening white matter grade on serial MRI scans in elderly is common, is associated with cognitive decline, and has complex relations with cardiovascular risk factors [28]. They studied a subgroup of 1919 patients from the Cardiovascular Health Study (CHS), a population-based longitudinal study of vascular disease, who underwent 2 MRI scans separated by 5 years and they found a worsening of the radiological status in 28% (538 patients). Also, scores on modified Mini-Mental State examination and Digit-Symbol Substitution test deteriorated significantly more in those with than without worsening on MR scores. Kuller et al. found that white matter hyperintensities were a risk factor for stroke: indeed Results the relative risk of stroke increased significantly as the disease increased [23]. The risk of stroke was 2.8% per year for participants with extensive white matter disease, compared with only 0.6% for participants with less disease. The relationship between leucoaraiosis and carotid stenosis has been open to debate: Streifler et al. studied 2618 patients from the NASCET study and found 493 with leucoaraiosis; they also found no relationship between severity of stenosis and severity of leucoaraiosis, however they later found that there seems to be a relationship between cerebrovascular disease, stroke and leucoaraiosis and patients with more extensive leucoaraisos seem to have a more severe prognosis overall [53]–[55]. Kuo et al. described a correlation between these white matter changes and severity of dysfunction with different geriatric syndromes such as falls, executive cognitive impairment, depressive symptoms, and urinary incontinence. They postulated that there was damage to associative pathways in frontal and subcortical regions due to hypoperfusion that may disrupt frontal executive, motor control, and other systems, resulting in these manifestations [24]. Neuroimaging has been recently revolutionized by the development of methods such as diffusion-weighted MRI and diffusion tensor imaging. Diffusion-weighted MRI has found its main application in the acute diagnosis of stroke whereas diffusion tensor imaging is used to investigate the structure and integrity of white matter [36]. Diffusion-weighted MRI has been used to monitor both stenting and endarterectomy of the carotid artery [7], [34] as well as to define age related ADC changes [30]. Diffusion tensor changes have been demonstrated to accompany the earliest changes in ischemia [68], [51]. O'Sullivan found that additionally hypoperfusion seems to play a role in the development of periventricular lesions in ischemic leucoaraiosis and may play a direct pathogenic role. They performed a study on twenty-one patients with ischemic leucoaraiosis using perfusion MRI, with an echo-planar sequence requiring paramagnetic contrast injection: they found that cerebral blood flow (CBF) was lower in the periventricular white matter than in other brain regions (e.g., centrum semi-ovale), attesting a role for hypoperfusion [40]. Helenius et al., using a more simple approach with diffusion-weighted MRI was able to detect increases in the ADC that corresponded to the leucoaraiotic areas [20]. In a further study Jones et al. using diffusion tensor technology in a small series of 9 patients with what they defined as ischemic leucoaraiosis (radiological presence of leucoaraiosis and clinical lacunar stroke [21], found that the characteristic pattern found on diffusion tensor imaging in this patient group was consistent with axonal loss and gliosis leading to impairment to and loss of directional diffusion with consequent loss of anisotropy. More and more, recently new MR technology such as diffusion tensor MRI (DTI) has been applied to the aging brain, especially with calculation of fractional anisotropy (FA) maps: with a decrease of the FA over time. In another study, O'Sullivan et al. found DTI to be more sensitive to brain changes that correlated with functional decrease than conventional MRI alone [41]. They further studied a collective of 36 patients with ischemic leucoaraiosis and found that on DTI, diffusivity was increased both within lesions and in normal appearing white matter. Also, they found that the mean diffusivity of normal appearing white matter correlated with full scale IQ and tests of executive function. They further determined that these correlations remained significant after controlling for age, sex, brain volume, and T1/T2 lesion volume, while there was less or no such good correlation between

T2 lesions and neuropsychological scores. Even in normal appearing white matter of patients with leucoaraiosis, O'Sullivan was able to detect changes in anisotropy that corresponded to areas of white matter disruption [39]. They also found that the DTI changes in the normal-appearing white matter correlated both with executive dysfunction and global cognitive impairment. O'Sullivan et al. found that the DTI changes corresponding to white matter tract disruption occurs in normal aging and would be consistent with the cortical disconnection hypothesis of age-related cognitive decline [39]. They studied twenty "normal" elderly (56 to 85 years old) volunteers with DTI and compared the findings to those in ten younger volunteers. The tests they performed included the Wisconsin Card Sorting Test, Reitan Trail Making Test, Verbal Fluency, and the Mini-Mental State Examination. On MRI, they found that whole white matter FA declined with age, whereas mean diffusivity increased overall.

Perfusion MR studies

The advent of fast imaging techniques such as echoplanar imaging and/or gradient-echo imaging has allowed acquiring quickly and repeatedly MR images that are sensitive to changes induced by contrast materials [27].

Perfusion of the brain with MRI is performed principally with 3 techniques: contrast-enhanced techniques [46], [44], [43], arterial spin-labeling techniques [13] and the blood oxygenation level-dependent (BOLD) principle. The BOLD technique is mainly used in functional activation imaging and will not be discussed here as will not the use of spin-labeling techniques, even if they have been used successfully in acute human stroke [8], [49]. The problem with contrast-derived MR perfusion techniques is that one measures variations in the magnetic field that represent extreme susceptibility artifacts, rendering quantification difficult (e.g., measurement of cerebral blood volume (CBV) and CBF) Also we are mainly facing relative values of the CBV and CBF since no clear arterial input function can be obtained easily.

However the MR perfusion images correlate well with the taste of the cerebral vasculature (Fig. 11). Studying the various various parameters obtained from MR T2* imaging, Sorensen found that lesion volumes on blood volume and diffusion maps correlated better with eventual infarct volumes than did those on blood flow and tracer mean transit time maps [50].

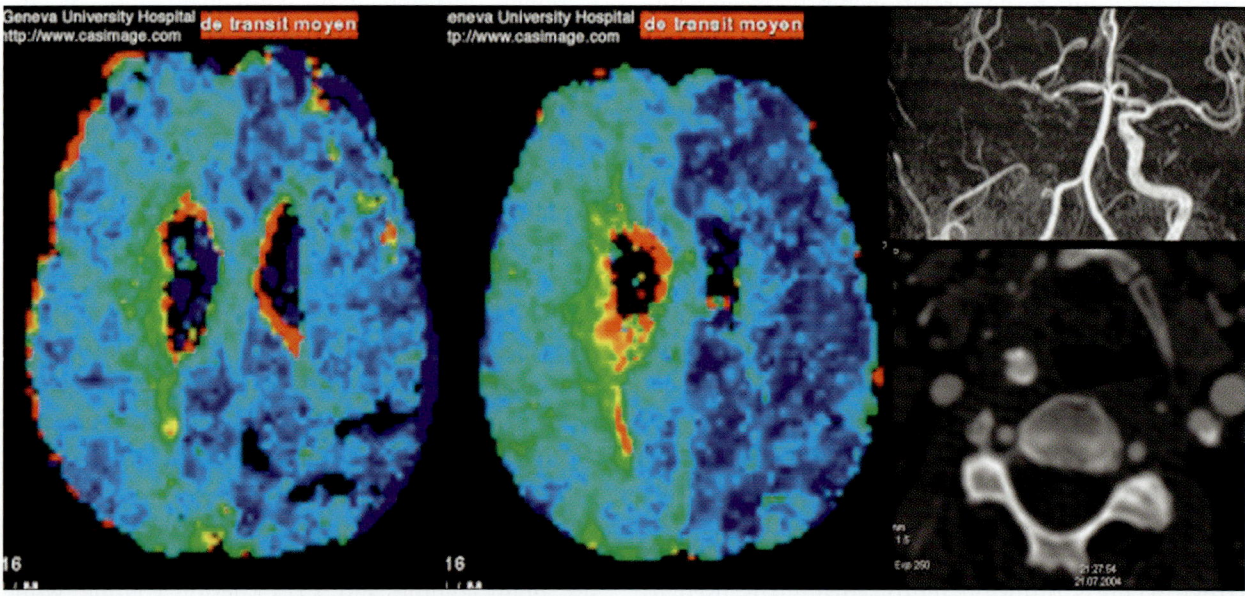

Fig. 11. Severe right-hemispheric hypoperfusion seen on perfusion MR images due to carotid occlusion.

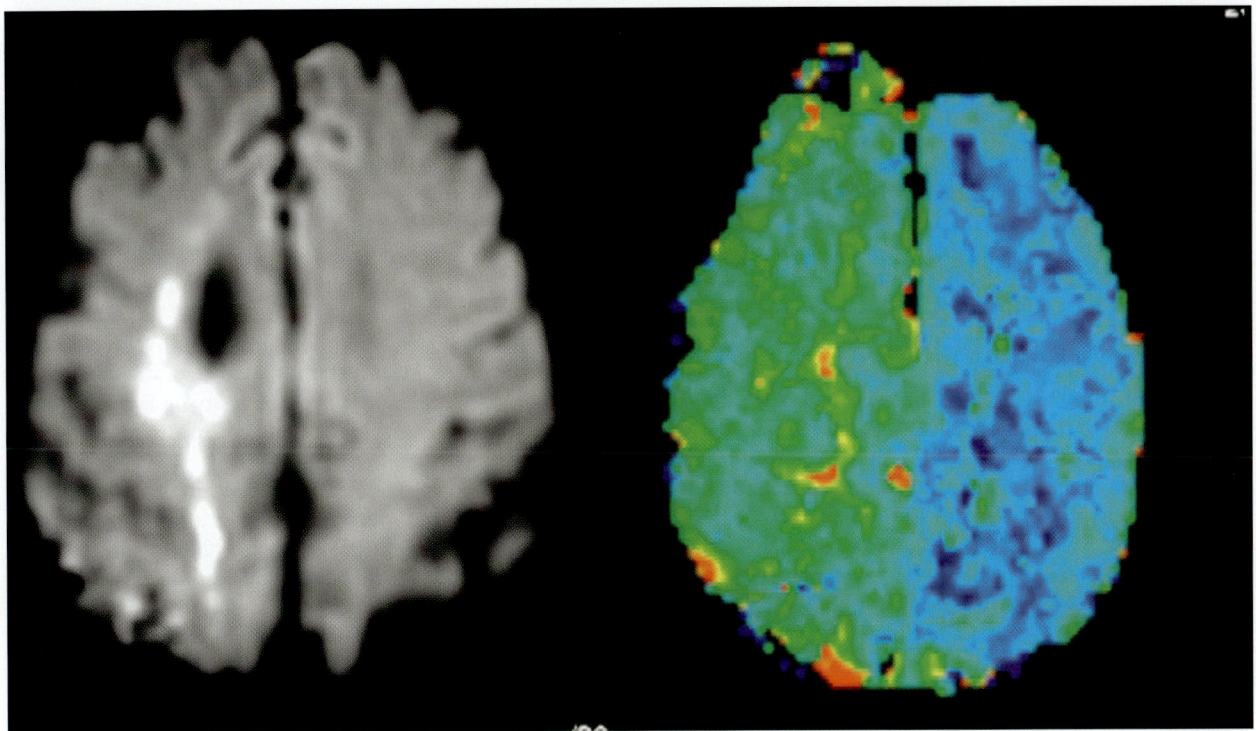

Fig. 12. White matter watershed lesion on the diffusion image (left) due to severe chronic hypoperfusion (right).

Also, T1-weighted MR perfusion imaging is possible and probably advantageous, but it has not yet established itself as a viable option [19].

However the use of perfusion-weighted imaging (PWI) in addition to DWI has allowed Steven Warach [64] among others to develop a model of penumbra that can be used in clinical practice: the central area of diffusion anomaly at the first time point corresponds to the ischemic core while the hypoperfused area surrounding it represents the penumbra, or tissue at risk of undergoing further infarction if nothing is undertaken (Fig. 12). This model has proven itself usable clinically since then by many authors [42], [57]. This penumbra however has been found to extend into the early diffusion lesions when imaging is done very early on.

Conclusions

In the work-up of patients with carotid disease, imaging of the brain parenchyma has a central role. Due to recent advances in technology MR imaging has taken a central role; indeed we can now not just study anatomy, but look for early pathological changes with diffusion imaging, investigate the hemodynamic parameters with perfusion imaging and look for vascular occlusion with MR angiography.

This work is supported by a grant from the Swiss National Science Foundation (Mapping the ischemic tissue at risk with diffusion and perfusion MRI) Grant No 3100-066348.01.

References

[1] Beneficial effect of carotid endarterectomy in symptomatic patients with high-grade carotid stenosis. North American Symptomatic Carotid Endarterectomy Trial Collaborators. N Engl J Med 325: 445–453 (1991).
[2] Endarterectomy for asymptomatic carotid artery stenosis. Executive Committee for the Asymptomatic Carotid Atherosclerosis Study. JAMA 273: 1421–1428 (1995).
[3] Randomized trial of endarterectomy for recently symptomatic carotid stenosis: final results of the MRC

European Carotid Surgery Trial (ECST). Lancet 351: 1379–1387 (1998).

[4] Baird AE, Benfield A, Schlaug G et al.: Enlargement of human cerebral ischemic lesions mesured by diffusion weighted magnetic resonance imaging. Ann Neurol 41: 581–589 (1997).

[5] Baird AE, Lövblad KO, Dashe JF et al.: Clinical correlations of diffusion and perfusion lesion volumes in acute stroke. Cerebrovasc Dis 10: 441–448 (2000).

[6] Baird AE, Lövblad KO, Schlaug G et al.: The multiple acute stroke syndrome – A marker of embolic disease? Neurology 54: 674–679 (2000).

[7] Barth A, Remonda L, Lövblad KO et al.: Silent cerebral ischemia detected by diffusion-weighted MRI after carotid endarterectomy. Stroke 31: 1824–1828 (2000).

[8] Chen Q, Siewert B, Bly BM et al.: STAR-HASTE: perfusion imaging without magnetic susceptibility artifact. Magn Reson Med 38: 404–408 (1997).

[9] Chien D, Kwong KK, Gress DR et al.: MR diffusion imaging of cerebral infarction in humans. AJNR 13: 1097–1102 (1992).

[10] Dardzinski BJ, Sotak CH, Fisher M et al.: Apparent diffusion coefficient mapping of experimental focal cerebral ischemia using diffusion-weighted echo-planar imaging. MRM 30: 318–325 (1993).

[11] de Leeuw FE, de Groota JC, Achten E et al.: Prevalence of cerebral white matter lesions in elderly people: a population based magnetic resonance imaging study. The Rotterdam Scan Study. J Neurol Neurosurg Psychiatry 70: 9–14 (2001).

[12] DeCarli C, van Fletcher E, Ramey V et al.: Anatomical Mapping of White Matter Hyperintensities (WMH). Stroke 36: 50 (2005).

[13] Edelman RR, Siewert B, Darby DG et al.: Qualitative mapping of cerebral blood flow and functional localization with echo-planar MR imaging and signal targeting with alternating radio frequency. Radiology 192: 513–520 (1994).

[14] Edelman RR, Wielopolski P, Schmitt F: Echo-planar MR imaging. Radiology 192: 600–612 (1994).

[15] El-Koussy M, Lövblad KO, Kiefer C et al.: Apparent diffusion coefficient mapping of infarcted tissue and the the penumbra in acute stroke. Neuroradiology 44: 812–818 (2002).

[16] Gillard JH, Papadakis NG, Martin K et al.: MR diffusion tensor imaging of white matter tract disruption in stroke at 3 T. Br J Radiol 74: 642–647 (2001).

[17] Hachinski VC, Potter P, Merskey H: Leuko-araiosis. Arch Neurol 44: 21–23 (1987)

[18] Hasegawa Y, Fisher M, Latour LL et al.: MRI diffusion mapping of reversible and irreversible injury in focal brain ischemia. Neurology 44: 1484–1490 (1994).

[19] Heid O: T1-gewichtete MR Perfusion. Dissertation, University of Bern,Switzerland.

[20] Helenius J, Soinne L, Salonen O et al.: Leukoaraiosis, Ischemic Stroke, and Normal White Matter on Diffusion-Weighted MRI. Stroke 33: 45–50 (2002).

[21] Jones DK, Lythgoe D, Horsfield MA et al.: Characterization of White Matter Damage in Ischemic Leukoaraiosis with Diffusion Tensor MRI. Stroke 30: 393–397 (1999).

[22] Khong PL, Zhou LJ, Ooi GC et al.: The Evaluation of Wallerian Degeneration in Chronic Paediatric Middle Cerebral Artery Infarction Using Diffusion Tensor MR Imaging. Cerebrovasc Dis 18: 240–247 (2004).

[23] Kuller LH, Longstreth WT Jr, Arnold AM et al.: Cardiovascular Health Study Collaborative Research Group. White matter hyperintensity on cranial magnetic resonance imaging: a predictor of stroke. Stroke 35: 1821–1825 (2004).

[24] Kuo HK, Lipsitz LA: Cerebral White Matter Changes and Geriatric Syndromes: Is There a Link? J. Gerontol. A Biol Sci Med Sci 59: 818–826 (2004).

[25] Le Bihan D, Breton E, Lallemand D et al.: MR Imaging of intravoxel incoherent motions: application to diffusion and perfusion in neurologic disorders. Radiology 161: 401–407 (1986).

[26] Le Bihan D, Mangin JF, Poupon C et al.: Diffusion tensor imaging: concepts and applications. J Magn Reson Imaging 13: 534–546 (2001).

[27] Le Bihan D: Theoretical principles of perfusion imaging Application to magnetic resonance imaging. Investigative Radiology 27: 6–11 (1992).

[28] Longstreth WT, Arnold AM, Beauchamp NJ et al.: Incidence, Manifestations, and Predictors of Worsening White Matter on Serial Cranial Magnetic Resonance Imaging in the Elderly: The Cardiovascular Health Study. Stroke 36: 56–61 (2005).

[29] Lövblad KO, Baird A, Schlaug G et al.: Ischemic lesion volumes in acute stroke by diffusion-weighted magnetic resonance imaging correlate with clinical outcome. Ann Neurol 42: 164–170 (1997).

[30] Lövblad KO, Delavelle J, Wetzel S et al.: ADC mapping of the aging frontal lobes in mild cognitive impairment. Neuroradiology 46: 282–286 (2004).

[31] Lövblad KO, Jakob PM, Baird AE et al.: Turbo-spin echo Diffusion-weighted MR of human stroke. Am J Neuroradiol 19: 201–208 (1998).

[32] Lövblad KO, Kiefer C, Oswald H et al.: Imaging the ischemic penumbra. Riv Neuroradiol 16: 833–838 (2003).

[33] Lövblad KO, Laubach HJ, Baird AE et al.: Clinical experience with diffusion weighted MR in patients with acute stroke. Am J Neuroradiol 19: 1061–1066 (1998).

[34] Lövblad KO, Plüschke W, Remonda L et al.: Diffusion-weighted MR imaging as a monitor of neurovascular intervention. Neuroradiology 42: 134–138 (2000).

[35] Lövblad KO, Remonda L, Heid O et al.: Clinical single-shot diffusion-weighted MR of the human brain

on a short-bore medium-field scanner. Neuroradiology 41: 889–894 (1999).
[36] Melhem ER, Mori S, Mukundan G et al.: Diffusion Tensor MR Imaging of the Brain and White Matter Tractography. AJR 178: 3–16 (2002).
[37] Minematsu K, Fisher M, Li L et al.: Effects of a novel NMDA antagonist on experimental stroke rapidly and quantitatively assessed by diffusion-weighted MRI. Neurology 43: 397–403 (1993).
[38] Moseley ME, Cohen Y, Mintorovitch J et al.: Early detection of regional cerebral ischemia in cats: Comparison of diffusion- and T2-weighted MRI and spectroscopy. MRM 14: 330–346 (1990).
[39] O'Sullivan M, Jones DK, Summers PE et al.: Evidence for cortical "disconnection" as a mechanism of age-related cognitive decline. Neurology 57: 632–638 (2001).
[40] O'Sullivan M, Lythgoe DJ, Pereira AC et al.: Patterns of cerebral blood flow reduction in patients with ischemic leucoaraiosis. Neurology 59: 321–326 (2002)
[41] O'Sullivan M, Morris RG, Huckstep B et al.: Diffusion tensor MRI correlates with executive dysfunction in patients with ischaemic leucoaraiosis. J Neurol Neurosur Ps 75: 441–447 (2004)
[42] Ostergaard L, Sorensen AG, Chesler DA et al.: Combined diffusion-weighted and perfusion-weighted flow heterogeneity magnetic resonance imaging in acute stroke. Stroke 31: 1097–1103 (2000).
[43] Ostergaard L, Sorensen AG, Kwong KK et al.: High resolution measurement of cerebral blood flow using intravascular tracer bolus passages. Part II: Experimental comparison and preliminary results. Magn Reson Med 36: 726–736 (1996).
[44] Ostergaard L, Weisskoff RM, Chesler DA et al.: High resolution measurement of cerebral blood flow using intravascular tracer bolus passages. Part I: Mathematical approach and statistical analysis. Magn Reson Med 36: 715–725 (1996).
[45] Pantoni and Garcia. Pathogenesis of Leukoaraiosis: A Review. Stroke 28: 652–659 (1997).
[46] Rosen BR, Belliveau JW, Vevea JM et al.: Perfusion Imaging with NMR contrast agents. Magn Reson Med 14: 249–265 (1990).
[47] Schlaug G, Benfield A, Baird A et al.: The ischemic penumbra of human stroke: using functional MRI parameters to define tissue at risk for infarct progression. Neurology 53: 1528–1537 (1999).
[48] Schlaug G, Siewert B, Benfield A et al.: Time course of the apparent diffusion coefficient (ADC) abnormality in human stroke. Neurology 49: 113–119 (1997).
[49] Siewert B, Schlaug G, Edelman RR et al.: Comparison of EPISTAR and T2*-weighted gadolinium-enhanced perfusion imaging in patients with acute cerebral ischemia. Neurology 48: 673–679 (1997).
[50] Sorensen AG, Copen WA, Ostergaard L et al.: Hyperacute stroke: simultaneous measurement of relative cerebral blood volume, relative cerebral blood flow, and mean tissue transit time. Radiology 210: 519–527 (1999).
[51] Sorensen AG, Wu O, Copen WA et al.: Human acute cerebral ischemia: detection of changes in water diffusion anisotropy by using MR imaging. Radiology 212: 785–792 (1999).
[52] Sotak CH: The role of diffusion tensor imaging in the evaluation of ischemic brain injury – a review. NMR Biomed 15: 561–569 (2002).
[53] Streifler JY, Eliasziw M, Benavente OR et al.: North American Symptomatic Carotid Endarterectomy Trial Group. Development and progression of leukoaraiosis in patients with brain ischemia and carotid artery disease. Stroke 34: 1913–1916 (2003).
[54] Streifler JY, Eliasziw M, Benavente OR et al.: North American Symptomatic Carotid Endarterectomy Trial Group. Prognostic importance of leukoaraiosis in patients with symptomatic internal carotid artery stenosis. Stroke 33: 1651–1655 (2002).
[55] Streifler JY, Eliasziw M, Benavente OR et al.: Lack of relationship between leukoaraiosis and carotid artery disease. The North American Symptomatic Carotid Endarterectomy Trial.: Arch Neurol 52: 21–24 (1995).
[56] Takano K, Carano RAD, Tatlisumak T et al.: Efficacy of intra-arterial and intravenous prourokinase in an embolic stroke model evaluated by diffusion-perfusion magnetic resonance imaging. Neurology 50: 870–875 (1998).
[57] Taleb M, Lövblad KO, El-Koussy M et al.: Reperfusion demonstrated by ADC mapping after intra-arterial thrombolysis for human ischemic stroke confirmed by cerebral angiography. Neuroradiology 43: 591–594 (2001).
[58] Tanner JE, Stejskal EO: Restricted self-diffusion of protons in colloidal systems by the pulsed-gradient, spin-echo method 1768–1777 (1968).
[59] Thomalla G, Glauche V, Koch MA et al.: Diffusion tensor imaging detects early Wallerian degeneration of the pyramidal tract after ischemic stroke. Neuroimage 22: 1767–1174 (2004).
[60] Tullberg M, Fletcher E, Decarlic, Mungas D, Reed BR, Harvey DJ, Weiner MW, Chui HC, Jagust WJ: White matter lesions impair frontal lobe function regardless of their location. Neurology 63: 246–253 (2004).
[61] Turner R, LeBihan D, Maier J et al.: Echo-planar imaging of intravoxel incoherent motion. Radiology 177: 407–414 (1990).
[62] Warach S, Chien D, Li W et al.: Fast magnetic resonance diffusion-weighted imaging of acute stroke. Neurology 42: 1717–1723 (1992).
[63] Warach S, Gaa J, Siewert B et al.: Acute human stroke studies by whole brain echo planar diffusion-weighted magnetic resonance imaging. Ann Neurol 37: 231–241 (1995).

[64] Warach S, Wielopolski P, Edelman RR: Identification and characterization of the ischemic penumbra of acute human stroke using echo planar diffusion and perfusion imaging. In: Proceedings of the 12th annual meeting of the Society of Magnetic Resonance in Medicine, Berkeley, Ca 263: (1993).

[65] Warach SJ, Dashe JF, Edelman RR: Clinical outcome in ischemic stroke predicted by early diffusion-weighted and perfusion magnetic resonance imaging: A preliminary analysis. J Cerebral Blood Flow and Metabolism 16: 53–59 (1996).

[66] Weber J, Mattle HP, Heid O et al.: Diffusion-weighted imaging in ischaemic stroke: a follow-up study. Neuroradiology 42: 184–191 (2000).

[67] Yadav JS, Wholey MH, Kuntz RE et al.: Stenting and Angioplasty with Protection in Patients at High Risk for Endarterectomy Investigators. Protected carotid-artery stenting versus endarterectomy in high-risk patients. N Engl J Med 351: 1493–1501 (2004).

[68] Yang Q, Tress BM, Barber PA et al.: Serial Study of Apparent Diffusion Coefficient and Anisotropy in Patients With Acute Stroke. Stroke 30: 2382–2390 (1999).

[69] Yue NC, Arnold AM, Longstreth WT Jr et al.: Sulcal, ventricular, and white matter changes at MR imaging in the aging brain: data from the cardiovascular health study. Radiology 202: 33–39 (1997).

Chapter 1.7

PET IMAGING IN CAROTID STENOSIS

C. P. Derdeyn

Mallinckrodt Institute of Radiology and The Departments of Neurology and Neurological Surgery,
Washington University School of Medicine, St. Lovis, WA, USA

Introduction

Positron Emission Tomography (PET) is a physiological, not anatomical imaging method: it is not used for the measurement or detection of carotid artery disease. It is primarily a research tool that has several important applications for the study of human carotid atherosclerotic disease. Functional imaging methods, including PET, have provided compelling data that embolic and hemodynamic factors have a synergistic effect on stroke risk. The foremost role of PET has been in studies of the assessment of the hemodynamic and metabolic effects of these lesions on the distal cerebral circulation. This information has proven prognostic value. In addition, molecular imaging applications have been described, allowing investigation of physiological aspects of the plaque itself. Finally, some radiotracers may be used to identify recent brain injury. This could help distinguish symptomatic from asymptomatic lesions, a critical distinction in carotid disease.

Carotid artery disease is a frequent cause of ischemic stroke. Up to one third of patients presenting with stroke or transient ischemic attack are found to have ipsilateral severe stenosis or occlusion of the carotid artery [55], [7]. Both embolic and hemodynamic mechanisms play a role in the pathogenesis of stroke in these patients [57], [8], [48]. These mechanisms may be synergistic in many patients [37]. Endarterectomy has been proven effective in patients with symptomatic stenosis [60], [73]. This procedure addresses both embolic and hemodynamic mechanisms.

There is no proven therapy for complete carotid occlusion, however [84], [37]. In addition, asymptomatic patients with carotid atherosclerotic disease have a much lower risk for future stroke with medical therapy than symptomatic patients with similar degrees of stenosis or occlusion [60], [25], [85], [68]. The benefit of endarterectomy in patients with asymptomatic stenosis is marginal [25], [85].

At present, evidence-based treatment decisions for patients with atherosclerotic carotid disease are made using anatomical information (the degree of stenosis) and clinical factors (symptoms and gender, for example) [73], [22]. The information gained from these research PET studies has no proven value on treatment decisions for patients with atherosclerotic carotid disease. One area of potential future importance lies in identifying subgroups of patients with higher or lower natural history risks for stroke based on the underlying physiology. These subgroups could then be evaluated in trials of specific therapy aimed at the underlying stroke mechanism. This would include patients with complete carotid occlusion, for whom hemodynamic impairment is a proven risk factor for future stroke [37], [91], patients with near-occlusion [73], [72], and patients with asymptomatic carotid stenosis, particularly women [74]. A randomized clinical trial of surgical revascularization for patients with symptomatic complete carotid occlusion is underway, utilizing a PET screen to identify those with severe hemodynamic impairment [37]. The natural history risk for stroke in asymptomatic stenosis patients is very low: a high-risk sub-group might be identified within this population owing to hemodynamic or physiologic plaque characteristics [81]. Endarterectomy or stenting might be more effective in this subgroup than in the greater population in whom there is no clear benefit currently.

This chapter focuses on knowledge gained from PET regarding atherosclerotic carotid disease. We will first discuss experimental studies, beginning with the basic principles of PET. Next, we will review normal cerebral hemodynamics and metabolism. We will then review the responses of the brain and its vasculature to reduced perfusion pressure, primarily autoregulatory vasodilation and increased oxygen extraction fraction. We will review recent PET molecular imaging studies of atherosclerotic plaque and brain ischemia. Following this discussion of experimental data, we will review the use of PET to investigate the effects of chronic hemodynamic compromise (Clinical Studies). We will conclude with a section on future applications and a brief summary.

PET physics and experimental studies

PET basics

PET imaging requires three components: a radiotracer, a system to detect and measure the quantity of radiation, and a mathematical model relating the physiological process under study to the detected radiation. One method for the measurement of cerebral blood flow, for example, uses a bolus injection of ^{15}O-labeled water. The PET camera measures the counts in the head during the circulation of the water through the brain. Finally, the PET image of raw counts is converted into a map of regional quantitative CBF using computer programs that require measurements of arterial blood counts and incorporate models and assumptions regarding the transit of water through the cerebral circulation. Radiotracers are radioactive molecules administered in such small quantities that they do not affect the physiologic process under study. PET radiotracers may be separated into two broad categories: normal biological molecules, such as ^{15}O-labeled water, or non-biologic elements attached to organic molecules as radiolabels, such as ^{18}F-labeled deoxy-glucose (FDG). By definition, these tracers decay by positron emission. Their half-lives range from a few minutes to a few hours. The most commonly used radiotracers, ^{18}F and ^{15}O, require a linear accelerator or cyclotron for production.

The PET imaging detection system uses the phenomenon of annihilation radiation to localize and measure physiologic processes in the brain. PET radionuclides decay by emission of a positively charged electron (a positron). The positron may travel a few millimeters within the tissue losing before encountering an electron. This encounter results in the annihilation of both the positron and electron and the consequent generation of two gamma photons of equal energy. These two photons are emitted in characteristic 180 degree opposite directions. A pair of detectors positioned on either side of the source of the annihilation photons detects them simultaneously. This allows localization of the point source of the radiation. The spatial resolution of a pair of annihilation coincidence detectors is nearly uniform for most of the region found between detectors. After the correction for attenuation, the data from the detector pairs is used to construct a series of projections, each representing the distribution of regional radioactivity viewed from a different angle. These projections are then combined by a computer to produce a two-dimensional reconstruction of the regional radioactivity within the combined field of view of all the detector pairs. Scanners with multiple rings of detectors are capable of generating several reconstructed slices of the imaged volume simultaneously, each depicting a different level of the brain and together providing a three-dimensional image.

The most important limitations of PET imaging of physiologic processes relates to the phenomenon of full-width, half-maximum (FWHM) and a related phenomenon of partial-volume averaging. Detected radiation is observed over a larger area than the actual source. The spread or distribution of activity is approximately Gaussian for a point source of radiation, with the maximum located at the original point. The FWHM describes the degree of smearing of radioactivity in a reconstructed image. The ability of a PET scanner to discriminate between two small adjacent structures or accurately measure the activity in a small region will depend on the FWHM of the system as well as the amount and distribution of activity within the region of interest and the surrounding areas. *Because of the smearing or redistribution of detected radioactivity, any given region in the reconstructed image will not contain all the activity actually within the region. Some of the activity will spill over into adjacent areas.* Similarly, activity in the surrounding tissue or structures will also be redistributed into the region of interest. This phenomenon is known as the partial volume effect. An important consequence of this principle is that PET will always measure a gradual change in activity where an abrupt change actually exists, such as in a vessel wall. Measurements made at the borders of such structures will not be accurate.

Third, the externally measured tissue concentration of the positron emitting radiotracer (PET counts) is quantitatively related to the physiologic variable under study by a mathematical model. The PET scanner measures the total counts in a volume of tissue. The models calculate how that measured activity reflects the physiologic parameter under study. These calculations account for several factors related to the tracer biomechanics and metabolism. These factors include the mode of tracer delivery to the tissue, the distribution and metabolism of the tracer within the tissue, the egress of the tracer and metabolites from the tissue, the recirculation of both the tracer and its labeled metabolites, and the amount of tracer and metabolites remaining in the blood. The validity of all the underlying assumptions and possible sources of error for each model when applied to the study of both normal physiology and disease states must be clearly understood.

An issue of great importance in the analysis of PET data is that of statistics. PET counts are statistical data by nature. Consequently, when comparing the data from several regions of interest to each other, a correction for the potential error introduced by multiple comparisons must be used. The selection of proper control subjects and regions of interest is also crucial to accurate data analysis.

Finally, a major advantage of PET over other physiological imaging techniques relates to signal to noise. This is particularly true for molecular imaging approaches. The only signal detected by the PET scanner is the radiation from the positron emitting isotopes. PET can provide very sensitive and quantitative measurements of the presence of any labeled molecule. Other methods such as CT or MR have better spatial resolution, but overcoming the background signal is a particular problem.

Physiological factors measured by PET

Cerebral blood flow (CBF) is the volume of blood delivered to a defined mass of tissue per unit time, generally in milliliters of blood per 100 grams of brain per minute (mLs/(100g · min)). ^{15}O-labeled water is the tracer used for measurements of CBF in our laboratory [69]. The tracer kinetic models treat water as a freely diffusible tracer. Counts are nearly linearly proportionally to CBF. As a consequence, relative CBF can be easily estimated as the ratio of PET counts between one brain region and another. Several other methods are in common use as well, including O-15 labeled butanol and continous $C^{15}O_2$ inhalation [50].

Cerebral blood volume (CBV) is the volume of blood within a given mass of tissue and is expressed as milliliters of blood per 100 grams of brain tissue. Regional CBV measurements may serve as an indicator of the degree of cerebrovascular vasodilatation, as discussed further in the text to follow. CBV can be measured by PET with either trace amounts of ^{15}O-labeled carbon monoxide or ^{11}CO [53]. Both carbon monoxide tracers label the red blood cells. Blood volume is calculated using a correction factor for the difference between peripheral vessel and cerebral vessel hematocrit.

Mean transit time (MTT) is usually calculated as the ratio of CBV/CBF. By the central volume theorem, this ratio yields mean transit time, the hypothetical mean time for a particle to pass through the cerebral circulation. MTT is not measured directly with PET. Increased MTT is used as an indicator of autoregulatory vasodilation. Some PET groups have advocated the use of the inverse of this ratio instead [80].

Oxygen extraction fraction (OEF) is measured by an O15O inhalation scan and independent measurements of CBF and CBV [56]. The CBF accounts for the amount of oxygen delivered to the brain. The CBV corrects for oxygen in the blood that is not extracted. An alternative count based method uses the ratio of the counts after an O15O inhalation scan to the counts from an O15O water scan, without CBV correction [46], [19]. Other similar methods are also in common use [4].

Cerebral metabolic rate of oxygen (CMRO2) can be calculated from an equation using OEF, CBF and arterial oxygen content (CaO$_2$) [56], [4]. CMRO$_2$ is equal to the CBF multiplied by OEF and the CaO$_2$ (delivery of oxygen times the fraction extracted times the amount of available oxygen).

Glucose metabolism (CMRGlu) is most frequently measured using the glucose analog ^{18}F-fluorodeoxyglucose (FDG). CMRglu measurements are limited in pathological conditions such as ischemia, however, because the ratio of tissue uptake of glucose and its analog, DG, varies with the severity of ischemia. Glucose metabolism can be measured directly with 1-^{11}C–D-glucose [6], [67].

Molecular imaging studies in patients with cerebrovascular disease have used several different labeled substances [13], [15], including 11-C-labeled FK506 (tacrolimus) [58] copper-60, and a host of other labeled neurotransmitters [1]. Studies specific to atherosclerotic occlusive disease will be reviewed at the end of the Experimental Studies section below.

Normal cerebral hemodynamics and metabolism

Whole brain mean CBF of the adult human brain is approximately 50 mL per 100 g per minute. Functional activation increases local or regional CBF, but global CBF remains unchanged [70]. CBF for any brain region is determined by the ratio of cerebral perfusion pressure (CPP) and cerebral vascular resistance (CVR) in that region. Cerebral perfusion pressure is the difference between the arterial pressure forcing blood into the cerebral circulation and intracranial pressure or the pressure in the venous system. The venous pressure is negligible under normal conditions, so for people with carotid atherosclerotic disease the CPP is generally equal to the systemic arterial pressure (CPP = MAP).

Under normal conditions any change in regional CBF must be caused by a change in regional CVR. Vascular resistance is mediated by alterations in the diameter of small arteries or arterioles. In the resting brain with normal CPP, CBF is also closely matched to the metabolic rate of the tissue. Regions with higher metabolic rates have higher levels of cerebral blood flow. For example, gray matter has a higher CBF than white matter owing to the differences in oxygen metabolism. While there is wide variation in levels of flow and metabolism, the ratio between CBF and metabolism is nearly constant in all areas of the brain. Consequently, the maps of OEF and glucose extraction (not metabolism) from the blood show little regional variation [5]. One exception to this is seen with physiological activation, where blood flow increases well beyond the metabolic needs of the tissue. This leads to a relative decrease of OEF and a reduction in local venous deoxyhemoglobin [30]. This phenomenon is the basis for the use of MR imaging as a means to map brain function.

Responses to reductions in cerebral perfusion pressure

An arterial stenosis or occlusion may cause a reduction in perfusion pressure if collateral sources of flow are not adequate [65]. The mere presence of arterial stenosis or occlusion does not equate with hemodynamic impairment: up to 50% of patients with complete carotid artery occlusion and prior ischemic symptoms have normal no evidence of reduced CPP [37]. It is the adequacy of collateral sources of flow that largely determine whether an occlusive lesion will cause a reduction in perfusion pressure. When perfusion pressure falls owing to an arterial stenosis or occlusion, and in most cases, an inadequate circle of Willis, the brain and its vasculature can maintain the normal delivery of oxygen and glucose through two mechanisms, autoregulatory vasodilation and increased oxygen extraction fraction [21]. The presence of these mechanisms has been extensively studied, primarily in animal models employing acute reductions in perfusion pressure. The extent to which these models are applicable to humans with chronic regional reductions in perfusion pressure is not completely known.

Changes in perfusion pressure have little effect on CBF over a wide range of pressure owing to vascular autoregulation. Increases in mean arterial pressure produce vasoconstriction of the pial arterioles, serving to increase vascular resistance and maintain CBF at a constant level [29]. Conversely, when the pressure falls, reflex vasodilation will maintain CBF at near normal levels [28], [71]. Two measurable parameters that indicate autoregulatory vasodilation are mean transit time and cerebral blood volume (Fig. 1). In addition, there is some slight reduction in CBF through the autoregulatory range, leading to a slight increase in oxygen extraction [21], [79].

At some point, however, the capacity for autoregulatory vasodilation can be exceeded. The threshold value for autoregulatory failure is variable between patients and can be shifted higher or lower by prior ischemic injury or long standing hypertension. Beyond this point, cerebral blood flow falls linearly as a function of pressure (Fig. 1). Direct measurements of arteriovenous oxygen differences have demonstrated the brain's capacity to increase OEF and maintain normal cerebral oxygen metabolism (CMRO2) while the oxygen delivery diminishes due to decreasing CBF [54]. The precise mechanism by which OEF increases is not completely understood. Oxygen passively diffuses from the blood to the tissue. Increases in the gradient between capillary and tissue partial pressures of oxygen and longer transit times that may allow for greater oxygen diffusion may be involved.

PET assessment of hemodynamic status

As discussed above, the hemodynamic effect of an arterial stenosis or occlusion depends on the adequacy of collateral circulation as well as the degree of stenosis. An occluded carotid artery, for example, often has no measurable effect on the distal cerebral perfusion pressure because the collateral flow through the circle of Willis is adequate. Many imaging techniques, such as arteriography, magnetic resonance imaging (MR), computed tomography angiography, and Doppler ultrasound, can identify the presence of these collaterals. These tools show us the highways for blood flow, but not the traffic on them.

It is important to recognize that a single measurement of flow is meaningless when investigating the effects of an arterial lesion. Normal values of CBF

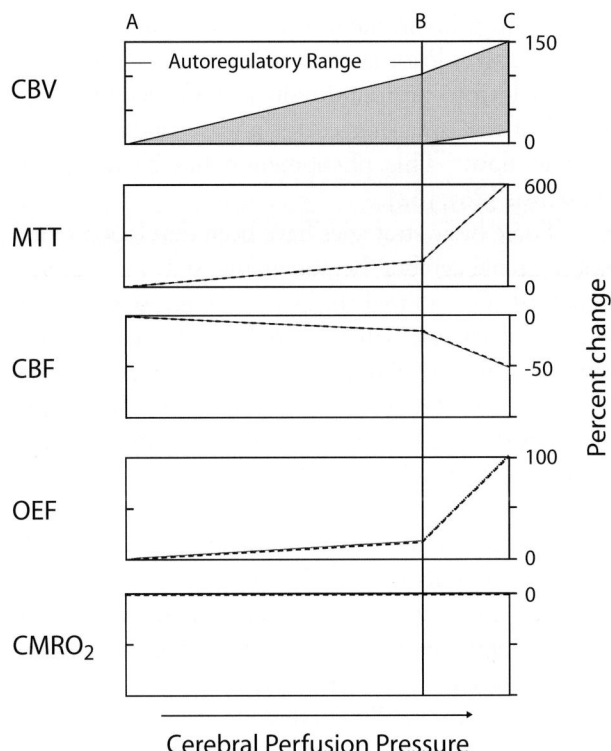

Fig. 1. Hemodynamic and metabolic responses to reductions in cerebral perfusion pressure modified after Powers [66] and Derdeyn et al [20]. Progressive reduction in perfusion pressue is shown from right to left on the x-axis. The autoregulatory range extends between points A and B. The region between points B and C is the region of autoregulatory failure where cerebral blood flow (CBF) begins to fall passively as a function of pressure. Point C represents the exhaustion of both compensatory mechanisms to maintain normal oxygen metabolism and the onset of true ischemia. CBV: Cerebral blood volume either remains unchanged or increases with autoreulatory vasodilation, depending largely on the methods used to measure CBV. With autoregulatory failure, most investigations have found further increases in CBV. CBF: Cerebral blood flow falls slightly through the autoregulatory range. Once autoregulatory capacity is exceeded, CBF falls passively as a function of pressure down to 50% of baseline values. OEF: Oxygen extraction fraction (OEF) increases slightly with the reductions in CBF through the autoregulatory range. After autoregulatory capacity is exceeded and flow falls up to 50% of baseline, OEF may increase up to 100% from baseline. CMRO2: The cerebral metabolic rate for oxygen consumption remains unchanged throughout this range of CPP reduction owing to both autoregulatory vasodilation and increased OEF.

do not exclude the presence of autoregulatory vasodilation and reduced CBF may be present with normal perfusion pressure. This second situation may occur with prior stroke in the region of interest or in a remote area. Prior lacunar stroke in the basal ganglia may lead to profound reduction in metabolic demand of the overlying cortex and secondary reduction in flow. This phenomenon has been termed diaschisis [26], [62].

Three basic strategies have been developed to assess regional cerebral hemodynamic status noninvasively [66]. The normal compensatory responses of the brain and its vasculature to reduced perfusion pressure, as outlined above, are assumed to be present. The first two strategies are used to indirectly identify the presence and degree of autoregulatory vasodilation. The third relies on direct measurements of oxygen extraction. It is important to note that these approaches are accurate only with normal or remotely infracted brain tissue [31].

The first strategy relies on paired blood flow measurements with the initial measurement obtained at rest and the second measurement obtained following a cerebral vasodilatory stimulus. Hypercapnia, acetazolamide, and physiologic tasks such as hand movement have been used as vasodilatory stimuli. Normally, each will result in a robust increase in CBF. If the CBF response is muted or absent, preexisting autoregulatory cerebral vasodilation due to reduced cerebral perfusion pressure is inferred. The blood flow or blood velocity responses to these vasodilatory stimuli have been categorized into several grades of hemodynamic impairment: (i) reduced augmentation (relative to the contralateral hemisphere or normal controls); (ii) absent augmentation (same value as baseline); and iii) paradoxical reduction in regional blood flow compared to baseline measurement. This final category, also called the "steal" phenomena, can only be identified with quantitative CBF techniques [51].

The second strategy uses either the measurement of regional cerebral blood volume (CBV), alone, or in combination with measurements of CBF in the resting brain in order to detect the presence of autoregulatory vasodilation. The CBV/CBF ratio (or, inversely, the CBF/CBV ratio), mathematically equivalent to the vascular mean transit time [66], may be more sensitive than CBV alone for the identification of autoregulatory vasodilation [79]. It may be less specific, however. The CBV/CBF ratio may increase in low flow conditions with normal perfusion pressure, such as hypocapnia [35]. Patients are identified as abnormal with these techniques based on comparison of absolute quantitative values or hemispheric ratios of quantitative values to the range observed in normal control subjects. One issue that remains unresolved is to what extent autoregulatory vasodilation of arterioles gives rise to measurable increases in the cerebral blood volume. Experimental data have produced conflicting results [34], [86]. Some studies have found minimal or no increase until autoregulatory capacity is exceeded [79], [96], while others have reported CBV increases within the autoregulatory range [34], [36], [27]. Thus, the sensitivity and specificity of CBV measurements for detecting reduced CPP is not known.

The third strategy relies on direct measurements of OEF to identify patients with increased oxygen extraction (Fig. 2). At present, regional measurements of OEF can be made only with PET using O-15 labeled radiotracers [56], [46], [3]. Both absolute values and side-to-side ratios of quantitative and relative OEF have been used for the determination of abnormal from normal [19].

Variability of CBV measurements in severe hemodynamic impairment

Measurements of CBV in patients with reduced CBF and increased OEF are often variable. Increased CBV is interpreted as evidence of autoregulatory vasodilation. Some patients, however, have normal or even reduced values of CBV in regions with increased OEF and reduced CBF. These patients appear to have a lower risk of stroke than those with increased CBV [21].

We reviewed data from 81 patients with symptomatic carotid occlusion enrolled in a prospective study of hemodynamic factors and stroke risk, the St. Louis Carotid Occlusion Study [37]. This was a blinded, prospective study designed to test the hypothesis that increased OEF predicts stroke risk. The results of the primary analysis of this study are presented below in the Clinical Studies section. Measurements of CBV, CBF, OEF and CMRO2 were

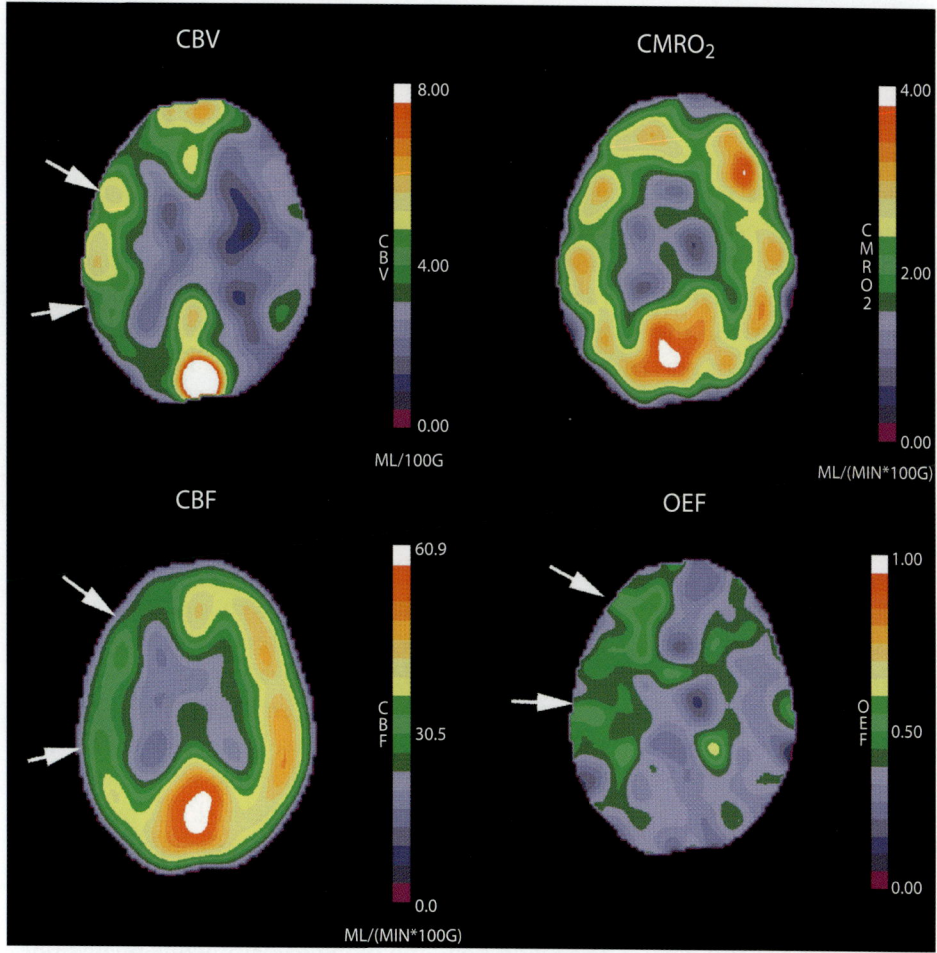

Fig. 2. PET study showing classic misery perfusion with increased OEF and preserved CMRO2. CBV is elevated. The PET examination was performed 2 days after a transient ischemic attack. CT examination was normal. The images show reduced blood flow (CBF, top left, arrows) and near normal oxygen metabolism (CMRO2, top middle) and increased OEF in the hemisphere distal to the occluded carotid. CBV and mean transit time (MTT) are elevated.

made on entry using PET. For the retrospective analysis of CBV variability, patients were divided into groups by hemispheric ratios and absolute ipsilateral values of OEF and CBV, based on comparison with normal controls [21]. Hemodynamic and metabolic values, risk factors, and stroke risk were compared between groups.

Based on hemispheric ratios, 45 patients had increased ipsilateral OEF; CBV was increased in 19 of these 45 patients. No differences in CBF, CMRO2, or clinical risk factors were found between these 19 patients and the remaining 26 patients with increased OEF and normal or reduced CBV. Thirteen ipsilateral strokes occurred during follow up, and 10 of the 13 occurred in the 19 patients with increased OEF and CBV (Log rank p < 0.0001). Thirty-two of the 68 patients with complete quantitative PET data had increased OEF by absolute ipsilateral values. CBV was increased in 20 of the 32 patients. No differences in CBF, CMRO2, or clinical risk factors were found between these 20 patients and the remaining 12 patients with increased OEF and normal CBV. Seven of the 9 ipsilateral strokes that occurred in the 68 patients occurred in the 20 patients with increased OEF and increased CBV (Log rank p = 0.003).

The higher risk of ischemic stroke in patients with increased OEF and CBV suggests that their degree of hemodynamic compromise is more severe than those with increased OEF and normal CBV. In patients with chronic carotid occlusion and increased OEF, increased CBV may indicate pronounced vasodilation due to exhausted autoregulatory vasodilation. The physiological explanation for the measurement of normal CBV in patients with increased OEF is less certain and may reflect preserved autoregulatory capacity.

Correlative studies between PET and other methods of hemodynamic assessment

Transcranial Doppler, MR and CT perfusion techniques, and SPECT are all capable of measuring relative, and in some situations, absolute cerebral blood flow [20]. These methods are often used to assess for impaired vasodilatory responses or increased mean transit time. Several of these methods have been compared to PET measurements of OEF. The correlation is inconsistent. A significant relationship between impaired vasodilatory responses and increased OEF is frequently found, but for any given patient, the sensitivity and specificity of an impaired vasodilatory response is not strong. Given this discordance, it is imperative to prove that an abnormal hemodynamic response by any particular method is clinically meaningful: that it predicts stroke risk, for example.

The results of paired-flow studies with vasodilatory stimuli in any given patient may differ. The effects of acetazolamide on blood flow are different from hypercapnia or physiologic activation. Inao and colleagues a discordance between results with acetazolamide and neural activation [45]. They found that CBF increased bilaterally with bimanual activation, but only contralaterally with acetazolamide. The exact mechanism by which acetazolamide causes an increase in flow is unknown. The evidence points to local, rather than systemic, effects on the cerebrovasculature [41]. Possible local mechanisms include direct vasodilatory actions or secondary local metabolic changes due to carbonic anhydrase inhibition [41]. The effect of acetazolamide can vary in response to the total dose, the timing of CBF measurement after the dose, and the age and sex of the patient [41], [11]. One possible explanation for the discordant results seen with acetazolamide and other vasodilatory stimuli was put forward by Inao et al. [45]. They suggested that regions with reduced baseline flow receive a lower dose of acetazolamide than regions with normal blood flow. The lower acetazolamide dose will result in a greater likelihood that a reduced or absent blood flow response will be seen with acetazolamide in these regions compared to hypercapnia alone, which produces a uniform stimulus throughout the brain.

An additional factor which may contribute to the discordance observed between acetazolamide and CO_2 or activation studies is the use of non-radioactive xenon as a blood flow tracer. The inhalation of xenon gas causes increases in blood flow [39]. The steal phenomena with acetazolamide is reported with much greater frequency with stable xenon blood flow methods than with O-15 labeled PET radiotracers [11]. It is possible that the pre-existing vasodilation due to xenon augments the dose-dependent effects of acetazolamide. Finally, absolute blood flow, relative blood flow, and blood velocity, while related phenomena, are not equivalent. Dahl and coworkers found no relationship between the increase in velocity (by TCD) and the increase in blood flow (by Xe-CT) after acetazolamide [43].

The correlation between methods that evaluate vasodilatory response or mean transit time and increased OEF by PET in patients with cerebrovascular disease has been inconsistent. One issue that remains unclear is to what extent maximal autoregulatory vasodilation persists when oxygen extraction fraction is elevated, particularly in humans with chronic reductions in perfusion pressure. As discussed above, many patients with increased OEF do not have increased CBV or MTT. Whether this later finding represents a variable vasodilatory capacity or some form of long-term compensatory response remains to be determined. Therefore, both the independence of the mechanisms of autoregulatory vasodilation and oxygen extraction and the changes occurring over time may be sources of difficulty in comparing the results of vasodilatory and oxygen extraction methods.

Several studies have investigated the relationship between acetazolamide reactivity and OEF. The most consistent results were published by Hirano et al. [44], who reported that all seven patients with acetazolamide responses below the normal range also had OEF values above normal. Some patients with increased OEF had normal acetazolamide responses, however. A sensitivity of 45% and a specificity of 98% of the steal phenomena after acetazolamide for increased OEF was reported by the same investigators [40], [93]. Similar data were reported by Narai and colleagues [59]. Other investigators have reported no significant relationship between changes in blood flow after acetazolamide and quantitative values of OEF [42].

Most recently, Yamauchi and colleagues examined 30 patients with symptomatic carotid occlusive disease with PET measurements of CBF before and after acetazolamide and compared this to OEF [92]. The baseline OEF value was inversely and non-linearly correlated with the percentage change in CBF during acetazolamide administration (p = 0.02). They reported an upward trend of OEF with diminishing acetazolamide response below a critical level around zero response. An post acetazolamide CBF response of less than 6.65% over baseline had a sensitivity 100%, specificity 89%, positive predictive value 50%, negative predictive value 100% for OEF beyond the normal range.

Two comparative studies of CO_2 reactivity and OEF found linear relationships between the change in quantitative flow after CO_2 and the absolute value of quantitative OEF [43], [47]. In both studies, however, a threshold value CO_2 reactivity which included all patients with increased OEF would also included many patients with normal OEF (low specificity). Sugimori and coworkers found no relationship between blood velocity changes after CO_2 and OEF [83].

The data for the correlation between the CBV/CBF or CBF/CBV ratios and OEF is variable. Two investigators found linear relationships [43], [33]. Two other studies found no correlation when all patients were included in the analysis [42], [64].

Borderzone hemodynamics

Acute reductions in perfusion pressure can cause ischemic infarction of the cortex and adjacent subcortical white matter located at the borderzones between major cerebral arterial territories, such as the middle and anterior cerebral arteries [2], [9]. Severe systemic hypotension is a well-recognized cause of multiple bilateral discrete cortical borderzone infarctions(70). The mechanism of cortical borderzone infarction in most patients with carotid atherosclerotic disease is likely embolic [15], [16], [87], [88].

In addition to this cortical arterial borderzone, there is good evidence for an arterial borderzone is present within the white matter of the centrum semi-ovale and corona radiata [97], [89]. This has been called the internal arterial borderzone (between lenticulostriate perforators and deep penetrating branches of the distal middle cerebral artery). There is a strong association between hemodynamic impairment of the hemisphere and prior stroke in the white matter borderzone [16].

We studied 110 patients with atherosclerotic carotid occlusion with PET measurements of CBF, CBV, and OEF [16]. MR and CT studies of all patients were reviewed. No borderzone-region infarctions were found in 35 asymptomatic patients. For 75 symptomatic patients, cortical borderzone-region infarction was found in 7 of 36 patients with increased OEF and in 2 of 39 patients with normal OEF (p = 0.08, ns). The pattern of multiple white matter lesions arranged parallel to the lateral ventricle was only observed in symptomatic patients with increased OEF (8 of 36, p = 0.002, sensitivity = 19%, specificity = 100%). This finding was more frequent with MR imaging (7 of 14) than with CT (1 of 22). We concluded that this pattern of infarction is likely due to a hemodynamic mechanism.

In study involving many of the same patients, we examined the structurally normal white matter regions for evidence of selective ongoing hemodynamic abnormalities [17]. Thirty-six patients with carotid occlusion and structurally normal deep white matter were studied with positron emission tomography (PET). Measurements of oxygen extraction fraction (OEF) were made in superficial (cortical and sub-cortical) regions in the middle cerebral artery territory and in deep white matter (internal borderzone) regions. The presence of selective ischemia of the deep white matter was assessed by the ratio of deep white matter to superficial OEF. Ipsilateral hemispheric ratios in patients were assessed as a group against contralateral hemispheric ratios and 15 normal controls. We found no difference in the degree of OEF elevation in the white matter compared to the overlying cortex. These findings suggest that these white matter infarctions may occur at the time of occlusion or soon after (when some selective increase in OEF is present) and not in the chronic situation. There is no good prospective data to support or refute this hypothesis, however.

Improvement in hemodynamics over time

In some patients with atherosclerotic carotid occlusion, hemodynamic impairment can improve over time, as collateral flow increases [18]. We repeated PET measurements in ten patients with complete atherosclerotic carotid artery occlusion with increased OEF by PET and no interval stroke 12 to 59 months after the initial examination. Quantitative regional measurements of CBF, CBV, CMRO2, and OEF were obtained. Regional measurements of the cerebral rate of glucose metabolism (CMRGlc) were also made on follow-up in 5 patients. As a group, the ratio of ipsilateral to contralateral OEF declined from a mean of 1.16 to 1.08 (p = 0.022). Greater reductions were seen with longer duration of follow-up (p = 0.023, r = 0.707). The cerebral blood flow ratio improved from 0.81 to 0.85 (p= 0.021). No change in cerebral blood volume or CMRO2 was observed. CMRGlc was reduced in the ipsilateral hemisphere (p = 0.001 compared with normal), but the CMRO2/CMRGlc ratio was normal.

This improvement in collateral sources of flow over time may be a factor that accounts for the reduction in stroke risk over time in all the major cerebral revascularization trials. The greatest risk for stroke in medically treated patients in the North American Symptomatic Carotid Stenosis Trial, the EC/IC bypass trial, the Warfarin versus Aspirin for Symptomatic Intracranial study, the European Carotid Stenosis Trial, as well as the St. Louis Carotid Occlusion Study was in the first two years after stroke (Fig. 3) [60], [84], [24], [10].

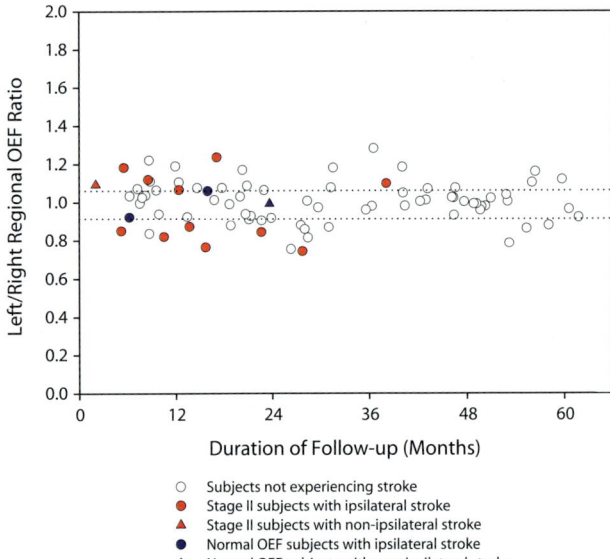

Fig. 3. Most strokes in patients with atherosclerotic carotid occlusion occurred during the first two years after enrollment. This may reflect interval improvement in hemodynamics. The circles indicate patients with increased OEF (left to right hemispheric ratios of OEF beyond the normal range (dotted lines from the y-axis). The red circles indicate patients suffering a stroke during follow up. The length of follow up is indicated on the x-axis.

Metabolic down-regulation

There are other possible mechanisms for the phenomenon of normal CBV in patients with increased OEF discussed above. One potential cause for normal or reduced CBV values is reduced metabolic demand. CBV falls when the metabolic activity of the tissue falls, due to either local or remote neuronal injury (diaschisis) [80], [6], [90]. In the study presented above, however, we found no significant difference in CMRO2 between patients with increased OEF and increased CBV and those with normal or reduced CBV.

Sette and colleagues noted the phenomenon of increased OEF associated with normal CBV and proposed a metabolically-mediated vasconstriction, associated with the vascular collapse that may occur with severe reductions in perfusion pressure, to account for their observations [80]. Based on CBF/CBV ratios, they considered these patients to have greater reductions in perfusion pressure than those with increased OEF and increased CBV. They studied 4 patients with carotid occlusion and found regions with reduced absolute ipsilateral values of CBF, increased OEF, and normal CBV. CMRO2 was slightly reduced in these areas as well. Importantly, the outcome data from our study suggests that patients with increased OEF and normal CBV have less severe hemodynamic impairment than those with increased OEF and increased CBV. If the normal CBV values in patients with increased OEF were caused by reductions in the diameter of previously dilated vessels, secondary to severe reductions in intraluminal pressure, one would expect a higher risk of stroke in the patients with increased OEF and normal CBV than those with increased OEF and increased CBV. In our data, patients with increased OEF and increased CBV had a higher risk of stroke, suggesting the degree of hemodynamic impairment is more, not less, severe in these patients.

Bilateral hemispheric reductions in absolute CMRO2 have been found in patients with unilateral carotid occlusion [33], [76]. Gibbs et al., reported hemodynamic and metabolic data for 32 patients with unilateral and bilateral carotid occlusions [33]. They grouped their data by anatomy – contralateral hemisphere and ipsilateral hemisphere for unilateral occlusions, and both hemispheres for bilateral occlusions. Absolute hemispheric values of CMRO2 were significantly lower than normal control values in all three groups. No difference between the three groups was seen, however. Additionally, improvement in CBF and CMRO2 in both hemispheres has been reported after EC/IC bypass or with increased mean arterial pressure in selected patients [76], [77]. The nature of this phenomenon remains unclear.

The phenomenon of reversible metabolic down-regulation due to long-standing hemodynamic impairment and a clinical correlate to improved cognitive function after revascularization are two unproven but attractive hypotheses [80], [78].

CMRO2 is frequently reduced patients with severe hemodynamic impairment. Whether this is a reversible compensation to reduced CBF or reflects underlying ischemic injury is unknown. Prospective randomized studies before and after revascularization will be required.

Molecular imaging studies of carotid atherosclerosis

As discussed above, there is more to carotid atherosclerosis than just vessel narrowing and limitation of flow. Growing evidence points to synergistic effects of embolic and hemodynamic factors [37], [67]. Patients with recent transient ischemic attack, stroke, or silent emboli in the middle cerebral artery by transcranial Doppler are at much higher risk for subsequent stroke than asymptomatic patients with identical degrees of carotid stenosis [57]. Molecular imaging techniques have great promise in the investigation of the biology of atherosclerosis and in identifying factors associated with the formation of thrombo-emboli [13].

The pathology of atherosclerosis is well described. Lipids and macrophages accumulate on the endothelium, initially as a fatty streak. Over time, a plaque develops with a central lipid core and a fibrous cap. The fibrous cap has an endothelial covering and contains vascular smooth muscle cells and collagen. In carotid disease, this plaque may expand to cause severe stenosis or occlusion. As discussed above, this limits flow only if collateral sources are not adequate. In addition, as there is no global increase in flow with neuronal activation, there is no angina-equivalent in the brain: you don't get a headache from thinking.

Thrombo-embolic phenomenon occurs when the fibrous cap ruptures. This exposes subendothelial structures that are very thrombogenic [32]. Circulating clotting factors VII and XI are activated through extrinsic and intrinsic pathways. Thrombin, fibrinogen and fibrin are generated. Platelet activation occurs via upregulation of glycoprotein IIb/IIIa receptors. The ultimate product of these events is thrombus formation.

Plaque formation and rupture is a consequence of multiple complex and inter-related factors. These factors include endothelial cell function (impaired in atherosclerotic disease, even in the absence of plaque) and inflammation. Atherosclerotic risk factors, smoking, elevated low-density lipoprotein (LDL) levels, and hypertension, are associated with impaired endothelial responses to hypoxia. This endothelial dysfunction likely predisposes to the accumulation of foam cells in the subendothelial layer. The vascular smooth muscle cells that migrate from the media create the collagen that forms the fibrous cap. The foam cells often die and leave behind the lipid that forms the core of the plaque. Lesions with a thin fibrous cap have a higher risk for future rupture [12]. Inflammation likely plays a role in this process [12], [52].

Much of the molecular imaging studies to date have utilized single-photon emission computed tomography (SPECT) tracers in animal models of atherosclerosis and will not be reviewed here. These labels have been aimed at the plaque itself, including LDL, endothelial peptides, and receptor site antibodies for macrophages, and at adherent thrombus, using labeled platelets, fibrin and other related molecules.

The only studies to date using PET radiotracers have employed 18F-Fluouro deoxyglucose (FDG). FDG is taken up by metabolically active cells as a glucose analog, but cannot be metabolized. Uptake is particularly high in anaerobic cells, such as most tumors and macrophages [49]. Yun and colleagues observed vascular FDG uptake in approximately 50% of 137 consecutive cancer patients undergoing PET [95]. This uptake was associated with risk factors for atherosclerosis [94]. Age and hypercholesterolemia had the strongest associations. Rudd et al., studied 8 patients with symptomatic carotid atherosclerosis with CT/PET image fusion [75]. They found uptake of FDG within the plaque in all patients. They also performed autoradiography of the removed plaques from 3 patients that underwent endarterectomy. Tritiated deoxyglucose (an analogue of FDG) accumulation was localized to macrophage-rich areas of the plaque.

Molecular imaging studies of stroke

The potential utility of this application of PET imaging is to confirm or exclude a cerebral ischemic event in a patient with a clinical history that is not definitive. The presence or absence of ischemic symptoms is a critical distinction in determining therapy for many patients with atherosclerotic disease, particularly women [74]. In some patients, it may not be clear from history or structural brain imaging if an ischemic event occurred in association with carotid disease.

DeReuck and colleagues have extensively investigated the use of Cobalt-55 as a label for recent (within two months) irreversible brain ischemia [15], [14] Cobalt-55 is a calcium analogue and may reflect calcium influx in ischemic tissue [82]. The degree of uptake appears to correlate with the severity of the ischemic damage within the first 2 months after stroke and then returns to normal levels [15].

Clinical studies

There is presently no proven indication for PET in patients with atherosclerotic carotid disease, other than as a predictor for future stroke risk [19], [37], [91]. A clinical trial of extracranial to intracranial bypass based on PET screening of patients with symptomatic carotid occlusion and hemodynamic failure – the carotid occlusion surgery study (COSS) - is underway [38]. If this trial shows that surgery is beneficial in this population, we will have proof of therapeutic efficacy for this application of PET. In this section we will review the current literature associating PET measurements of hemodynamics with the risk of future stroke.

Patients with complete atherosclerotic occlusion of the carotid artery are at high risk for future stroke [48]. A randomized trial of extracranial to intracranial arterial bypass (the EC/IC Bypass Trial) failed to show a benefit of surgical revascularization in over 800 patients randomized to surgery or aspirin [84]. One possible reason for the failure of this study to show a benefit was the lack of an effective tool to establish whether flow was normal or impaired. A

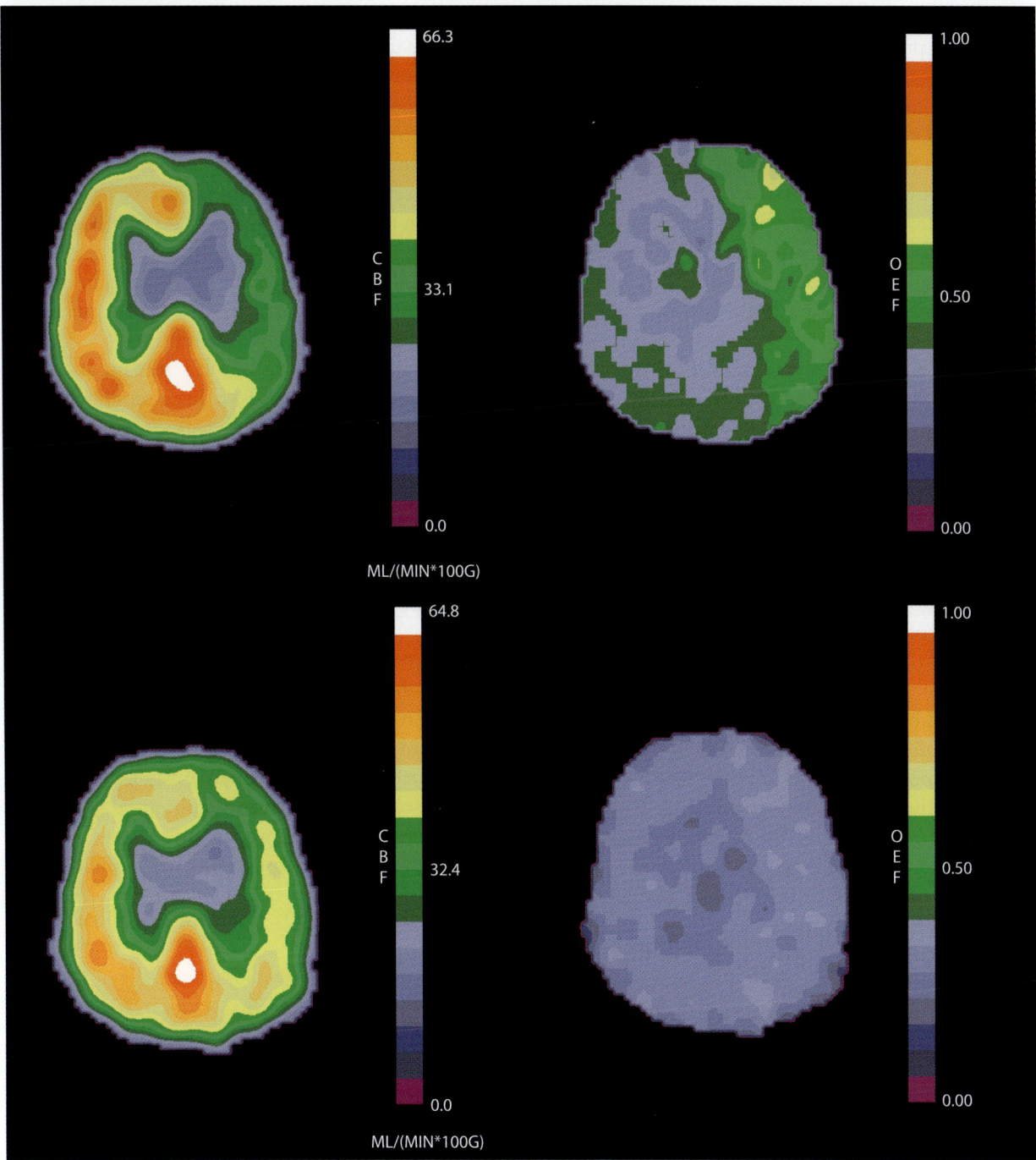

Fig. 4. Reversal of increased OEF after extracranial to intracranial arterial bypass. The top row shows reduced CBF and increased OEF in the hemisphere distal to an occluded carotid artery. The bottom row was performed within 7 days after extracranial to intracranial arterial bypass. The OEF abnormality has normalized. Some persistent reduction in CBF is present, likely due to permanent ischemic injury.

procedure intended to improve flow if flow is normal is unlikely to provide any benefit. It is possible that a benefit of bypass was missed for a subgroup at high risk due to hemodynamic factors.

The St. Louis Carotid Occlusion Study was designed to determine if such a subgroup existed [37]. This was a blinded, prospective study of stroke risk designed to test the hypothesis that increased OEF in patients with symptomatic atherosclerotic carotid occlusion predicted future stroke risk. All together, 81 patients with complete carotid occlusion and ipsilateral ischemic symptoms were enrolled. At baseline, 17 clinical, epidemiologic, and laboratory stroke risk factors were recorded. PET measurements of oxygen extraction were obtained. Thirty-nine of the 81 patients had increased OEF. All 81 patients were followed for a mean duration of 3.1 years. Fifteen total and thirteen ipsilateral ischemic strokes occurred during this period. Eleven of the 13 ipsilateral strokes occurred in the 39 patients with increased OEF. Multivariate analysis found only age and OEF as predictors of stroke risk. Log rank analysis demonstrated increased OEF to be a powerful predictor of subsequent stroke ($p = 0.004$). Similar results were reported by Yamauichi and coworkers [91].

Prior studies with PET have shown that the superficial temporal artery to middle cerebral artery bypass procedure is capable of reversing the OEF abnormality [63], [3] (Fig. 4). Based on these facts, the Carotid Occlusion Surgery Study was funded by the National Institutes of Health and is underway. Patients with complete atherosclerotic carotid artery occlusion and recent (120 days) ipsilateral cerebral ischemic symptoms are eligible for enrollment. PET studies are obtained on enrollment. Patients with increased OEF are randomized to surgery or best medical therapy.

Future applications

PET remains a unique research tool, capable of quantitative and accurate in vivo measurements of physiological processes in humans. The O-15 radiotracers necessary for the measurement of CBF, OEF and CMRO2 will remain limited to academic centers with on-site cyclotrons. These methods will continue to be used to define human cerebrovascular disease and responses to treatment, but will not become widely used in community practice. PET molecular imaging methods, on the other hand, have much greater potential for wide usage. Dedicated CT/PET scanners for oncological FDG imaging are in common use. If some PET method of plaque imaging is proven as a predictor of stroke risk and future clinical trials demonstrate improvement in patient outcome with this approach, this PET application could become a routine clinical study.

Research applications of PET remain abundant. Most of these applications have been described in the chapter above. Brain hemodynamic and metabolic imaging and molecular plaque imaging both have great promise for defining high-risk or low risk subgroups of patients with carotid atherosclerotic disease.

Summary

The determination of the hemodynamic status of the brain has proven prognostic value in patients with atherosclerotic carotid occlusion. A clinical trial is underway to determine if this information has therapeutic value. PET remains, at this point, a unique research tool with great potential to investigate the embolic and hemodynamic factors involved in stroke pathogenesis in patients with atherosclerotic carotid disease.

Support: NINDS RO1 NS39864, P01 NS35966, R01 NS39526

References

[1] Abe K, Kashiwagi Y, Tokumura M et al.: Discrepancy between cell injury and benzodiazepine receptor binding after transient middle cerebral artery occlusion in rats. Synapse 53: 234–239 (2004).

[2] Adams J, Brierley J, Connor R, Treip C: The effects of systemic hypotension upon the human brain. Clinical and neuropathological observations in 11 cases. Brain 89: 235–268 (1966).

[3] Baron JC, Bousser MG, Rey A et al.: Reversal of focal "misery perfusion syndrome" by extra-intracranial artery bypass in hemodynamic cerebral ischemia. A case

study with 0-15 positron emission tomography. Stroke 12: 454–459 (1981).
[4] Baron JC, Steinling M, Tanaka T et al.: Quantitative measurement of CBF, oxygen extraction fraction (OEF) and CMRO2 with the O-15 continuous inhalation technique positron emission tomography (PET): experimental evidence and normal values in man. J Cereb Blood Flow and Metab 1: S5–S6 (1981).
[5] Baron JC, Rougemont D, Soussaline F et al.: Local interrelationships of cerebral oxygen consumption and glucose utilization in normal subjects and in ischemic stroke patients: a positron tomography study. J Cereb Blood Flow Metab 4: 140–149 (1984).
[6] Baron JC, Frackowiak RSJ, Herholz K et al.: Use of PET methods for measurement of cerebral energy metabolism and hemodynamics in cerebrovascular disease. J Cereb Blood Flow Metab 9: 723–742 (1989).
[7] Bogousslavsky J, Hachinski VC, Boughner DR et al.: Cardiac and arterial lesions in transient ischemic attacks. Arch Neurol 43: 223–228 (1986).
[8] Bozzao L, Fantozzi LM, Bastianello S et al.: Ischaemic supratentorial stroke: angiographic findings in patients examined in the very early phase. J Neurol 236: 340–342 (1989).
[9] Brierley JB, Excell BJ: The effects of profound systemic hypotension upon the brain of M. Rhesus: Physiological and pathological observations. Brain 89: 269–298 (1986).
[10] Chimowitz MI, Lynn MJ, Howlett-Smith H et al.: Comparison of warfarin and aspirin for symptomatic intracranial arterial stenosis. N Engl J Med 352: 1305–1316 (2005).
[11] Dahl AL, Russell D, Nyberg-Hansen R et al.: Simultaneous assessment of vasoreactivity using transcranial Doppler ultrasound and cerebral blood flow in healthy subjects. J Cereb Blood Flow Metab 14: 974–981 (1994).
[12] Davies MJ: Stability and instability: two faces of coronary atherosclerosis-The Paul Dudley White Lecture 1995. Circulation 94: 2013–2020 (1996).
[13] Davies JR, Rudd JH, Weissberg PL: Molecular and metabolic imaging of atherosclerosis. J Nucl Med 45: 1898–1907 (2004).
[14] De Reuck J, Vonck K, Santens P et al.: Cobalt-55 positron emission tomography in late-onset epileptic seizures after thrombo-embolic middle cerebral artery infarction. J Neurol Sci 181: 13–18 (2000).
[15] De Reuck J, Paemeleire K, Santens P et al.: Cobalt-55 positron emission tomography in symptomatic atherosclerotic carotid artery disease: borderzone versus territorial infarcts. Clin Neurol Neurosurg 106: 77–81 (2004).
[16] Derdeyn CP, Khosla A, Videen TO et al.: Severe hemodynamic impairment and border zone–region infarction. Radiology 220: 195–201 (2001).
[17] Derdeyn CP, Simmons NR, Videen TO et al.: Absence of selective deep white matter ischemia in chronic carotid disease: a positron emission tomographic study of regional oxygen extraction. AJNR 21: 631–638 (2000).
[18] Derdeyn CP, Videen TO, Fritsch SM et al.: Compensatory mechanisms for chronic cerebral hypoperfusion in patients with carotid occlusion. Stroke 30: 1019–1024 (1999).
[19] Derdeyn CP, Videen TO, Simmons NR et al.: Count-based PET method for predicting ischemic stroke in patients with symptomatic carotid arterial occlusion. Radiology 212: 499–506 (1999).
[20] Derdeyn CP, Grubb RL Jr., Powers WJ.: Cerebral hemodynamic impairment: methods of measurement and association with stroke risk. Neurology 53: 251–259 (1999).
[21] Derdeyn CP, Videen TO, Yundt KD et al.: Variability of cerebral blood volume and oxygen extraction: stages of cerebral haemodynamic impairment revisited. Brain 125: 595–607 (2002).
[22] Derdeyn CP.: Conventional angiography remains an important tool for measurement of carotid arterial stenosis. Radiology 235: 711–712; author reply 712–713 (2005).
[23] De Reuck JL: Pathophysiology of carotid artery disease and related clinical syndromes. Acta Chir Belg 104: 30–34 (2004).
[24] European Carotid Surgery Trialists' Collaborative Group.: MRC European Carotid Surgery Trial: interim results for symptomatic patients with severe (70–99%) or with mild (0–29%) carotid stenosis. Lancet 337: 1235–1243 (1991).
[25] Executive Committee of the Asymptomatic Carotid Atherosclerosis Study.: Endarterectomy for asymptomatic carotid artery stenosis. JAMA 273: 1421–1428 (1995).
[26] Feeney DM, Baron JC: Diaschisis. Stroke 17: 817–830 (1986).
[27] Ferrari M, Wilson DA, Hanley DF et al.: Effects of graded hypotension on cerebral blood flow, blood volume, and mean transit time in dogs. Am J Physiol 262: H1908–H1914 (1992).
[28] Fog M. Cerebral circulation.: The reaction of the pial arteries to a fall in blood pressure. Arch Neurol and Psychiatry 24: 351–364 (1937).
[29] Forbes HS.: The cerebral circulation, I: observation and measurement of pial vessels. Arch Neurol Psych 19: 751–761 (1928).
[30] Fox PT, Raichle ME.: Focal physiological uncoupling of cerebral blood flow and oxidative metabolism during somatosensory stimulation in human subjects. Proc Natl Acad Sci USA 83: 1140–1144 (1986).
[31] Frackowiak RS: The pathophysiology of human cerebral ischaemia: a new perspective obtained with positron tomography. Q J Med 57: 713–727 (1985).
[32] Fuster V, Fallon JT, Nemerson Y.: Coronary thrombosis. Lancet 348: S7–S10 (1996).

[33] Gibbs JM, Wise RJS, Leendeers KL, Jones T.: Evaluation of cerebral perfusion reserve in patients with carotid artery occlusion. Lancet 1: 310–314 (1984).
[34] Grubb RL Jr, Phelps ME, Raichle ME et al.: The effects of arterial blood pressure on the regional cerebral blood volume by X-ray fluorescence. Stroke 4: 390–399 (1973).
[35] Grubb RL, Jr., Raichle ME, Eichling JO et al.: The effects of changes in PaCO2 on cerebral blood volume, blood flow, and vascular mean transit time. Stroke 5: 630–639 (1974).
[36] Grubb RL, Jr., Raichle ME, Phelps ME, Ratcheson RA: Effects of increased intracranial pressure on cerebral blood volume, blood flow, and oxygen utilization in monkeys. J Neurosurg 43: 385–398 (1975).
[37] Grubb RL, Jr., Derdeyn CP, Fritsch SM et al.: Importance of hemodynamic factors in the prognosis of symptomatic carotid occlusion. JAMA 280: 1055–1060 (1978).
[38] Grubb RL, Jr., Powers WJ, Derdeyn CP et al.: The carotid occlusion surgery study. Neurosurg Focus 14: e9 (2003).
[39] Hartmann A, Dettmers C, Schuier FJ et al.: Effect of stable Xenon on regional cerebral blood flow and the electroencephalogram in normal volunteers. Stroke 22: 182–189 (1991).
[40] Hasegawa Y, Minematsu K, Matsuoka H et al.: CBF responses to acetazolamide and CO2 for the prediction of hemodynamic failure: a PET study [abstract]. Stroke 28: 242 (1997).
[41] Hauge A, Nicolaysen G, Thoresen M: Acute effects of acetazolamide on cerebral blood flow in man. Acta Physiol Scand 117: 233–239 (1983).
[42] Hayashida K, Hirose Y, Tanaka Y et al.: Stratification of severity by cerebral blood flow, oxygen metabolism and acetazolamide reactivity in patients with cerebrovascular disease. In: Ishii Y, ed. Recent Advances in Biomedical Imaging: Elsevier Science BV, (1997).
[43] Herold S, Brown MM, Frackowiak RSJ, Mansfield AO, Thomas DJ, Marshall J: Assessment of cerebral haemodynamic reserve: correlation between PET and CO2 reactivity measured by the intravenous 133 xenon injection technique. J Neurol Neurosurg Psychiatry 51: 1045–1050 (1988).
[44] Hirano T, Minematsu K, Hasegawa Y et al.: Acetazolamide reactivity on I-IMP single photon emission computed tomography in patients with major cerebral artery occlusive disease: correlation with positron emission tomography parameters. J Cereb Blood Flow Metab 14: 763–770 (1994).
[45] Inao S, Tadokoro M, Nishino M et al.: Neural activation of the brain with hemodynamic insufficiency. J Cereb Blood Flow and Metab 18: 960–967 (1998).
[46] Jones T, Chesler DA, Ter-Pogossian MM: The continuous inhalation of Oxygen-15 for assessing regional oxygen extraction in the brain of man. Brit J Radiol 49: 339–343 (1976).
[47] Kanno I, Uemura K, Higano S et al.: Oxygen extraction fraction at maximally vasodilated tissue in ischemic brain estimated from regional CO2 responsiveness measured by positron emission tomography. J Cereb Blood Flow Metab 8: 227–235 (1988).
[48] Klijn CJM, Kappelle LJ, Tulleken CAF et al.: Symptomatic carotid artery occlusion: a reappraisal of hemodynamic factors. Stroke 28: 2084–2093 (1997).
[49] Kubota R, Kubota K, Yamada S et al.: Micro-autoradiographic study for the differentiation of intratumoral macrophages, granulation tissues and cancer cells by the dynamics of fluorine-18-fluorodeoxyglucose uptake. J Nucl Med 35: 104–112 (1994).
[50] Lammertsma AA, Wise RJS, Heather JD et al.: Correction for the presence of intravascular Oxygen-15 in the steady-state technique for measuring regional oxygen extraction ratio in the brain: 2. Results in normal subjects and brain tumour and stroke patients. J Cereb Blood Flow Metab 3: 425–431 (1983).
[51] Lassen NA, Palvolgyi R: Cerebral steal during hypercapnia and the inverse reaction during hypocapnia observed with the 133xenon technique in man (abstract). Scand J Clin Lab Invest 22(102): 13D (1968).
[52] Libby P: Molecular bases of the acute coronary syndromes. Circulation 91: 2844–2850 (1995).
[53] Martin WRW, Powers WJ, ME R: Cerebral blood volume measured with inhaled C15O and positron emission tomography. I Cereb Blood Flow and Metab 7: 421–426 (1987).
[54] McHenry LC Jr, Fazekas JF, Sullivan JF.: Cerebral hemodynamics of syncope. Am J Med Sci 80: 173–178 (1961).
[55] Mead GE, Murray H, Farrell A et al.: Pilot study of carotid surgery for acute stroke. Br J Surg 84: 990–992 (1997).
[56] Mintun MA, Raichle ME, Martin WRW et al.: Brain oxygen utilization measured with O-15 radiotracers and positron emission tomography. J Nuc Med 25: 177–187 (1984).
[57] Molloy J, Markus HS: Asymptomatic embolization predicts stroke and TIA risk in patients with carotid artery stenosis. Stroke 30: 1440–1443 (1999).
[58] Murakami Y, Takamatsu H, Noda A et al.: Pharmacokinetic animal PET study of FK506 as a potent neuroprotective agent. J Nucl Med 45: 1946–1949 (2004).
[59] Nariai T, Suzuki R, Hirakawa K et al.: Vascular reserve in chronic cerebral ischemia measured by the acetazolamide challenge test: comparison with psotiron emission tomography. AJNR 16: 563–570 (2005).
[60] North American Symptomatic Carotid Endarterectomy Trial (NASCET) Collaborators. Beneficial effect of carotid endarterectomy in symptomatic patients with

high-grade carotid stenosis. N Engl J Med 325: 445–453 (1991).

[61] Omae T, Mayzel-Oreg O, Li F et al.: Inapparent hemodynamic insufficiency exacerbates ischemic damage in a rat microembolic stroke model. Stroke 31: 2494–2499 (2000).

[62] Pantano P, Baron JC, Samson Y et al.: Crossed cerebrellar diaschisis. Further studies. Brain 109: 677–694 (1986).

[63] Powers WJ, Martin WR, Herscovitch P et al.: Extracranial-intracranial bypass surgery: hemodynamic and metabolic effects. Neurology 34: 1168–1174 (1984).

[64] Powers WJ, Raichle ME, Grubb RL Jr.: Positron Emission Tomography to assess cerebral perfusion [letter]. Lancet 1: 102–103 (1985).

[65] Powers WJ, Tempel LW, Grubb RL Jr et al.: Clinical correlates of cerebral hemodynamics. Stroke 18: 284 (1987).

[66] Powers WJ: Cerebral hemodynamics in ischemic cerebrovascular disease. Ann Neurol 29: 231–240 (1991).

[67] Powers WJ, Dagogo-Jack S, Markham J et al.: Cerebral transport and metabolism of 1-11C-D-glucose during stepped hypoglycemia. Ann Neurol 38: 599–609 (1995).

[68] Powers WJ, Derdeyn CP, Fritsch SM et al.: Benign prognosis of never-symptomatic carotid occlusion. Neurology 54: 878–882 (2000).

[69] Raichle ME, Martin WR, Herscovitch P et al.: Brain blood flow measured with intravenous H2(15)O. II. Implementation and validation. J Nucl Med 24: 790–798 (1983).

[70] Raichle ME.: Behind the scenes of functional brain imaging: a historical and physiological perspective. PNAS 95: 765–772 (1998).

[71] Rapela CE, Green HD: Autoregulation of canine cerebral blood flow. Circ Res 15: I205–I211 (1964).

[72] Rothwell PM, Warlow CP: Low risk of ischemic stroke in patients with reduced internal carotid artery lumen diameter distal to severe symptomatic carotid stenosis: cerebral protection due to low poststenotic flow? On behalf of the European Carotid Surgery Trialists' Collaborative Group. Stroke 31: 622–630 (2000).

[73] Rothwell PM, Eliasziw M, Gutnikov SA et al.: Analysis of pooled data from the randomised controlled trials of endarterectomy for symptomatic carotid stenosis. Lancet 361: 107–116 (2003).

[74] Rothwell PM, Goldstein LB: Carotid endarterectomy for asymptomatic carotid stenosis: asymptomatic carotid surgery trial. Stroke 35: 2425–2427 (2004).

[75] Rudd JH, Warburton EA, Fryer TD et al.: Imaging atherosclerotic plaque inflammation with [18F]-fluorodeoxyglucose positron emission tomography. Circulation 105: 2708–2711 (2002).

[76] Samson Y, Baron JC, Bousser MG et al.: Effects of extra-intracranial arterial bypass on cerebral blood flow and oxygen metabolism in humans. Stroke 16: 609–615 (1985).

[77] Samson Y, Baron JC, Pappata S et al.: Angiotensin II infusion improves perfusion and oxygen consumption in both cerebral hemispheres in patients with bilateral carotid artery obstruction. J Cereb Blood Flow Metab 7: S177 (1987).

[78] Sasoh M, Ogasawara K, Kuroda K et al.: Effects of EC-IC bypass surgery on cognitive impairment in patients with hemodynamic cerebral ischemia. Surg Neurol 59: 455–460; discussion 460–453 (2003).

[79] Schumann P, Touzani O, Young AR et al.: Evaluation of the ratio of cerebral blood flow to cerebral blood volume as an index of local cerebral perfusion pressure. Brain 121: 1369–1379 (1998).

[80] Sette G, Baron JC, Mazoyer B et al.: Local brain haemodynamics and oxygen metabolism in cerebrovascular disease. Brain 113: 931–951 (1989).

[81] Silvestrini M, Vernieri F, Pasqualetti P et al.: Impaired cerebral vasoreactivity and risk of stroke in patients with asymptomatic carotid artery stenosis. Jama 283: 2122–2127 (2000).

[82] Stevens H, Jansen HML, De Reuck J et al.: 55Cobalt (Co) as a PET-tracer in stroke, compared with blood flow, oxygen metabolism, blood volume and gadolinium-MRI. Journal of the Neurological Sciences 171: 11–18 (1999).

[83] Sugimori H, Ibayashi S, Fujii K et al.: Can transcranial Doppler really detect reduced cerebral perfusion states? Stroke 26: 2053–2060 (1995).

[84] The EC/IC Bypass Study Group.: Failure of extracranial-intracranial arterial bypass to reduce the risk of ischemic stroke: results of an international randomized trial. N Engl J Med 313: 1191–2000 (1985).

[85] The European Carotid Surgery Trialists Collaborative Group. Risk of stroke in the distribution of an asymptomatic artery. Lancet 345: 209–212 (1995).

[86] Tomita: Significance of cerebral blood volume. In: Tomita M, Sawada T, Naritomi H, Heiss W-D (eds.) Cerebral hyperemia and ischemia: From the standpoint of cerebral blood volume: Elsevier Science Publishers BV, (1988).

[87] Torvik A, Skellerud K: Wastershed infarcts in the brain caused by microemboli. Clin Neuropath 1: 99–105 (1982).

[88] Torvik A: The pathogenesis of watershed infarctions in the brain. Stroke 15: 221–223 (1984).

[89] Wodarz R: Watershed infarctions and computed tomography.: A topographical study in cases with stenosis or occlusion of the carotid artery. Neuroradiol 19: 245–248 (1980).

[90] Yamauchi H, Fukuyama H, Kimura J, Ishikawa M, Kikuchi H: Crossed cerebellar hypoperfusion indicates

the degree of uncoupling between blood flow and metabolism in major cerebral arterial occlusion. Stroke 25: 1945–1951 (1994).
[91] Yamauchi H, Fukuyama H, Nagahama Y et al.: Significance of increased oxygen extraction fraction in five-year prognosis of major cerebral arterial occlusive disease. J Nucl Med 40: 1992–1998 (1999).
[92] Yamauchi H, Okazawa H, Kishibe Y, Sugimoto K, Takahashi M: Oxygen extraction fraction and acetazolamide reactivity in symptomatic carotid artery disease. J Neurol Neurosurg Psychiatry 75: 33–37 (2004).
[93] Yokota C, Hasegawa Y, Minematsu K et al.: Effect of Acetazolamide Reactivity and Long-term Outcome in Patients With Major Cerebral Artery Occlusive Diseases. Stroke 29: 640–644 (1998).
[94] Yun M, Jang S, Cucchiara A et al.: 18F FDG uptake in the large arteries: a correlation study with the atherogenic risk factors. Semin Nucl Med 32: 70–76 (2002).
[95] Yun M, Yeh D, Araujo LI et al.: F-18 FDG uptake in the large arteries: a new observation. Clin Nucl Med 26: 314–319 (2001).
[96] Zaharchuk G, Mandeville JB, Bogdanov AA et al.: Cerebrovascular dynamics of autoregulation and hypoperfusion: An MRI study of CBF and changes in total and microvascular cerebral blood volume during hemorrhagic hypotension. Stroke 30: 2197–2205 (1999).
[97] Zulch KJ: Über die Entstehung und Lokalisation der Hirn-Infarkte. Zentralbl Neurochir 21: 158–178 (1961).

SPECIFIC PATHOLOGIC PROBLEMS IN CAROTID ARTERY IMAGING

Chapter 2.1

ATHEROSCLEROTIC PLAQUE CHARACTERISATION BY IMAGING

S. P. S. Howarth, J. U. King-Im, and J. H. Gillard

University Department of Radiology and Department of Neurosurgery, Addenbrooke's Hospital, Cambridge, UK

Background

Carotid artery stenosis is known to be a significant risk factor for stroke and indeed extracranial atheroma is the single most important contributor to non-haemorrhagic stroke in the developed world. Studies such as the European Carotid Surgery Trial (ECST) [63], [11] and North American Symptomatic Carotid Endarterectomy Trial (NASCET) [25], despite some methodological differences, demonstrated a significant benefit for endarterectomy in symptomatic carotid stenosis of more than 70%. More recently, evidence has been published in the form of the Asymptomatic Carotid Surgery Trial (ACST) [34], that intervention in the asymptomatic population with a stenosis of 70% or more may be of benefit providing the associated risks and likely morbidity of the intervention is low.

Atherosclerosis as a whole is a silent killer and patients with clinically significant atheroma in one organ system, are almost certain to be afflicted with it in other vascular beds. Thus, the 65 year old with stable angina may well have an asymptomatic carotid plaque from which he might eventually develop symptoms. It is of course this group of patients in whom identification of increased risk of stroke would be most useful, so that appropriate evidence based treatment and secondary prevention could be instituted in a timely manner.

Any screening process for such a cohort of patients would have to involve an investigation that is non-invasive, highly sensitive and specific and acceptable to the patients themselves. Whilst the commonly used clinical imaging methods fulfil some of these criteria, they all suffer from the same limitation.

X-ray angiography is currently considered the gold standard in terms of the assessment of luminal stenosis and has been used as such in most of the major trials concerning risk assessment in carotid stenosis such as NASCET and ECST. This technique is of course uncomfortable for the patient and carries with it a small risk of morbidity and mortality. This has lead to other measures of luminal stenosis by techniques much less invasive than conventional angiography.

Current clinical measures of atheroma burden by either duplex ultrasonography, CT angiography, or MR angiography (with or without IV contrast medium), although less invasive and better tolerated than conventional angiography, also only measure the degree of luminal stenosis and give no information about plaque morphology, physiology or biomechanics. There is a great deal of evidence to suggest that luminal stenosis alone is an inadequate predictor of risk, partly due to the process of arterial remodelling and partly due to the fact that none of the investigations used to measure it give any indication of plaque composition. This chapter will outline current imaging methods which are being used to characterise these plaque components and discuss the potential applications for them in a clinical setting.

Problems with luminal stenosis

Although luminal stenosis percentage is the most commonly used clinical measure of plaque risk, it is not at all clear how to measure it in the first place, as evidenced by the two different systems adopted by the two major clinical trials in this area, ECST and NASCET. ECST determined the fractional stenosis by using the luminal diameter at the point of maximal stenosis at angiography as the numerator and the projected diameter of the artery at that same

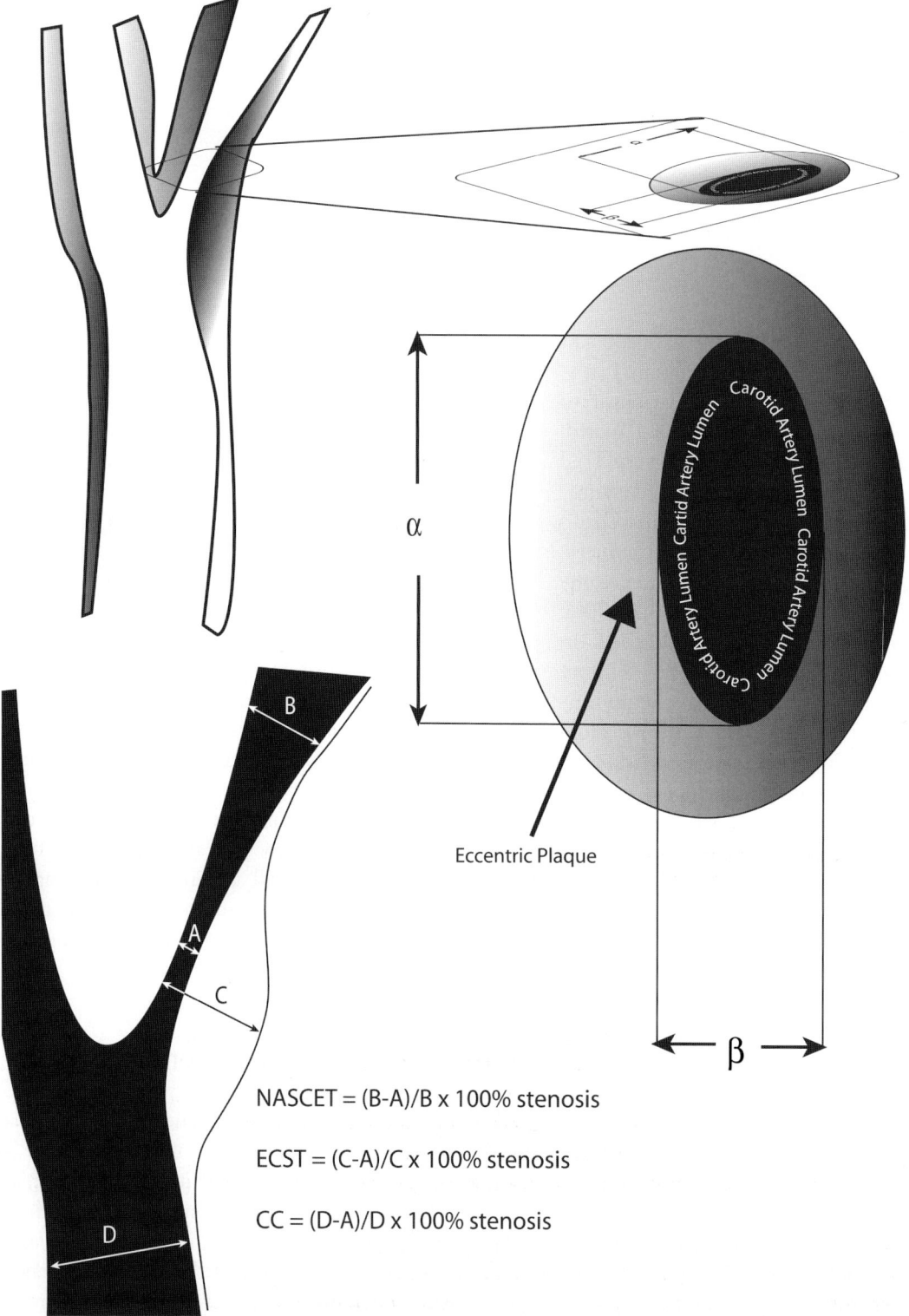

Fig. 1. Diagram showing the problems with luminal measurement and the methods of measurement of luminal stenosis most frequently discussed in the literature; namely NASCET, ECST and common carotid (CC) techniques.

point were it to be undiseased as the denominator. NASCET however used the luminal diameter of the undiseased internal carotid artery above the diseased portion as the denominator (Fig. 1). It has recently been shown that ECST measurements have a linear correlation with plaque risk whereas NASCET measurements need to be transformed before showing such a direct relationship [38].

A third method of using the diameter of the undiseased common carotid artery as the denominator has also been investigated and was thought by some to be superior to the two previous measurements [62], [49]. There remains no consensus in the literature, thus far, as to the gold standard measurement that should be adopted when assessing luminal stenosis using X-ray angiography.

One further factor, not controlled for in any angiographic study is one of projection. As shown in Fig. 1, an angiographic measure of stenosis is based on a 2D projection in the longitudinal direction of the point of maximal stenosis. Unless the luminal morphology is entirely round, this point of maximal stenosis should be better considered to be described by not one measurement, describing a circle but by two, describing an ellipse. Although more recent advances in X-ray angiography have addressed this problem with the advent of 3D rotational angiography, this is at the expense of significantly increased radiation exposure to both the patient and the radiologist. Increasingly, luminal morphology has been shown to be critical in the biomechanics of plaque rupture and thus should be taken into consideration in any model of plaque rupture risk [30], [4], [55], [66], [56], [51].

Plaque morphology

Stary et al. in 1995 set out to define what histological characteristics of atheromatous plaque made it vulnerable [50]. They defined a number of types and characteristics, detailed in Table 1.

It is now well described that the vulnerable atherosclerotic plaque has a thin, fibrous cap, extensive and necrotic lipid core and a significant amount of associated inflammation with infiltration of T lymphocytes and activated macrophages [28], [40], [5], [31], [52], [37], [46]. These inflammatory cells are found predominantly in the shoulders of the plaque in the fibrous cap, usually at its weakest point. Once activated, these inflammatory cells secrete proteolytic enzymes such as matrix metalloprotienases (MMPs) which degrade the collaginous extracellular matrix and serve to weaken the cap further, tending to increase its risk of rupture. Direct interactions with the vascular smooth muscle cells (VSMCs) may lead to promotion of VSMC apoptosis, further weakening the cap [7], [29], [53], [71].

Thus the non-invasive detection of these components is key to the ability to risk stratify patients

Table 1. American Heart Association (AHA) histological definitions of atherosclerosis (after [50])

Lesion Type	Histological Classification	Other terms used for the same lesions often based on appearance with the unaided eye	Progression
Type I	Initial lesion		Early lesions
Type IIa	Progression-prone type II lesion	Fatty dot or streak	
Type IIb	Progression-resistant type II lesion		
Type III	Intermediate lesion (preatheroma)		
Type IV	Atheroma	Atheromatous plaque	Intermediate lesions
Type Va	Fibroatheroma (type V lesion)	Fibrolipid plaque, fibrous plaque, plaque	
Type Vb	Calcific lesion (type VII lesion)	Calcified plaque	Advanced lesions
Type Vc	Fibrotic lesion (type VIII lesion)	Fibrous plaque	Raised lesions
Type VI	Lesion with surface defect, and/or haematoma-haemorrhage, and/or thrombotic deposit	Complicated lesion, complicated plaque	

with carotid atheroma, which conventional techniques of luminology are unable to address.

Why fibrous cap thickness?

As early as 1992, Loree et al. published a study simulating stress on idealised eccentric atheroma [30], using an engineering method, Finite Element Analysis, to determine the effect on the overall stress on the plaque when varying the overall degree of stenosis and thickness of fibrous cap. They postulated that the final link in the chain of plaque rupture was likely to be mechanical stress on a chronically weakened fibrous cap leading finally to rupture. Their simulations found that circumferential stress on the plaque was exquisitely linked to the thickness of the fibrous cap and degree of arterial remodelling (according to the law of Laplace); the thinner the cap, the greater the stress even at relatively low levels of stenosis. Further, increasing the simulated stenosis from 70 to 99% by increasing the thickness of the fibrous cap only, keeping the lipid core constant, served to decrease the overall stress, quite contrary to the accepted thinking at the time.

More evidence comes from cardiological post-mortem studies looking at culprit coronary lesions for sudden cardiac death. These showed that responsible lesions could be split broadly into three groups; one, the so-called fibroatheroma, with a very thin ruptured fibrous cap and extensive lipid core with associated intraluminal thrombus formation; two, the erosion, with no evidence of plaque rupture or intraplaque haemorrhage but a denuded fibrous cap with no overlying vascular endothelium and an associated overlying thrombus; three, a thrombus overlying a superficial calcified nodule. The fibroatheroma lesion with thin fibrous cap was by far the most common.

More recently, clinical studies histologically assessing symptomatic carotid atheroma following endarterectomy have shown these patients to show vulnerable plaque morphologies. Fig. 2 shows two plaques with both MR imaging and corresponding histology; one from an asymptomatic individual with a thick, fibrous cap and one from a symptomatic, showing a thin, vulnerable fibrous cap.

Why lipid core and inflammation?

The lipid core, once thought to be an inert deposition of lipid is now known to be a highly biologically active area. The core itself is predominantly composed of foamy macrophages that are dead or dying with more viable cells usually found at the interface between the core and the fibrous cap, particularly at the shoulders of the plaque. As macrophages translocate across the intimal endothelium as a result of endothelial dysfunction, they take up oxidised LDL cholesterol which activates them and encourages them to continue to do this. Activated macrophages secrete proteolytic enzymes such as matrix metalloproteinases (e.g., MMP-7, MMP-9) which degrade proteins and collagens making up the extracellular matrix of the fibrous cap, so weakening it and ultimately increasing its risk of rupture.

The AHA Classification of atheroma by Stary et al. was an early attempt to correlate plaque morphological characteristics with risk and ultimately outcome. Although this was undoubtedly a major step forward for the field of atherosclerosis, two omissions have led the classification to be modified. These two include the most common form of fibroatheroma with a thin fibrous cap at high risk of rupture and the histological characteristic of plaque erosions. Further, since its publication, atherosclerosis has been shown in numerous studies to be an active inflammatory systemic disease rather than the inert deposition of cholesterol that it was originally assumed to be [8], [14], [16], [18], [20], [27].

Thus, a larger lipid core represents a more active atherosclerotic process and likewise a greater macrophage burden most likely reflects a greater risk of fibrous cap weakening and ultimately plaque rupture.

Imaging modalities for plaque characterisation

Intravascular ultrasound (IVUS)

The use of an intravascular ultrasound catheter for in-vivo use in humans was first reported by Nissen et al. in 1991 [39]. They reported the use of this technology to assess the wall morphology in the

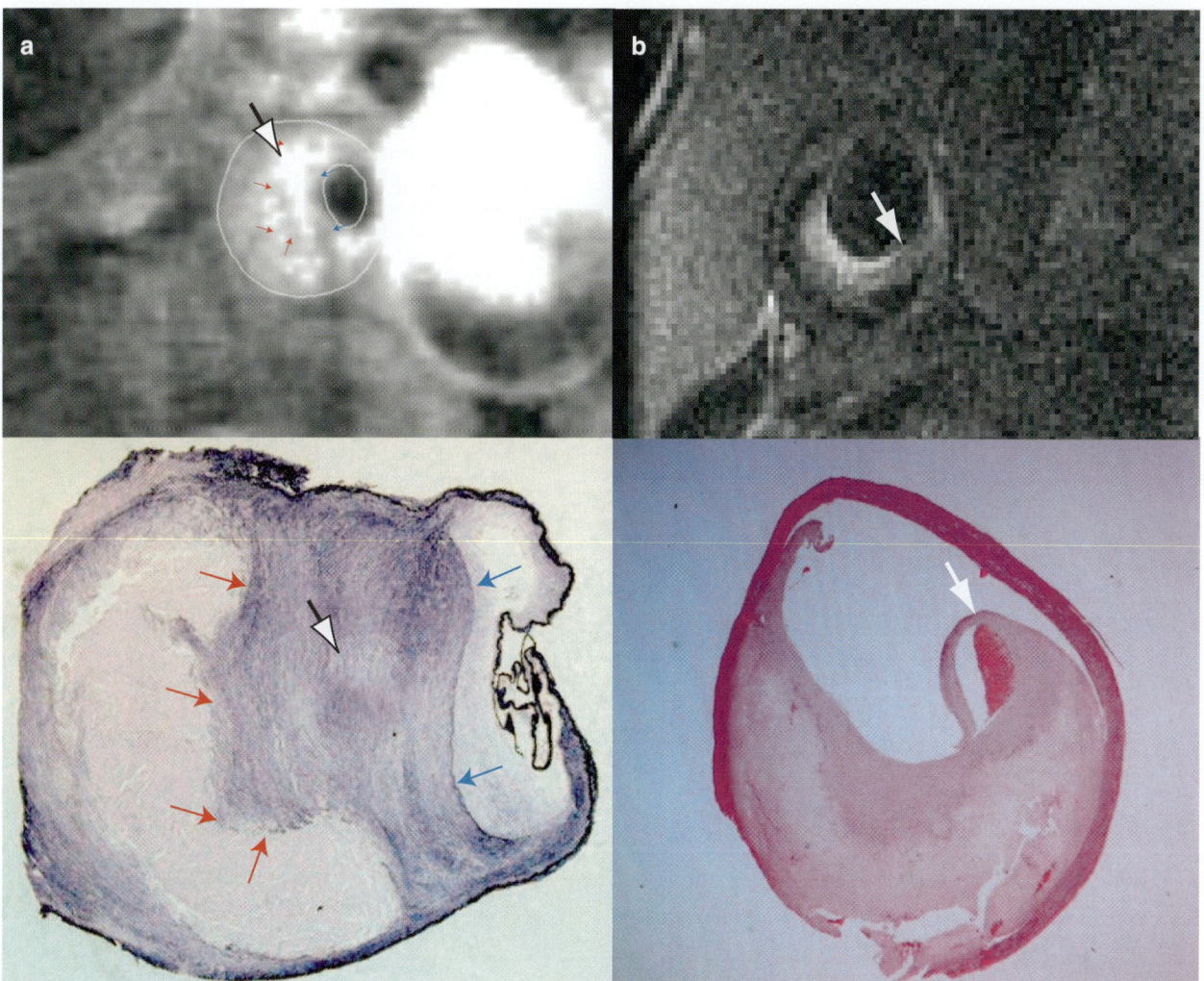

Fig. 2. Thick and thin fibrous cap: **a** intermediate T2 weighted MR imaging of an asymptomatic carotid plaque with coregistered histology below showing a thick fibrous cap (white arrow and between red and blue arrows) and fibrous cap/lipid core interface (red arrows); **b** STIR sequence of a symptomatic carotid plaque with coregistered histology below showing a thin fibrous cap, clearly resolved using the STIR sequence *in-vivo*.

coronary arteries of both normal patients and those with coronary artery atheroma. Whist this technology is very promising in the assessment of atheroma, it is highly interventional and, as such unsuitable for screening applications. Its use has also been reported intraoperatively to determine the extent of the carotid atheroma and help plan not only arteriotomy but also safe and accurate placement of a vascular shunt [21].

More recent studies have followed atheroma progression using IVUS particularly in the context of coronary atheroma. A combination of angiography and IVUS known as ANGUS has been described to reconstruct luminal and wall morphology in 3 dimensions using a "pull back" technique [48]. The technique was first described in coronary arteries by Slager et al. In 16 patients who were investigated 6 months following coronary stent implantation, a sheath-based catheter was used to acquire IVUS images during an R-wave-triggered, motorized stepped pullback. First, a single set of end diastolic biplane images were obtained to document the location of the catheter at the beginning of pullback. From these images, the 3D pullback trajectory was predicted. Contours of the lumen obtained from IVUS were fused with this trajectory. Reconstructions were obtained in 12 patients. Geometric measurements in silhouette images of the 3D reconstructions showed high correlation (kappa 0.84 to 0.97) with corresponding measurements in the actual biplane angiographic images. Thus, using ANGUS, they concluded that 3D reconstructions of coronary arteries can be successfully and accurately obtained in the majority of patients.

Examples of coronary IVUS imaging are given in Fig. 3.

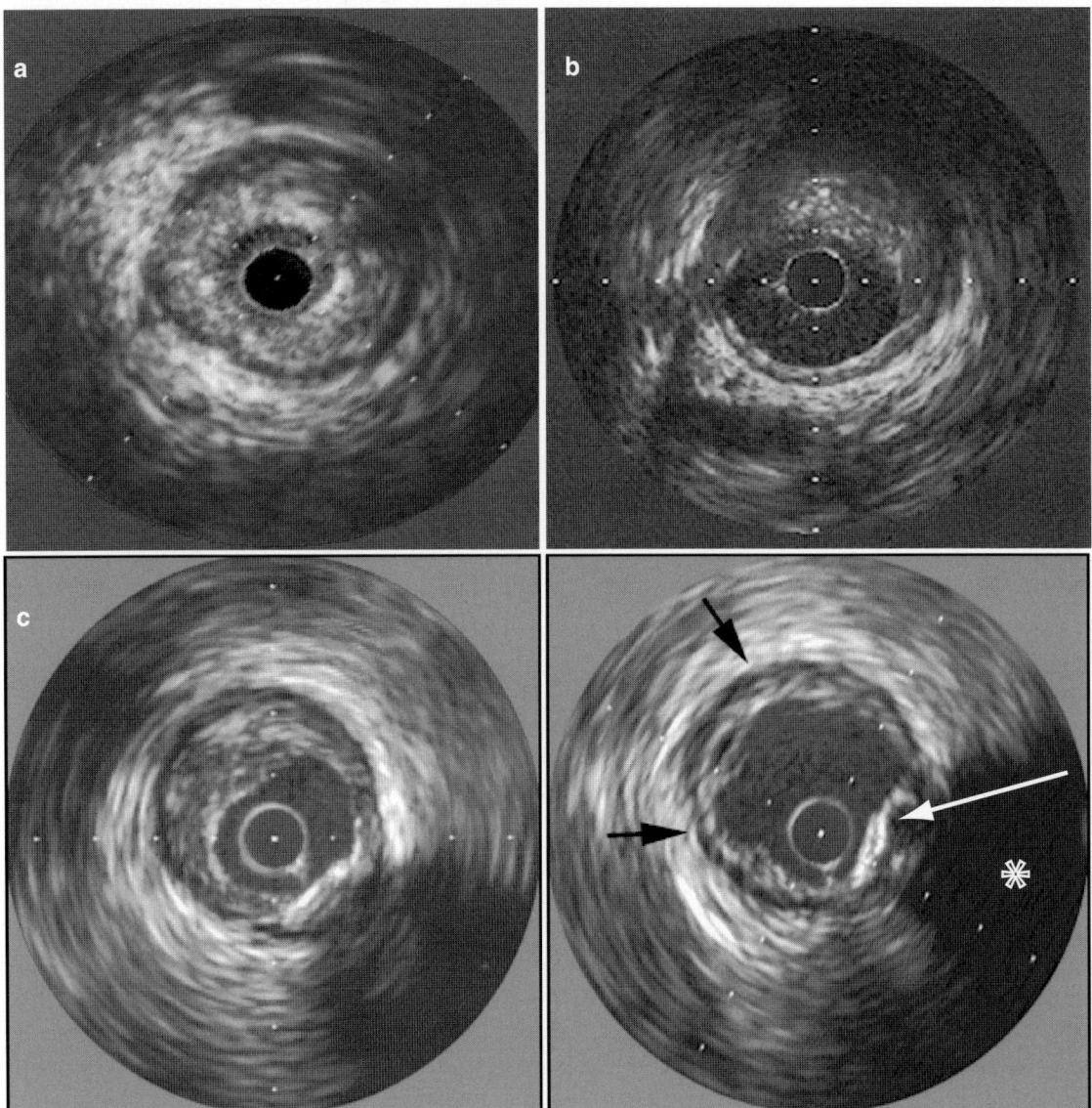

Fig. 3. a Intravascular ultrasound (IVUS) of a concentric, large coronary plaque with some "fibrotic" elements but no calcification; **b** IVUS of an eccentric and "soft" coronary plaque, not significantly stenotic but may be vulnerable; **c** Eccentric but circumferential involvement "mixed" coronary plaque with a small deposit of calcium (white arrow) with shadowing behind (white star). The internal elastic lamina of the vessel is delineated by the black arrows (courtesy Dr Murat E Tuzcu and Dr Steven Nissen).

CT plaque imaging

Attempts at using CT to image the components of carotid atheroma have been described by Porsche et al. [41], [42]. Fifty five patients undergoing carotid endarterectomy were imaged preoperatively using single-slice spiral CT angiography. A total of 165 histological sections were available for analysis. Plaque density was measured (in Hounsfield units) on axial CT sections and the presence or absence of ulceration was noted. The CT images were co-registered with the appropriate histological sections. ANOVA testing revealed a statistically significant decrease in CT attenuation values as total lipid content of the plaque increased, but the standard deviation of these values was very high. The authors were unable to demonstrate any other histological factors that showed a statistically significant correlation with CT attenuation. Plaque ulceration was detected by CT with a sensitivity and specificity of 60% and 74%, respectively. The authors concluded, therefore, that single-slice CT was unable to give useful information regarding plaque composition and is insufficiently robust to be a useful tool for characterisation of carotid plaque morphology. Thus, as a technique, CT is unable to accurately resolve the difference between fibrous cap and lipid core with the plaque but can still be used to assess overall plaque burden.

Magnetic resonance imaging

Magnetic Resonance Imaging (MRI) is an attractive non-invasive imaging modality for the assessment of plaque morphology in-vivo, as it allows exquisite resolution and using multi-sequence techniques allows good discrimination between fibrous cap and lipid core [17], [57], [59], [15]. It is usually well tolerated by patients and has few contraindications. Its other disadvantages in the context of atheroma relate to relatively long imaging time and availability of technology such as dedicated surface radiofrequency coils to maximise signal to noise ratio (Fig. 4).

Black-blood imaging

One of the major problems associated with vessel wall imaging until fairly recently has been the ar-

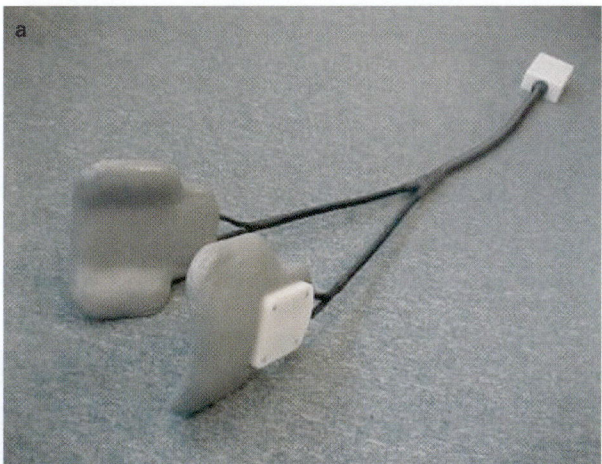

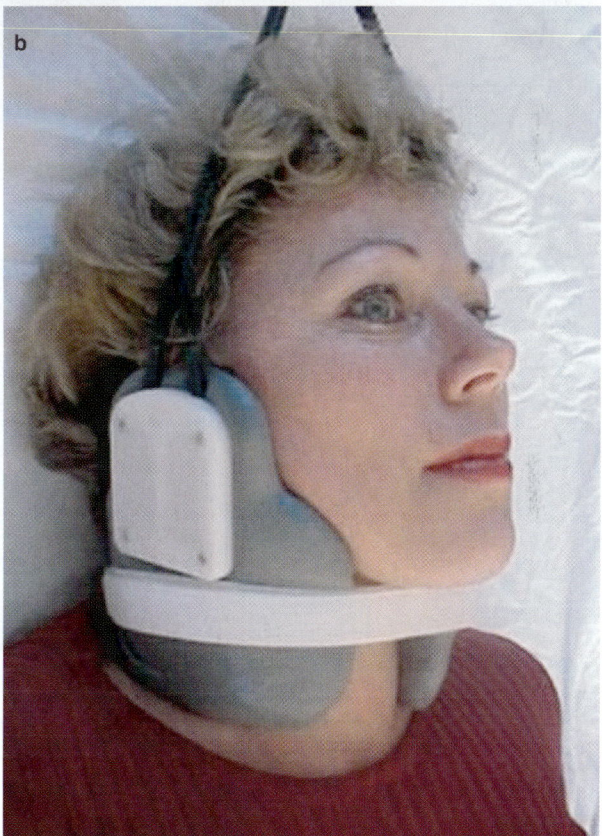

Fig. 4. Four-channel phased array surface coil dedicated to carotid imaging to maximise signal to noise at a 12 × 12 cm field of view (Flick Engineering).

tefact and bright signal from the moving blood pool. "Black-blood" imaging allows the use of a 90 degree pulse and a 180 degree rephasing pulse to

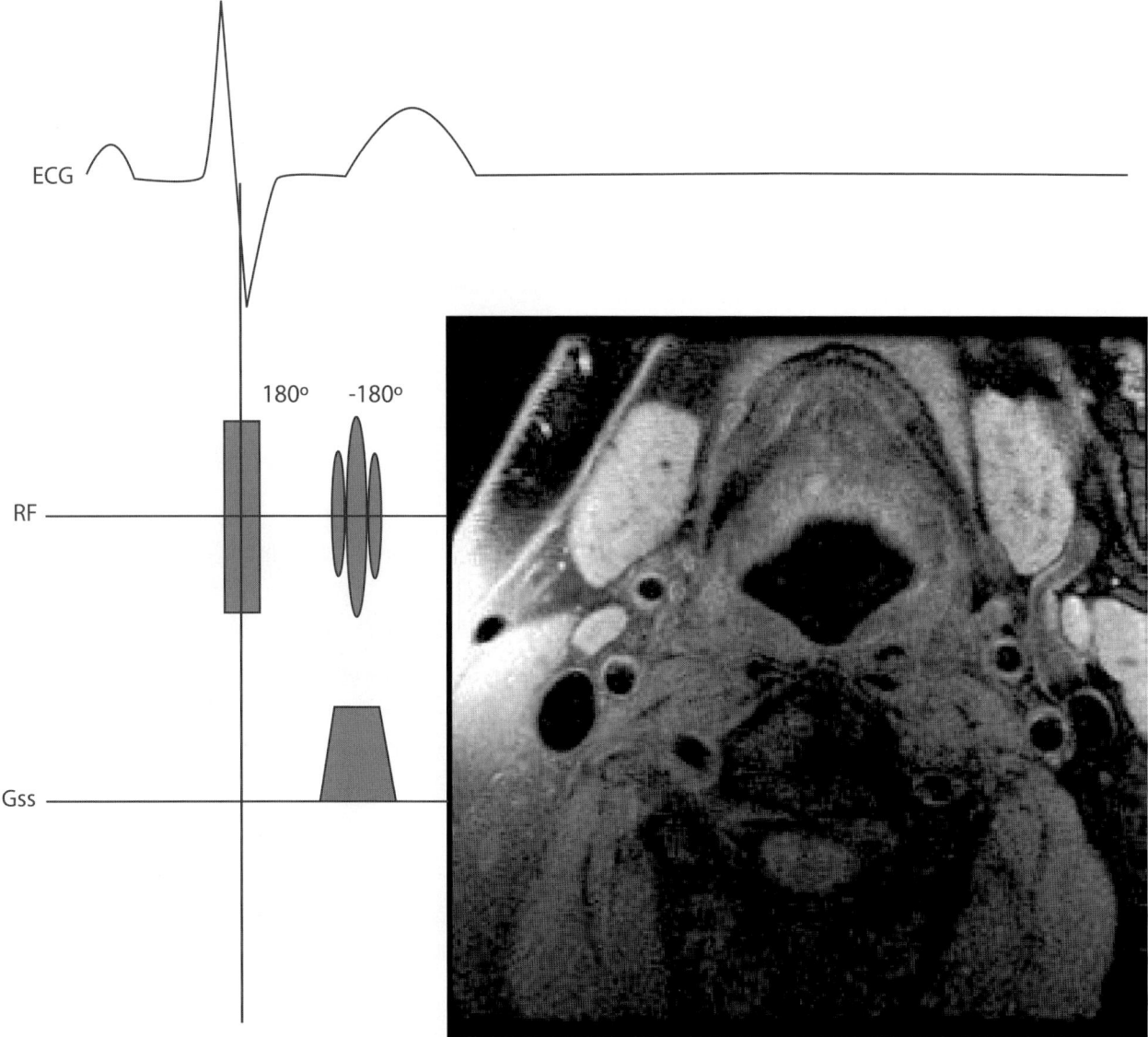

Fig. 5. (Black blood imaging) Partial sequence showing the use of two 180 degree RF pulses to allow the nulling of flowing blood. Inset: an example of carotid black blood imaging. Vessel outlines can clearly be delineated.

null the blood (Fig. 5). Since the spins in the blood are moving though the slice, the chances of them being hit by both pulses is very small and therefore their signal will be nulled providing that the readout is at the point where the blood signal crosses zero magnetization. To further enhance this pulse sequence the use of saturation pulses above and below the slice can ensure that the blood pool remains dark.

Multi-sequence imaging

Since different components of the plaque have inherently different signal characteristics on multi-spectral imaging, by using a number of different sequences including T_1 weighted, T_2 weighted, Short tau inversion recovery (STIR) and proton density (PD) sequences they can be distinguished from each other in axial section. These signal characteristics are out-

Table 2. Signal characteristics of different plaque components in different MR sequences. + is used to indicate enhancement, − is used to indicate signal loss and +/− is used to indicate variable signal characteristics

	T_1 Weighted	Intermediate T_2 Weighted	Long T_2	STIR
Fibrous Cap	+	++	++	+++
Lipid Core	+	+/−	+/−	−
Calcium	−	−	−	−
Haemorrhage	++	+/−	+/−	+/−

lined in Table 2. A number of articles have been published comparing the accuracy of this type of segmentation with histology following endarterectomy showing good correlation between the two. Yuan et al. and Trivedi et al. published the most recent papers on this topic with over 200 cases in total [57], [59], [67]–[70].

Trivedi et al. imaged 40 consecutive patients scheduled for endarterectomy using a multi-sequence high resolution MR protocol. Fibrous cap and lipid core thicknesses were measured on MR and histology images. Bland-Altman plots were generated to determine the level of agreement between the two methods and in all, 133 corresponding MR and histology slices were identified for analysis. MR and histology derived fibrous-cap to lipid-core thickness ratios showed strong agreement with a mean difference between MR and histology ratios of 0.02 (+/− 0.04). The intra-class correlation coefficient between two readers for measurements was 0.87 (95% confidence interval, 0.73 and 0.93). Thus, multi-sequence imaging accurately quantified the relative thickness of fibrous-cap and lipid-core components of carotid atheromatous plaques.

Lipid core and total plaque burden consistently show the closest correlation with fibrous cap thickness assessment pushing the limits of MR resolution achievable in a reasonable imaging time.

In order to maximise signal to noise ratio and maintain imaging time for a unilateral carotid examination to approximately 45 minutes, many designs of surface coils have been used. The authors currently use a dedicated 4 channel phased array surface coil (Flick Engineering Ltd., Holland) (see Fig. 4).

Many methods of image segmentation have been published including manual segmentation and fully automatic algorithms based on probabilistic analysis. These have always been shown to work well on high resolution ex-vivo data, imaging the plaque either in a microcoil on a standard 1.5 T clinical machine, or in a high-field machine (9.8 T). The semi-automated algorithms appear to be less robust when dealing with in-vivo data since resolution and SNR are must less optimal in the in-vivo setting.

From plaque morphology to function

Plaque haemorrhage and direct thrombus imaging

Although plaque structure is key to determination of individual risk, plaque physiology and function also plays a pivotal role. Histologically, atheromatous plaque has been shown not only to have a thin fibrous cap with extensive lipid core but also neovessel formation within the plaque [32], [33], [54] and associated plaque haemorrhage [3]. From post mortem coronary studies, haemorrhage is thought to be either associated with plaque rupture as the tissue factor and pro-coagulative cytokines in the lipid core are exposed to flowing blood following rupture of the fibrous cap, or de-novo thrombus overlying a denuded area of fibrous cap as previously described. It is likely that weak walled neovascularisation ruptures to create intraplaque haemorrhage and it is this that leads to further plaque vulnerability. Since blood itself has very specific signal characteristics on MR imaging, this can be taken advantage of in an attempt to image intraplaque haemorrhage.

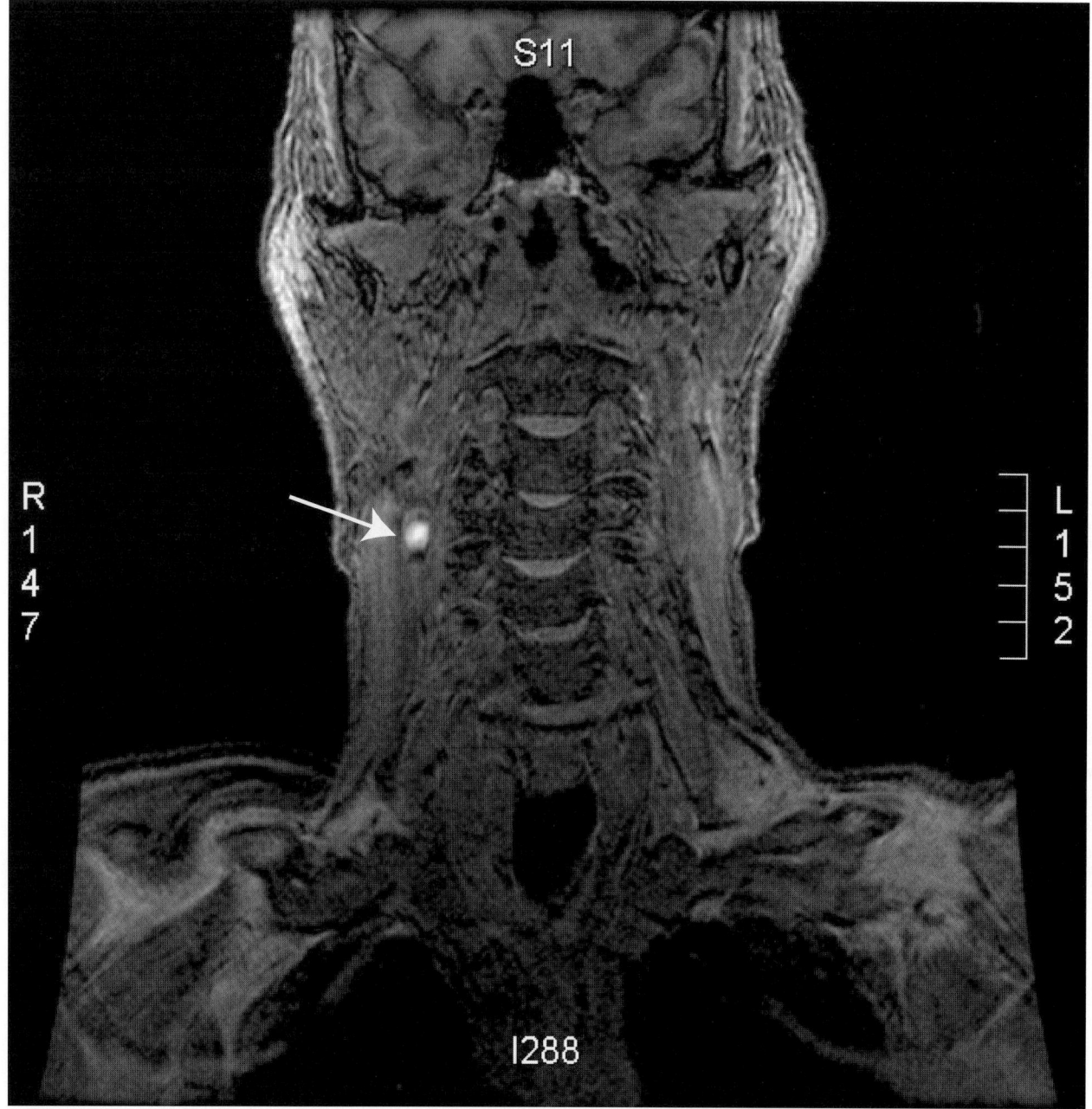

Fig. 6. (DTI) Direct Thrombus Imaging of the carotid arteries of a patient with a right sided symptomatic stenosis of 90% by NASCET criteria (courtesy of Dr Alan R Moody). The high signal indicating an acute thrombus is indicated with a white arrow. This was confirmed to be an acute thrombus in the plaque at histology following endarterectomy (image courtesy Dr Alan Moody).

As blood clots, methaemaglobin is formed. This shortens T_1 of the clot significantly leading to bright signal on T_1 weighted imaging. Unfortunately, this haemorrhage is usually found within the lipid core and since fat is usually high signal on T_1 imaging, the very short T_1 species of the clot are obscured. Moody et al. reported the use of a T_1 weighted sequence known as direct thrombus imaging (DTI)

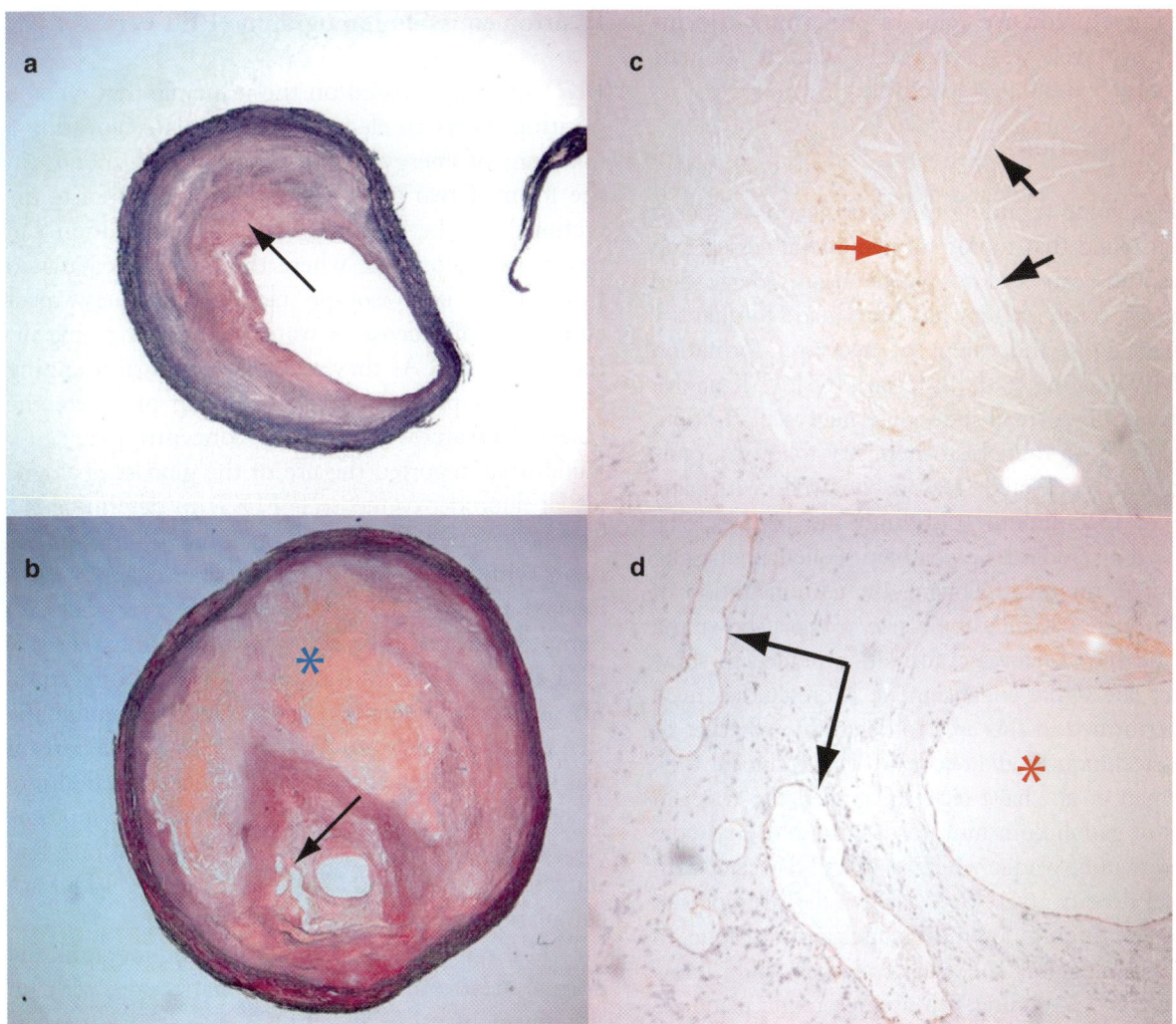

Fig. 7. Low power light microscopy (×10) of Elastin Van Gieson (EVG) stained plaque from an asymptomatic (**a**) and symptomatic (**b**) individual. The symptomatic plaque has a much more extensive lipid core (blue star) and relatively small fibrous cap in relation to this; **c** anti CD-31 (immunohistochemical stain) high power microscopy (×40) of the symptomatic plaque in A showing extensive neovessel formation (black arrows) close to the lumen (red star); **d** anti CD-31 (immunohistochemical stain) high power microscopy (×40) of the symptomatic plaque at the fibrous cap/lipid core (black arrows) interface showing weak positivity (red arrow) suggesting a small condensation of neovasculature.

that overcame this problem [22], [36], [35]. Their approach was to use a selective water excitation pulse to null the fat in the lipid core, so allowing the T_1 effect of the methaemaglobin to been seen. Fig. 6 shows an example of this sequence.

They imaged 63 patients with symptomatic carotid stenosis using this technique and compared MR imaging to postoperative histology. There was said to be a correlation if the artery showed high signal on MR imaging within 1 cm of the point of maximal stenosis and histology showed a Type IV plaque according to the AHA Classification of vulnerable plaque by Stary et al., first published in 1995.

DTI was shown to have an 84% sensitivity and specificity with a positive predictive value of 93%

and negative predictive value of 70%. Intra and interobserver error was acceptable with a Cohen's kappa of 0.75 and 0.9, respectively.

Neovascularisation

Work is ongoing regarding this difficult topic. Since it has been found that rupture of neointimal vessels and vasa-vasorum can lead to plaque haemorrhage and thrombosis, some attempt has been made to quantify and characterise the extent of neovessel formation using MR imaging [68], [23], [64], [65]. U-King-Im et al. showed in a small study that neovescularisation, as assessed by immunohistochemistry following end-arterectomy, correlated reasonably well with late uptake of Gadolinium (Gd) into the plaque [61]. They used a standard T_1 weighted sequence, imaging 0, 8 and 12 minutes following the administration of Gd. Although a small sample size, plaques showing a greater degree of neovessel formation tended to show a greater late signal enhancement. More studies need to be performed in this area to determine whether or not this technique could become a viable clinical tool. Wasserman et al. have recently studied the wash-in kinetics of gadolinium into fibrous cap and lipid core of atheromatous plaque which may well correlate with neovessel density [64]. Fig. 7 shows the histology of neovascularisation in a symptomatic carotid plaque on CD-31 staining (an endothelial marker) and at low power on EVG staining. An asymptomatic plaque is presented for comparison.

In-vivo imaging of inflammation

One of the major components of plaque pathophysiology that has been shown to be closely related to plaque vulnerability is the inflammatory milieu within. This has been shown to be comprised of monocyte macrophages, T cells and dendritic cells. Until relatively recently, there has been no way to image these cells or quantify the extent of the inflammatory component within the plaque. There are two techniques reported in the literature now capable of doing just that; positron emission tomography (PET) and ultrasmall superparamagnetic iron oxide (USPIO) enhanced MR imaging.

Positron emission tomography (PET)

PET imaging is based on the principle that when a positron meets an electron, it annihilates emitting a quantum of energy in the process. This energy (in the form of two gamma rays going in opposite directions) can be detected and this information can be used to determine where the positron emanated from. PET uses isotope tagged analogues, most commonly of glucose or water that decay giving off these positrons. As they annihilate with surrounding electrons, a picture can be made up of where the glucose or water was in highest concentration.

Rudd et al. reported the use of the glucose analogue [18F]-fluorodeoxyglucose (^{18}FDG) to determine the metabolic activity or carotid atheroma [44]. Eight patients with symptomatic carotid atherosclerosis were imaged using ^{18}FDG-PET and co-registered CT. Symptomatic carotid plaques were visible in ^{18}FDG-PET images acquired 3 hours post-^{18}FDG injection. Six of the 8 patients had contralateral asymptomatic stenoses ranging from 35% to 75%. A comparison was made between the net ^{18}FDG accumulation rate in symptomatic plaques and contralateral asymptomatic lesions. In all cases, symptomatic lesions had statistically significantly higher estimated ^{18}FDG accumulation rates than asymptomatic lesions.

The 2 remaining patients had angiographically normal arteries on the asymptomatic side, with no significant uptake of ^{18}FDG into those vessels. There was no measurable ^{18}FDG uptake into normal carotid arteries.

In a separate autoradiographic study, 3 carotid plaques from symptomatic patients were incubated whole with ^{50}Ci tritiated deoxyglucose (an in vitro analogue of ^{18}FDG) in 5 mL Medium 199 (Sigma) for 60 minutes at 37° C. Paraffin sections of 5 μm thickness were coated with autoradiographic emulsion (LM-1, Amersham), exposed for 6 weeks, developed, and counterstained with hematoxylin and eosin. Control slides were prepared without radioactivity. Autoradiography of these excised plaques confirmed accumulation of deoxyglucose in macrophage-rich areas of the plaque, predominately at the lipid core/fibrous cap border of the lesions. There was little or no uptake in other areas of the plaques

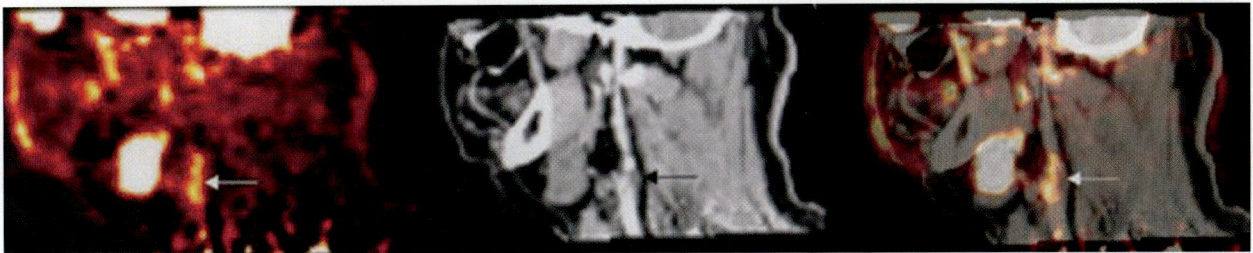

Fig. 8. (PET) Left to right shows PET, contrast CT, and co-registered PET/CT images in the sagittal plane, from a 63-year-old man who had experienced 2 episodes of left-sided hemiparesis. Angiography demonstrated stenosis of the proximal right internal carotid artery; this was confirmed on the CT image (black arrow). The white arrows show 18FDG uptake at the level of the plaque in the carotid artery. As expected, there was high 18FDG uptake in the brain, jaw muscles, and facial soft tissues (image courtesy Dr James Rudd).

and control sections showed no development of silver grains. Thus, this study demonstrated that atherosclerotic plaque inflammation can be imaged with ^{18}FDG-PET, and that symptomatic, unstable plaques accumulate more ^{18}FDG than asymptomatic lesions, having a higher metabolic rate.

An example of a PET ^{18}FDG study of carotid atheroma can be seen in Fig. 8.

PET is of course limited by the physics of the process and the resolution can never be greater than the minimum distance that a positron can travel in the body before meeting another electron. Thus, current resolution is between 2.5–5 mm. In order to improve spatial analysis, PET is often co-registered with either CT or MR. Whilst a powerful tool, metabolic activity is still only a surrogate for macrophage burden and since the resolution is limited to millimetres, spatial localisation of macrophages within the plaque is not possible using this technique. Further, the need for on-site cyclotron support for some isotopes (though FDG specifically does not require this) and extensive infrastructure required for PET imaging relegates the technique to a powerful research tool and unlikely to be used to any great extent in the clinical arena.

MR imaging of inflammation

The use of USPIO enhanced MR plaque imaging has been reported in a number of studies and takes advantage of the phagocytotic activity of human monocyte macrophages. Although a number of different USPIO compounds have been synthesised, they all share the same basic structure; that of a ferrous core surrounded by a dextran coating. It is this coating that allows the USPIO particles, when administered, to be phagocytosed by the macrophages and since inflammation within atheroma is a dynamic process, with transit of macrophages to the plaque, replacing dying cells in the lipid core, after approximately 24–36 hours, these peripheral iron-loaded cells will make their way to the site of any inflammation, including inflammatory plaque [10], [13], [19], [43]. Figure 9 shows USPIO accumulated within the lysosomes of a macrophage on transmission electron microscopy.

The USPIO particles themselves emit a tiny magnetic field around them and this serves to dephase the MR signal, leading to a susceptibility artefact most clearly seen on T_2^* imaging. Thus, USPIO-laden macrophages produce a region of signal drop on T_2^* imaging. Of course, since other plaque components can display very little signal, most notably calcium deposits, a pre USPIO imaging dataset needs to be obtained to ensure that the signal drop demonstrated is *new* following USPIO infusion. Originally developed for the imaging of metastatic disease [2], [1], [6], [24], [45] this technology has now also been successfully employed in the imaging of inflammatory carotid atheroma [9], [26], [58], [60]. Trivedi et al. showed that maximal signal loss is seen at between 24 and 36 hours following USPIO infusion [58]. Eight symptomatic patients

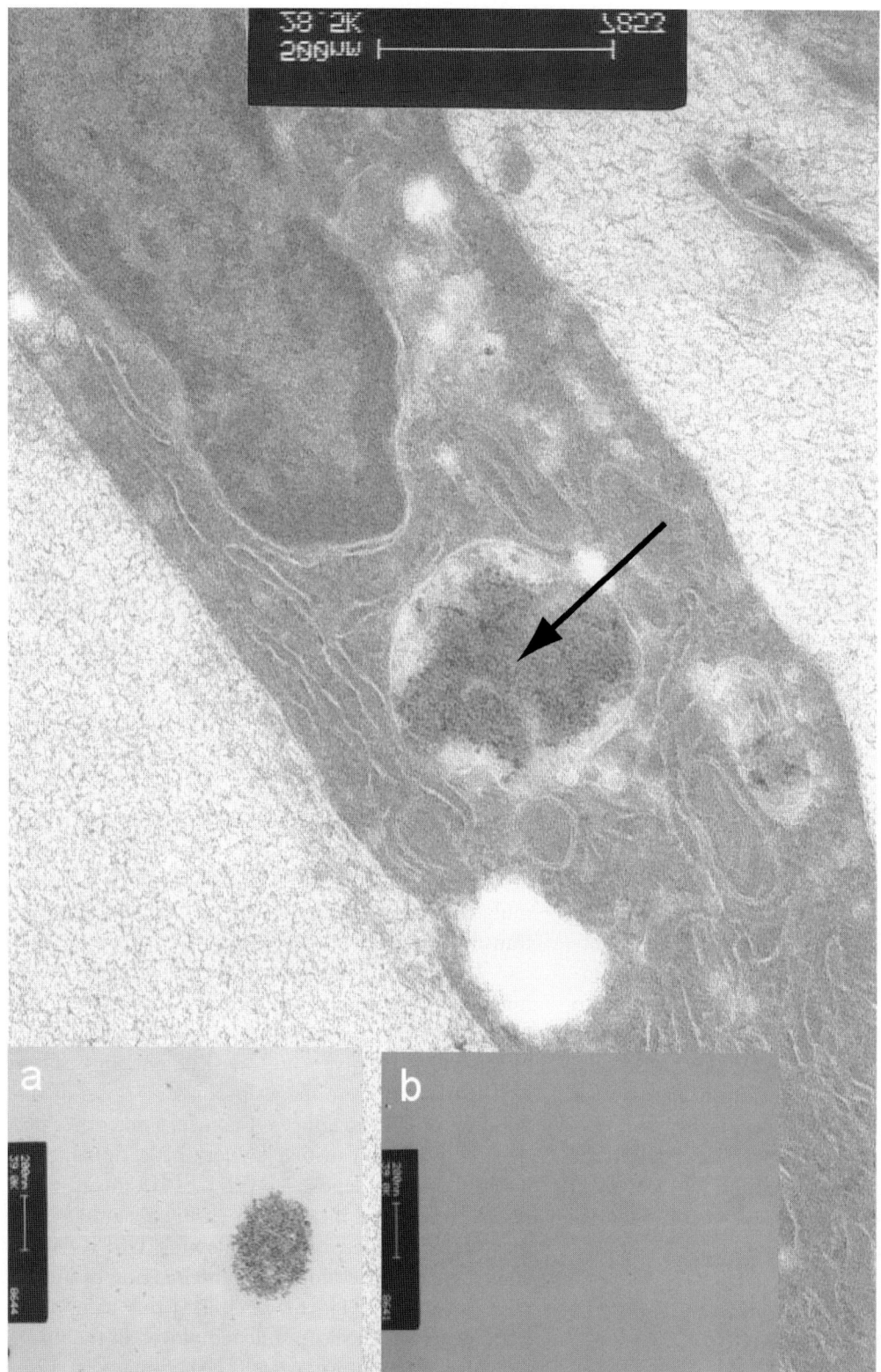

Fig. 9. Main image shows transmission electron micrograph of USPIO accumulation within a human monocyte macrophage. Accumulation is confined to the lysosomes of the macrophage (black arrow). Inset **a** and **b** shows the tendency of USPIO to clump together when present in high concentration (**a**) when compared with low concentration (**b**) (images courtesy Dr Jeremy Skepper).

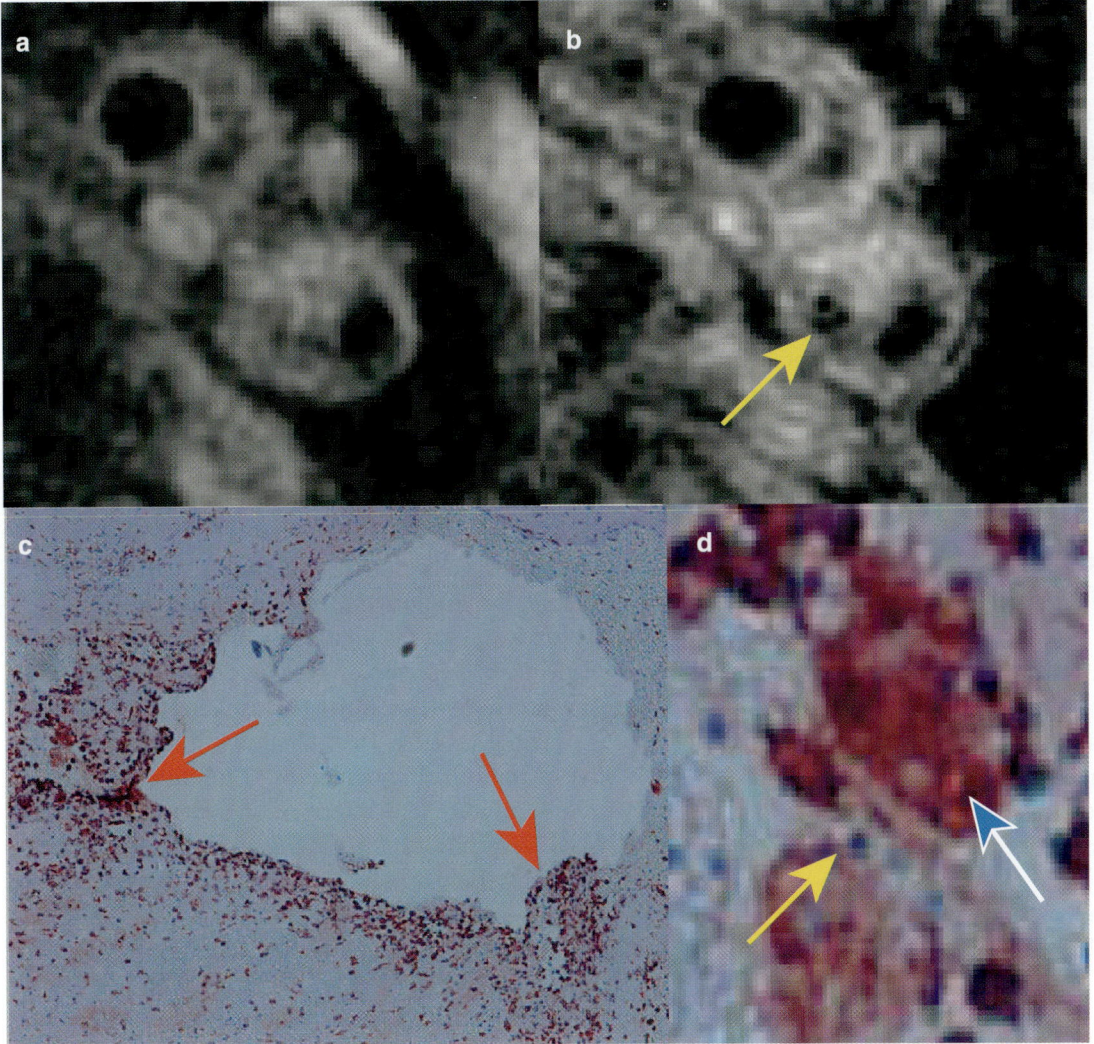

Fig. 10. (USPIO) **a** and **b** Symptomatic inflamed carotid plaque pre and 36 hours post USPIO infusion, respectively. Signal drop secondary to the T_2^* susceptibility effect of USPIO can be easily seen (yellow arrow). **c** and **d** Corresponding histology double-stain of Perls (blue Iron stain) and CD-68 (for macrophages) at two magnifications ×10 and ×40 which show USPIO being taken up by cells in the shoulder regions of the plaque (red arrows) and that USPIO (yellow arrow) co-localises to CD-68 positive cells (blue and white arrow).

were imaged at 8, 10, 24, 26 and 72 hours following infusion of the USPIO contrast agent. The following ECG-gated, fat-suppressed pulse sequences using double-inversion blood suppression were used on each occasion: 2D T_1-weighted fast spin-echo (repetition time [TR]/echo time [TE] eff 1 R-R/7.8 ms; voxel size 0.4 × 0.4 × 3 mm; echo train length = 12 matrix: 256 × 256 and 2 signal averages) and 2 2D T_2^*-weighted spiral acquisitions using spectral-spatial excitation pulses, 1 with a TE of 5.6 ms and 1 with a TE of 15 ms; both sequences used a TR of 1 R-R. The inversion time of the postinfusion T_1-weighted sequence was adjusted to counter the USPIO shortening effect in blood. The multi-shot spiral sequence involved the acquisition of 22 spiral interleaves, each of 4096 data points, resulting in an effective in-plane pixel size of 0.42 × 0.42 mm; 2 signal averages were performed. Signal loss was determined from the pre and post signal when normalised to the surrounding muscle to attempt to eliminate at much signal variation as possible across the coil between the various time points. Following this, plaques were excised and underwent Perls histological staining for iron in an attempt to co-localise macrophages with USPIO. Transmission electron microscopy was utilised to visualise the USPIO particles within the phagolysosomes of the macrophages (Fig. 9) 7 of the 8 plaques displayed signal loss in regions of interest following USPIO infusion and once co-registered with as many histological slices as possible, Perls staining correlated with regions of signal loss on MR. Double staining with anti-CD68 and Perls confirmed Perls positivity within CD68 positive macrophages (Fig. 10).

Other MR contrast agents for plaque imaging

Although not yet used in-vivo in humans, early rabbit models of atheroma suggest that the new contrast agent, gadoflourine has a high affinity for lipid rich and improves vessel wall delineation in T_1 weighted sequences. Sirol et al. published data on gadoflourine enhanced imaging in a rabbit model of atheroma [47].

Twelve rabbits with aortic plaque and 6 controls underwent MRI before and up to 24 hours after gadofluorine injection (50 micromol/kg). Two T_1-weighted, segmented gradient-echo sequences (TFL) were compared to enhance vessel wall delineation after injection: (1) an inversion-recovery prepulse (IR-TFL) or (2) a combination of inversion-recovery and diffusion-based flow suppression prepulses (IR-DIFF-TFL). At 1 hour and 24 hours after injection, the contrast-to-noise ratio was higher with the use of IR-DIFF-TFL than with IR-TFL. There was no enhancement in the vessel wall after gadofluorine injection in the control group. A strong correlation was found ($r^2 = 0.87$; $P < 0.001$) between the lipid-rich areas in histological sections and signal intensity in corresponding MR images.

Although these are promising results, there is some question over the safety of the compounds use in the context of human studies and further work needs to be done in this area.

Positive MR contrast agents are being developed that are much more targeted than the first generation agents such as simple gadolinium or even USPIO. Work thus far in humans has been limited to fibrin targeted gadolinium-based imaging [12]. However, molecular targeting of contrast agents to either membrane bound receptors or free proteins will eventually allow "in-vivo microscopy" at an exquisite resolution with the use of high-field clinical systems. Such potential targets could include IL-1 receptors, MMP-7, MMP-9 and TNFalpha to name but a few. Receptors involved in the apoptotic pathway in VSMCs are also under scrutiny as potential targets although, as yet, no useable agents have come forth from this research. Macrophage markers, well known in histological circles such as MAC387 and CD68 could well be used as targeted moieties for specific USPIOs to further aid localisation of USPIOs to these cells.

It is quite clear that luminal stenosis alone is an inadequate predictor of risk in carotid stenosis. The accurate in-vivo assessment of risk in carotid atheroma is essential to the correct targeting of interventions in the asymptomatic population, so minimising population morbidity. As interventions eventually become more pharmaceutical in nature, in-vivo follow up imaging using standardised measures of plaque risk will be required to assess stabilisation over time.

A combination of detailed plaque morphology and plaque physiology will need to be used to assess risk in the asymptomatic population and to inform subsequent intervention.

Acknowledgements

Mr Peter J Kirkpatrick, Consultant Neurosurgeon, Addenbrooke's Hospital
Mr Martin J Graves, Senior MR Physicist, Addenbrooke's Hospital
Mr Rikin Trivedi, Specialist Registrar, Department of Neurosurgery, Addenbrooke's Hospital.

References

[1] Anzai Y, Piccoli CW, Outwater EK et al.: Evaluation of neck and body metastases to nodes with ferumoxtran 10-enhanced MR imaging: phase III safety and efficacy study. Radiology 228: 777–788 (2003).

[2] Anzai Y: Superparamagnetic iron oxide nanoparticles: nodal metastases and beyond. Top Magn Reson Imaging 15: 103–111 (2004).
[3] Arapoglou B, Kondi-Pafiti A, Katsenis K et al.: The clinical significance of carotid plaque haemorrhage. Int Angiol 13: 323–326 (1994).
[4] Baldewsing RA, Schaar JA, Mastik F et al.: Assessment of vulnerable plaque composition by matching the deformation of a parametric plaque model to measured plaque deformation. IEEE Trans Med Imaging 24: 514–528 (2005).
[5] Bang OY, Lee PH, Yoon SR et al.: Inflammatory markers, rather than conventional risk factors, are different between carotid and MCA atherosclerosis. J Neurol Neurosurg Psychiatry 76: 1128–1134 (2005).
[6] Bellin MF, Beigelman C, Precetti-Morel S: Iron oxide-enhanced MR lymphography: initial experience. Eur J Radiol 34: 257–264 (2000).
[7] Bennett MR, Boyle JJ: Apoptosis of vascular smooth muscle cells in atherosclerosis. Atherosclerosis 138: 3–9 (1998).
[8] Cai H, Song C, Lim IG et al.: Importance of C-reactive protein in regulating monocyte tissue factor expression in patients with inflammatory rheumatic diseases. J Rheumatol 32: 1224–1231 (2005).
[9] Clinical alert: benefit of carotid endarterectomy for patients with high-grade stenosis of the internal carotid artery. National Institute of Neurological Disorders and Stroke Stroke and Trauma Division. North American Symptomatic Carotid Endarterectomy Trial (NASCET) investigators. Stroke 22: 816–817 (1991).
[10] Dousset V, Ballarino L, Delalande C et al.: Comparison of ultrasmall particles of iron oxide (USPIO)-enhanced T_2-weighted, conventional T_2-weighted, and gadolinium-enhanced T_1-weighted MR images in rats with experimental autoimmune encephalomyelitis. AJNR 20: 223–227 (1999).
[11] Ferro JM, Oliveira V, Melo TP et al.: Role of endarterectomy in the secondary prevention of cerebrovascular accidents: results of the European Carotid Surgery Trial (ECST). Acta Med Port 4: 227–228 (1991).
[12] Flacke S, Fischer S, Scott MJ et al.: Novel MRI contrast agent for molecular imaging of fibrin: implications for detecting vulnerable plaques. Circulation 104: 1280–1285 (2001).
[13] Fleige G, Seeberger F, Laux D et al.: In vitro characterization of two different ultrasmall iron oxide particles for magnetic resonance cell tracking. Invest Radiol 37: 482–488 (2002).
[14] Gori AM, Corsi AM, Fedi S et al.: A proinflammatory state is associated with hyperhomocysteinemia in the elderly. Am J Clin Nutr 82: 335–341 (2005).
[15] Hatsukami TS, Ross R, Polissar NL et al.: Visualization of fibrous cap thickness and rupture in human atherosclerotic carotid plaque in vivo with high-resolution magnetic resonance imaging. Circulation 102: 959–964 (2000).
[16] Heller EA, Liu E, Tager AM et al.: Inhibition of atherogenesis in BLT1-deficient mice reveals a role for LTB4 and BLT1 in smooth muscle cell recruitment. Circulation 112: 578–586 (2005).
[17] JM UK-I, Trivedi RA, Sala E et al.: Evaluation of carotid stenosis with axial high-resolution black-blood MR imaging. Eur Radiol 14: 1154–1161 (2004).
[18] Jude B, Zawadzki C, Susen S et al.: Relevance of tissue factor in cardiovascular disease. Arch Mal Coeur Vaiss 98: 667–671 (2005).
[19] Kanno S, Wu YJ, Lee PC et al.: Macrophage accumulation associated with rat cardiac allograft rejection detected by magnetic resonance imaging with ultrasmall superparamagnetic iron oxide particles. Circulation 104: 934–938 (2001).
[20] Karatzis EN: The role of inflammatory agents in endothelial function and their contribution to atherosclerosis. Hell J Cardiol 46: 232–239 (2005).
[21] Kawamata T, Okada Y, Kondo S et al.: Extravascular application of an intravascular ultrasound (IVUS) catheter during carotid endarterectomy to verify distal ends of stenotic lesions. Acta Neurochir (Wien) 146: 1205–1209 (2004).
[22] Kelly J, Hunt BJ, Moody A: Magnetic resonance direct thrombus imaging: a novel technique for imaging venous thromboemboli. Thromb Haemost 89: 773–782 (2003).
[23] Kerwin W, Hooker A, Spilker M et al.: Quantitative magnetic resonance imaging analysis of neovasculature volume in carotid atherosclerotic plaque. Circulation 107: 851–856 (2003).
[24] Kim JY, Harisinghani MG: MR imaging staging of pelvic lymph nodes. Magn Reson Imaging Clin N Am 12: 581–586 (2004).
[25] Kita MW: Carotid endarterectomy in symptomatic carotid stenosis: NASCET comparative results at 30 months of follow-up. J Insur Med 24: 42–46 (1992).
[26] Kooi ME, Cappendijk VC, Cleutjens KB et al.: Accumulation of ultrasmall superparamagnetic particles of iron oxide in human atherosclerotic plaques can be detected by in vivo magnetic resonance imaging. Circulation 107: 2453–2458 (2003).
[27] Laberge MA, Moore KJ, Freeman MW: Atherosclerosis and innate immune signaling. Ann Med 37: 130–140 (2005).
[28] Lendon CL, Davies MJ, Born GV et al.: Atherosclerotic plaque caps are locally weakened when macrophages density is increased. Atherosclerosis 87: 87–90 (1991).
[29] Littlewood TD, Bennett MR: Apoptotic cell death in atherosclerosis. Curr Opin Lipidol 14: 469–475 (2003).

[30] Loree HM, Kamm RD, Stringfellow RG et al.: Effects of fibrous cap thickness on peak circumferential stress in model atherosclerotic vessels. Circ Res 71: 850–858 (1992).

[31] Mauriello A, Sangiorgi G, Fratoni S et al.: Diffuse and active inflammation occurs in both vulnerable and stable plaques of the entire coronary tree: a histopathologic study of patients dying of acute myocardial infarction. J Am Coll Cardiol 45: 1585–1593 (2005).

[32] McCarthy MJ, Loftus IM, Thompson MM et al.: Angiogenesis and the atherosclerotic carotid plaque: an association between symptomatology and plaque morphology. J Vasc Surg 30: 261–268 (1999).

[33] McCarthy MJ, Loftus IM, Thompson MM et al.: Vascular surgical society of great britain and ireland: angiogenesis and the atherosclerotic carotid plaque: association between symptomatology and plaque morphology. Br J Surg 86: 707–708 (1999).

[34] Mohammed N, Anand SS: Prevention of disabling and fatal strokes by successful carotid endarterectomy in patients without recent neurological symptoms: randomized controlled trial. MRC asymptomatic carotid surgery trial (ACST) collaborative group. Lancet 363: 1491–502 (2004), Vasc Med 10: 77–78 (2005).

[35] Moody AR, Murphy RE, Morgan PS et al.: Characterization of complicated carotid plaque with magnetic resonance direct thrombus imaging in patients with cerebral ischemia. Circulation 107: 3047–3052 (2003).

[36] Moody AR: Magnetic resonance direct thrombus imaging. J Thromb Haemost 1: 1403–1409 (2003).

[37] Newby AC: Dual role of matrix metalloproteinases (matrixins) in intimal thickening and atherosclerotic plaque rupture. Physiol Rev 85: 1–31 (2005).

[38] Nicolaides AN, Kakkos SK, Griffin M et al.: Severity of asymptomatic carotid stenosis and risk of ipsilateral hemispheric ischaemic events: results from the ACSRS study. Eur J Vasc Endovasc Surg 30: 275–284 (2005).

[39] Nissen SE, Gurley JC, Grines CL et al.: Intravascular ultrasound assessment of lumen size and wall morphology in normal subjects and patients with coronary artery disease. Circulation 84: 1087–1099 (1991).

[40] Pasqui AL, Bova G, Maffei S et al.: Immune factors in atherosclerosis. Ann Ital Med Int 20: 81–89 (2005).

[41] Porsche C, Walker L, Mendelow AD et al.: Assessment of vessel wall thickness in carotid atherosclerosis using spiral CT angiography. Eur J Vasc Endovasc Surg 23: 437–440 (2002).

[42] Porsche C, Walker L, Mendelow D et al.: Evaluation of cross-sectional luminal morphology in carotid atherosclerotic disease by use of spiral CT angiography. Stroke 32: 2511–2515 (2001).

[43] Raynal I, Prigent P, Peyramaure S et al.: Macrophage endocytosis of superparamagnetic iron oxide nanoparticles: mechanisms and comparison of ferumoxides and ferumoxtran-10. Invest Radiol 39: 56–63 (2004).

[44] Rudd JH, Warburton EA, Fryer TD et al.: Imaging atherosclerotic plaque inflammation with [18F]-fluorodeoxyglucose positron emission tomography. Circulation 105: 2708–2711 (2002).

[45] Saini S, Sharma R, Baron RL et al.: Multicentre dose-ranging study on the efficacy of USPIO ferumoxtran-10 for liver MR imaging. Clin Radiol 55: 690–695 (2000).

[46] Schmeisser A, Marquetant R, Illmer T et al.: The expression of macrophage migration inhibitory factor 1alpha (MIF 1alpha) in human atherosclerotic plaques is induced by different proatherogenic stimuli and associated with plaque instability. Atherosclerosis 178: 83–94 (2005).

[47] Sirol M, Itskovich VV, Mani V et al.: Lipid-rich atherosclerotic plaques detected by gadofluorine-enhanced in vivo magnetic resonance imaging. Circulation 109: 2890–2896 (2004).

[48] Slager CJ, Wentzel JJ, Schuurbiers JC et al.: True 3-dimensional reconstruction of coronary arteries in patients by fusion of angiography and IVUS (ANGUS) and its quantitative validation. Circulation 102: 511–516 (2000).

[49] Staikov IN, Arnold M, Mattle HP et al.: Comparison of the ECST, CC, and NASCET grading methods and ultrasound for assessing carotid stenosis. European Carotid Surgery Trial. North American Symptomatic Carotid Endarterectomy Trial. J Neurol 247: 681–686 (2000).

[50] Stary HC, Chandler AB, Dinsmore RE et al.: A definition of advanced types of atherosclerotic lesions and a histological classification of atherosclerosis. A report from the Committee on Vascular Lesions of the Council on Arteriosclerosis, American Heart Association. Circulation 92: 1355–1374 (1995).

[51] Stehbens WE: The fatigue hypothesis of plaque rupture and atherosclerosis. Med Hypotheses 58: 359–360 (2002).

[52] Stintzing S, Heuschmann P, Barbera L et al.: Overexpression of MMP9 and tissue factor in unstable carotid plaques associated with Chlamydia pneumoniae, inflammation, and apoptosis. Ann Vasc Surg 19: 310–319 (2005).

[53] Stoneman VE, Bennett MR: Role of apoptosis in atherosclerosis and its therapeutic implications. Clin Sci (Lond) 107: 343–354 (2004).

[54] Sun L, Wei LX, Shi HY et al.: Angiogenesis in coronary atherosclerotic plaques and its relationship to plaque stabilization. Zhonghua Bing Li Xue Za Zhi 32: 427–431 (2003).

[55] Tang D, Yang C, Kobayashi S et al.: Effect of a lipid pool on stress/strain distributions in stenotic arteries: 3-D fluid-structure interactions (FSI) models. J Biomech Eng 126: 363–370 (2004).

[56] Tang D, Yang C, Kobayashi S et al.: Effect of stenosis asymmetry on blood flow and artery compression: a

three-dimensional fluid-structure interaction model. Ann Biomed Eng 31: 1182–1193 (2003).

[57] Trivedi RA, J UK-I, Graves MJ et al.: Multi-sequence in vivo MRI can quantify fibrous cap and lipid core components in human carotid atherosclerotic plaques. Eur J Vasc Endovasc Surg 28: 207–213 (2004).

[58] Trivedi RA, JM UK-I, Graves MJ et al.: In vivo detection of macrophages in human carotid atheroma: temporal dependence of ultrasmall superparamagnetic particles of iron oxide-enhanced MRI. Stroke 35: 1631–1635 (2004).

[59] Trivedi RA, JM UK-I, Graves MJ et al.: MRI-derived measurements of fibrous-cap and lipid-core thickness: the potential for identifying vulnerable carotid plaques in vivo. Neuroradiology 46: 738–743 (2004).

[60] Trivedi RA, JM UK-I, Graves MJ et al.: Noninvasive imaging of carotid plaque inflammation. Neurology 63: 187–188 (2004).

[61] U-King-Im JM TR, Higgins N, Cross JJ et al.: Characterisation of carotid atheroma in symptomatic and asymptomatic patients using gadolinium-enhanced MRI. European Congress of Radiology, Vienna (2005).

[62] Wardlaw JM, Lewis S: Carotid stenosis measurement on colour Doppler ultrasound: Agreement of ECST, NASCET and CCA methods applied to ultrasound with intra-arterial angiographic stenosis measurement. Eur J Radiol (2005).

[63] Warlow CP: Symptomatic patients: the European Carotid Surgery Trial (ECST). J Mal Vasc 18: 198–201 (1993).

[64] Wasserman BA, Casal SG, Astor BC et al.: Wash-in kinetics for gadolinium-enhanced magnetic resonance imaging of carotid atheroma. J Magn Reson Imaging 21: 91–95 (2005).

[65] Wasserman BA, Smith WI, Trout HH 3rd et al.: Carotid artery atherosclerosis: in vivo morphologic characterization with gadolinium-enhanced double-oblique MR imaging initial results. Radiology 223: 566–573 (2002).

[66] Yamamoto K, Ikeda U, Shimada K: Role of mechanical stress in monocytes/macrophages: implications for atherosclerosis. Curr Vasc Pharmacol 1: 315–319 (2003).

[67] Yuan C, Beach KW, Smith LH Jr et al.: Measurement of atherosclerotic carotid plaque size in vivo using high resolution magnetic resonance imaging. Circulation 98: 2666–2671 (1998).

[68] Yuan C, Kerwin WS, Ferguson MS et al.: Contrast-enhanced high resolution MRI for atherosclerotic carotid artery tissue characterization. J Magn Reson Imaging 15: 62–67 (2002).

[69] Yuan C, Mitsumori LM, Beach KW et al.: Carotid atherosclerotic plaque: noninvasive MR characterization and identification of vulnerable lesions. Radiology 221: 285–299 (2001).

[70] Yuan C, Mitsumori LM, Ferguson MS et al.: In vivo accuracy of multispectral magnetic resonance imaging for identifying lipid-rich necrotic cores and intraplaque hemorrhage in advanced human carotid plaques. Circulation 104: 2051–2056 (2001).

[71] Zhang QJ, Goddard M, Shanahan C et al.: Differential gene expression in vascular smooth muscle cells in primary atherosclerosis and in stent stenosis in humans. Arterioscler Thromb Vasc Biol 22: 2030–2036 (2002).

Chapter 2.2

IMAGING FINDINGS IN CAROTID ARTERY DISSECTION

C. Chaves and G. Lee

Department of Neurology and Department of Neuroradiology, Lahey Clinic, Burlington, MA, USA

Internal carotid artery (ICA) dissections are an increasingly recognized cause of stroke, particularly due to the development of non-invasive imaging techniques in the last few years. Most reported dissections involve the extracranial portion of the ICA, even though dissection of its intracranial portion has been more recognized and described recently.

Dissection is one of the most frequent etiologies of ischemic strokes in patients younger than 50, with no male/female preponderance.

Experimental knowledge

Dissections can be traumatic or spontaneous in origin. Most of the dissections are probably traumatic in origin, with minor or trivial trauma observed in 40% of the cases [90]. Such trivial traumas such as rapid head turning, unusual positions of the neck and head, prolonged bouts of coughing, vomiting and sneezing are often forgotten or not considered relevant by the patient and careful questioning is necessary to elicit them.

Connective tissue disorders (Ehlers-Danlos, Marfan syndrome, pseudoxanthoma elasticum), fibromuscular dysplasia, cystic medial necrosis, intimal fibroelastic aberrations have been associated with carotid dissections [40], [17] [42]. Intracranial aneurysms, polycystic kidney disease, widened aortic root and arterial redundancies (kinks, coils and loops) are also commonly associated with dissections suggesting an underlying generalized arteriopathy [17], [42], [10].

Migraines are more prevalent in patients with arterial dissections than in the general population [92]. The development of local vascular edema during a migrainous attack has been posited as a potential mechanism to the development of intracranial dissection in those patients [84].

Dissections usually involve the mobile portions of the arteries: the upper cervical segment of the extracranial ICA and the supraclinoid segment of its intracranial portion.

Dissections are produced by the penetration of circulating blood into the vessel wall. The dissection can involve the subintimal and intramedial layers causing stenosis or occlusion of the artery, or the subadventitial layer leading to an aneurysm formation. The hemorrhage can rupture back through the intima to the vessel lumen, producing a false lumen.

Okamoto et al. recently reported a study where experimental dissections were created in the common carotid arteries of mongrel dogs. Morphologic changes were closely related to the size of the intimal entry zone with small lesions resulting in spontaneous healing, medium lesions inducing aneurysm formation and large lesions causing stenosis or occlusion of the artery [72].

Clinical knowledge

Extracranial ICA dissection

Clinical presentation

Patients with extracranial ICA dissection usually present with ipsilateral sharp pain in the neck, jaw and pharynx associated with a throbbing unilateral headache [73], [35], [78], [16], [41], [86], [40], [20]. The pain usually precedes the development of ischemic strokes or transient ischemic attacks (TIAs) for a few days or weeks. A partial ipsilateral Horner syndrome (ptosis and miosis) is commonly observed and caused by involvement of the sympathetic fibers traveling along the ICA wall. Ipsilateral pulsatile tinnitus and lingual paresis can also be seen in some patients.

TIAs are common and can involve the ipsilateral eye or middle cerebral artery (MCA) territory. Most of them are felt to be secondary to distal cerebral hypoperfusion. Ischemic strokes usually involve the MCA territory and most of those patients have evidence of intra-arterial emboli from a thrombus on the site of the dissection [78], [41], [20].

The most common clinical presentation in patients with pseudoaneurysm formation is dysfunction of the lower cranial nerves (IX, X, XI, XII) at the skull base.

Approximately 5% of the patients with arterial dissection are asymptomatic and discovered incidentally [78].

Imaging studies

The diagnosis of extracranial ICA dissection can be made by noninvasive vascular imaging techniques such as ultrasonography, computed tomography angiography (CTA), and combined magnetic resonance imaging (MRI) and magnetic resonance angiography (MRA). Catheter angiography has been considered the gold standard for the diagnosis of arterial dissection [66], but in recent years its use has become limited to selected cases when the diagnosis of dissection is still indeterminate after non-invasive methods were used.

Ultrasound techniques
Ultrasound techniques, including extracranial Doppler, color-coded duplex ultrasonography and transcranial Doppler are usually abnormal in most patients with ICA dissection, but are rarely specific (Fig 1).

Common findings on Doppler are the presence of high-resistance bidirectional flow pattern along the ICA up to the mandibular region and reduced velocity in both proximal ICA and common carotid artery (CCA) reflecting a distal ICA obstruction [89], [45], [87].

With Duplex examination the most common direct sign is a tapering ICA lumen occurring in about 2/3 of the cases, while a double lumen and intimal flap are less commonly seen. Presence of a patent bulb despite an absent flow signal, stump flow, lack of wall pulsations and absent atheromatous plaque are commonly seen in patients with carotid dissection, but are less specific [89].

Transcranial Doppler can show compromise of the intracranial blood flow in the cerebral arteries distal to the ICA involved [87], [51] as well as high-intensity transient signals suggestive of intracranial microembolism from the dissected artery in the neck [85], [51], [8] (Fig. 2). Taken together, the overall sensitivity of those techniques to detect arterial dissection is approximately 95% [89].

The main limitations of this technique include suboptimal visualization of dissections in the distal ICA which is the most common location and pseudoaneurysms as well as technical difficulties associated with the presence of a short and/or large neck, poor transtemporal windows and high cervical bifurcations.

Magnetic resonance
Magnetic resonance imaging (MRI) and magnetic resonance angiography (MRA) of the neck can provide morphological details as well as document intraluminal blood flow, respectively, in patients with ICA dissection and is frequently the first choice of imaging studies in the work-up.

The typical MRI appearance of a dissected artery in cross-section is an increased diameter of the artery with an eccentric narrowed lumen caused by the presence of an intramural hematoma [36], [97], [74]. The hematoma can be crescent, oval or circumferential and can be detected on spin-echo T1- and T2-weighted images and fat suppressed T1-weighted techniques [37] (Fig. 3). The lumen containing a flow void indicating patency is usually the true lumen.

The signal intensity on T1- and T2-weighted images depends on the age of the hemorrhage [57]. In the acute phase the intramural hematoma appears isointense on T1 and hypointense on T2 (deoxyhemoglobin phase) and then becomes hyperintense in

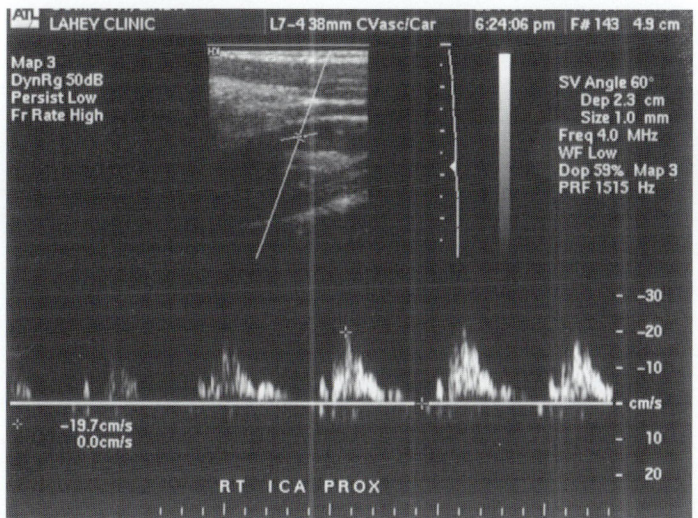
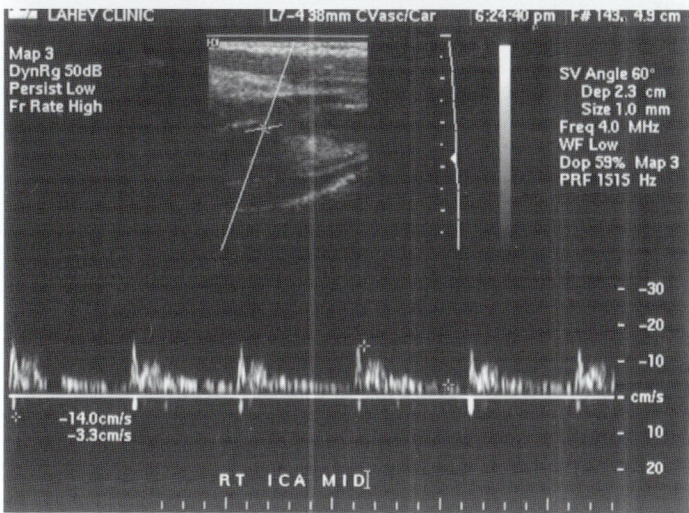
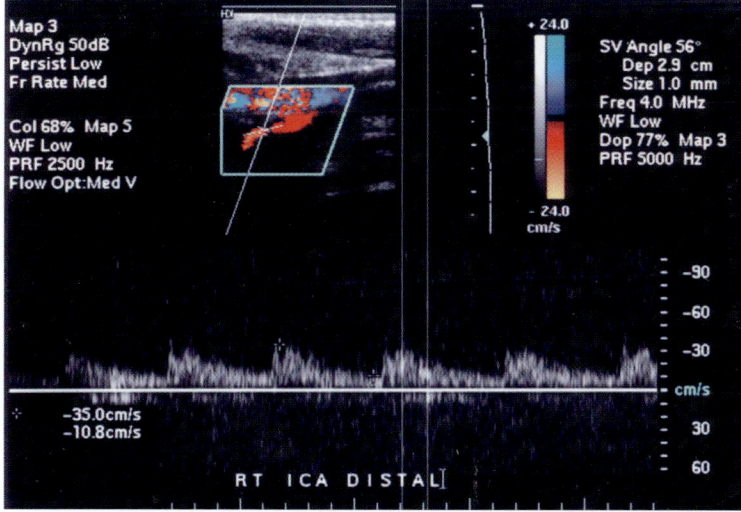

Fig. 1. Doppler scan showing reduced velocity in the proximal, mid and distal portions of the RICA in a patient with RICA dissection. Color Duplex scan (bottom) in the same patient showing the presence of diffuse narrowing of the submandibular portion of the RICA.

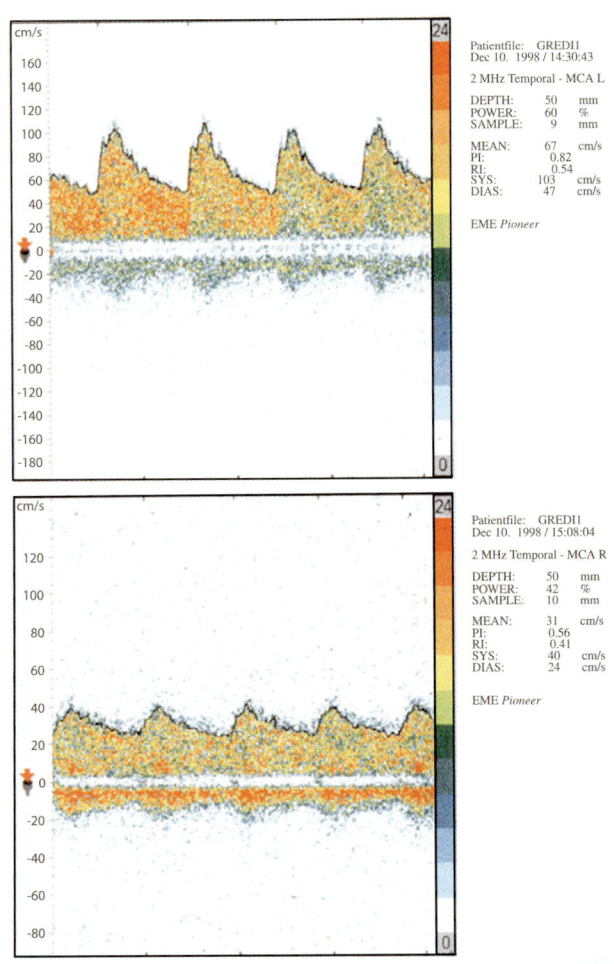
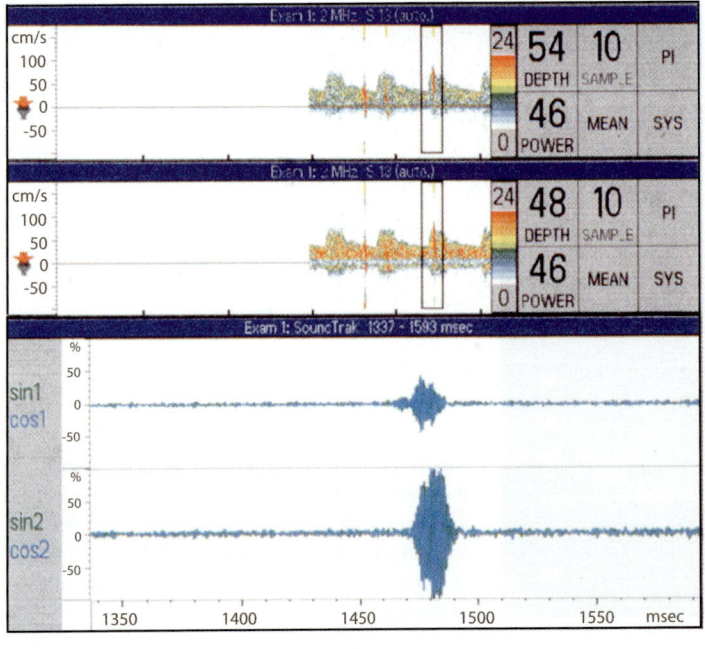

Fig. 2. Top: TDC in a patient with RICA dissection showing decreased velocity with blunted waveform in the ipsilateral MCA reflecting the compromised cerebral blood flow distal to the occlusion. Bottom: Presence of high intensity transit signals in a patient with RICA dissection suggestive of intracranial embolism.

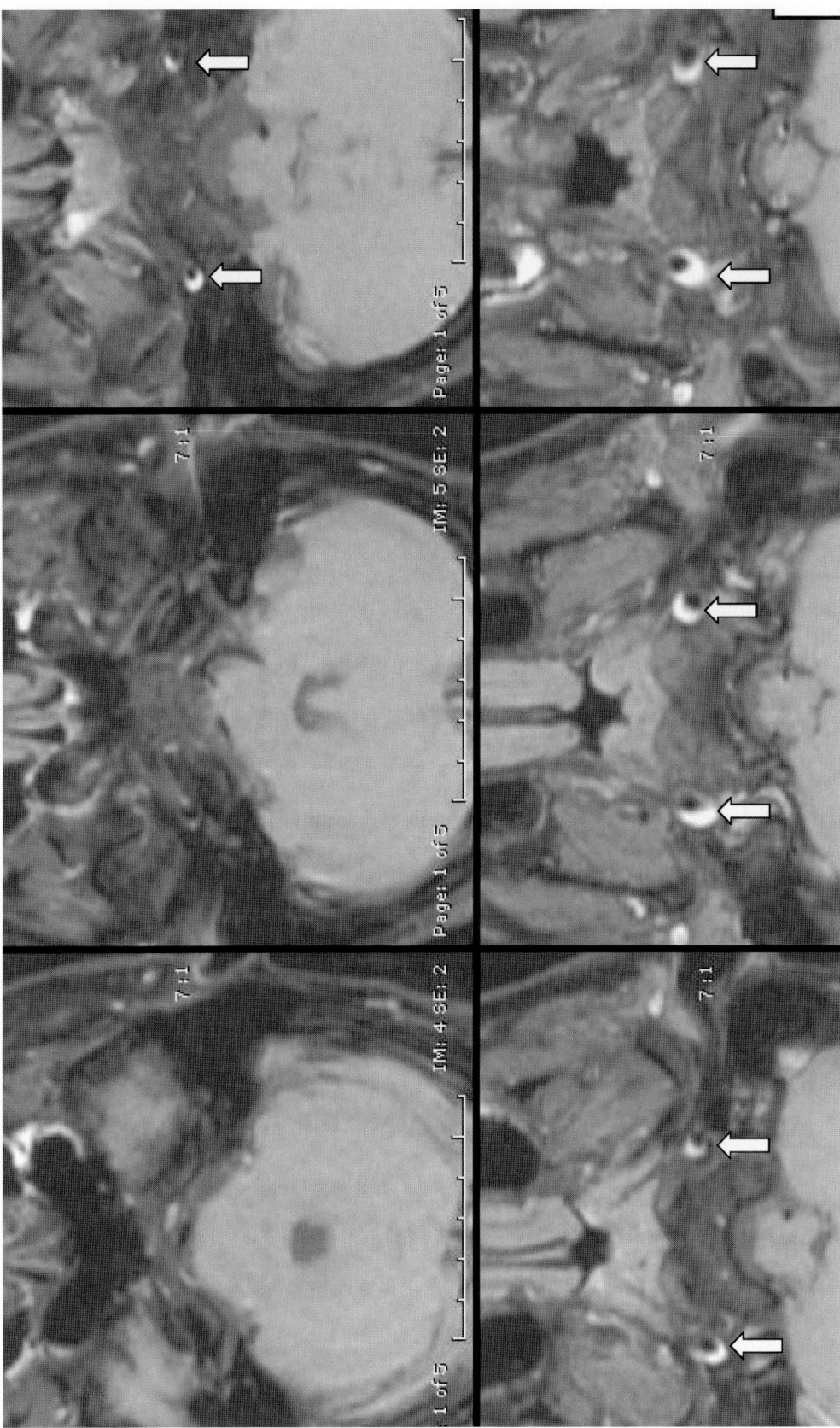

Fig. 3. Fat-suppressed T1-weighted imaging showing eccentric narrowed lumen and the presence of an intramural hematoma in both distal ICA suggestive of bilateral ICA dissection.

the subacute stage (methemoglobin phase). Because the high signal seen on T1-weighted images in the subacute stages of the hematoma can blend in with surrounding fat, fat-suppressed T1-weighted techniques are used to better delineate the subacute intramural hematoma, vessel wall thickening and overall vessel diameter [74]. The length of the dissection can also be estimated [36]. The abnormal signal can persist for several months and may be detected in 70% to 100% of dissected vessels [88], [97], [55], [89]. Other MRI findings include stenosis or occlusion of the carotid artery, but these markers lack specificity.

Three-dimensional time-of-flight magnetic resonance angiography (3D TOF MRA) without gadolinium can show the presence of a double-lumen, string sign, wall irregularity and aneurysmal dilatation, not usually seen on segmental MRI (33) (Figs. 4 and 5). Levy et al. showed 84% and 95% sensitivity for MRI and 3D TOF MRA respectively and 99% specificity for both techniques as compared with 4-vessel angiography. Two-dimensional time-of-flight (2D TOF) MRA can be used to cover a larger area although is more susceptible to artifacts from turbulent flow.

An important aspect of the axially acquired 2D TOF or 3D TOF MRA studies is the close inspection of the axial source data that can often demonstrate a double lumen as well as the intimal flap.

Limitations of MRI and MRA include: artifacts from swallowing or patient's movement, tendency to overestimate the degree of stenosis and difficulties detecting an acute hematoma and distinguishing it from slow flow or intraluminal thrombus [97], [7], [26]. MRI and MRA are also less sensitive than conventional angiography for detection of fibromuscular dysplasia [55], [26], [69] and aneurysmal dissection [55], [89].

Important advances have been made recently with the advent of MRA with contrast. MRA with gadolinium infusion allows a quick evaluation of the full extent of the cervical vessels from the arch to the intracranial segment as well as provides a high-quality image with less flow-related artifacts and in-plane saturation allowing a better evaluation of tortuous arteries, a more precise assessment of the degree of arterial stenosis and better detection of pseudoaneurysms [53] (Figs. 6 and 7). Slight luminal abnormalities may not be as well detected as compared with angiography [53] and subadventitial hematomas can also be missed [4].

Computed tomography (CT)
Conventional CT using dynamic CT technique (axial images at a single level during contrast administration) or dynamic incremental CT (dynamic CT with multilevel slices) has been used in patients in patients with cervical arterial dissection [97], [28], [76]. Narrowed eccentric lumen, mural thickening and thin annular contrast enhancement were the most common signs suggestive of arterial dissection using this technique.

With the advent of multidetector CT scanners, computed tomography angiography (CTA) has emerged as a non-invasive alternative for the diagnosis of cerebrovascular disease (Figs. 8–10). Leclerc et al. [54] found that a narrowed eccentric lumen at the upper segment of the ICA was a sensitive and specific finding in patients with a stenotic type of dissection, while an increase in external diameter was the most common finding in patients with occlusive-type dissection. Arterial wall thickening was very specific but less sensitive, while thin annular contrast enhancement was a less reliable sign. Since CTA is independent of flow phenomena, even small residual lumen and pseudoaneurysms causing slow or turbulent flow can be detected [71], [70], [33], [6]. However, subtle intimal flaps and intramural thrombi can escape detection with CTA [54], [70]. Also, the external wall of the vessel can be difficult to visualize accurately.

Angiography
Angiography has made it possible to classify carotid dissection into 3 patterns: stenotic, occlusive and aneurysmal types. The stenotic type [76], [6], [67], [15], [32] is the most frequent one and is characterized by a luminal narrowing usually irregular and ta-

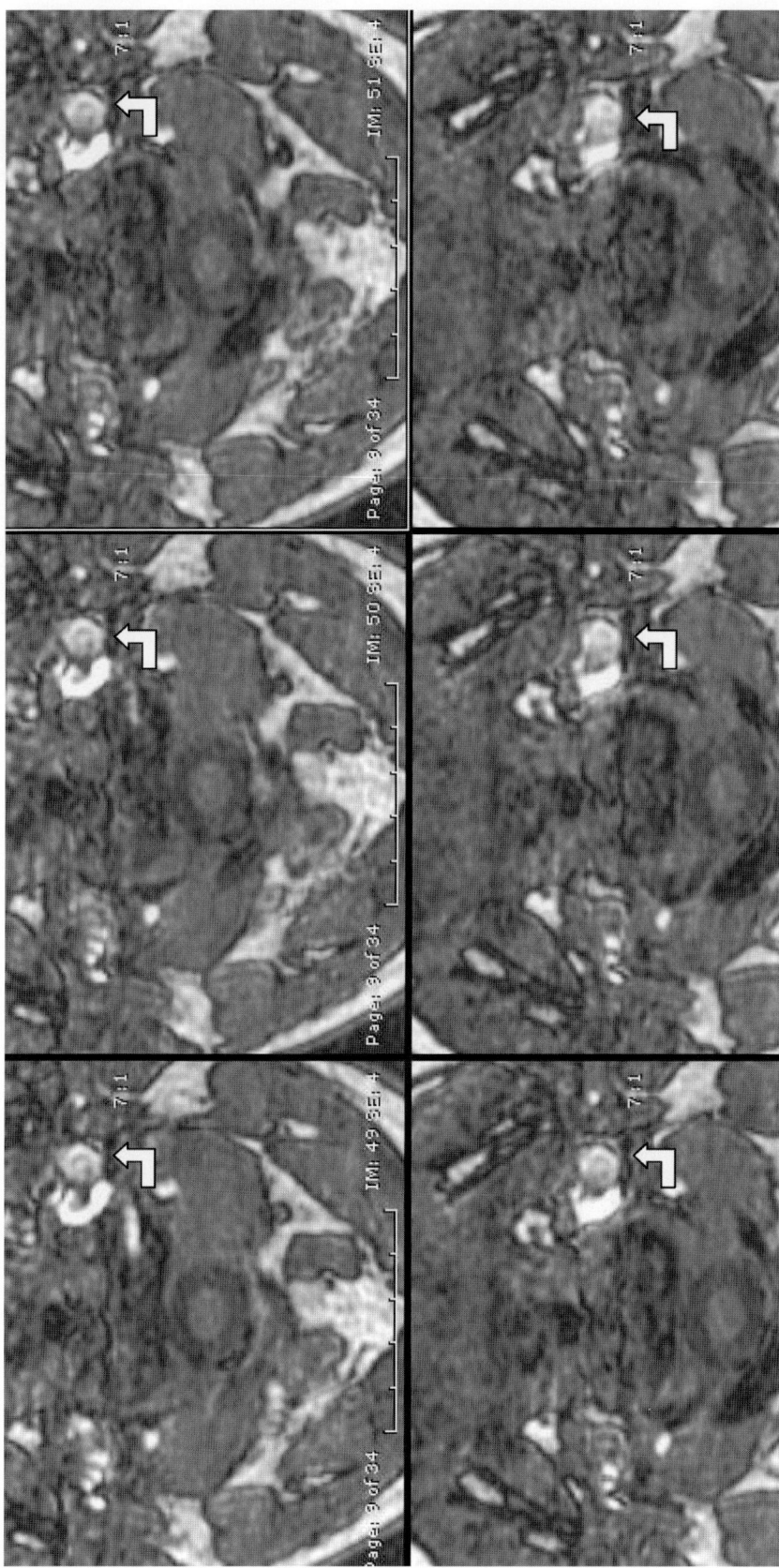

Fig. 4. Cross-section images of a 3D-TOF MRA showing a LICA pseudoaneurysm (bent-up arrow).

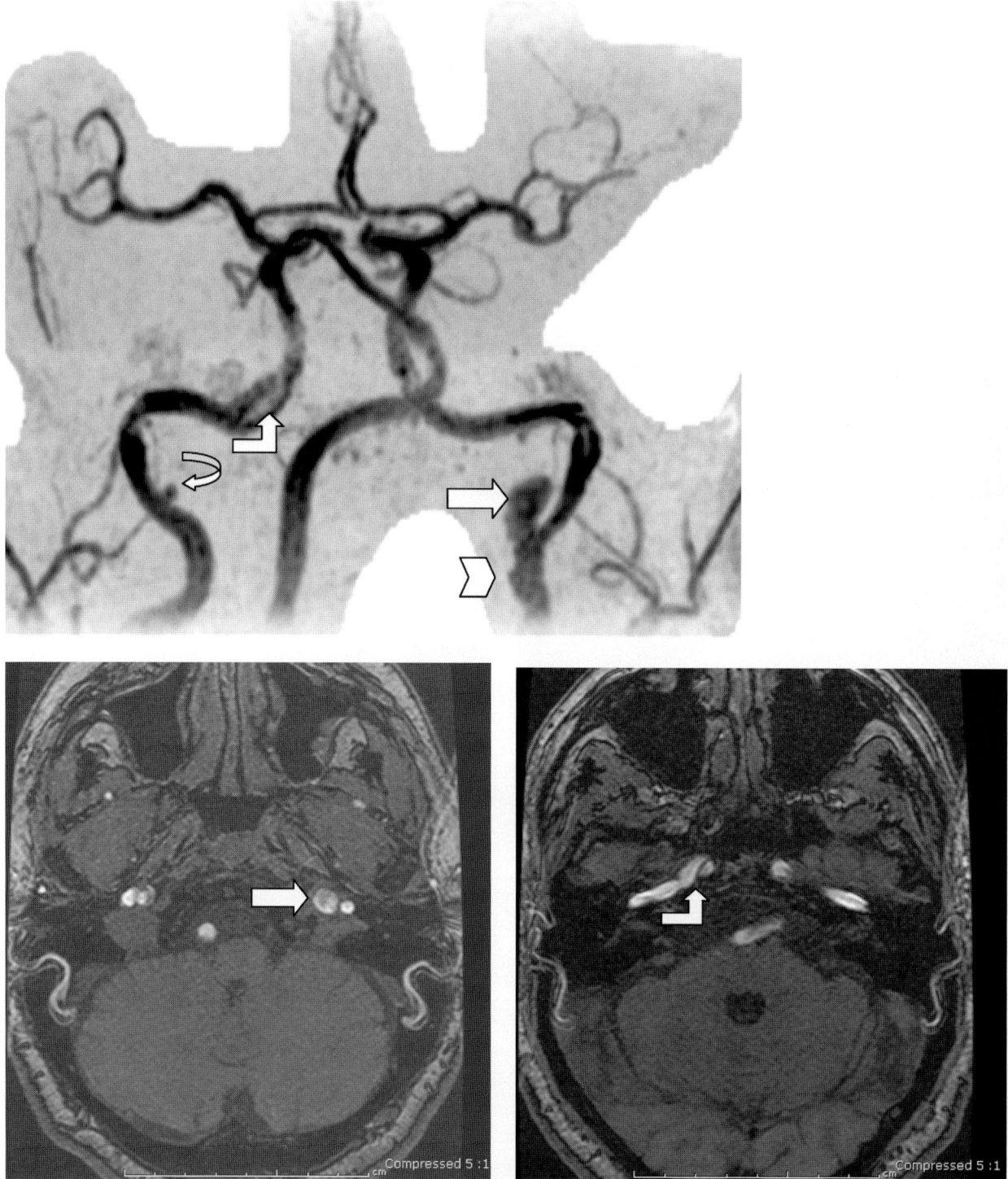

Fig. 5. 3D TOF MRA of the intracranial vessels, showing a large pseudoaneurysm (arrow) arising from the distal ICA below the level of entry in to the skull base with presence of irregularity proximal to this segment (arrow head). A small pseudoaneurysm in the RICA is also seen below the entry into the skull base (curved arrow). Presence of an intimal flap in the distal horizontal segment of the RICA (bent-up arrow).

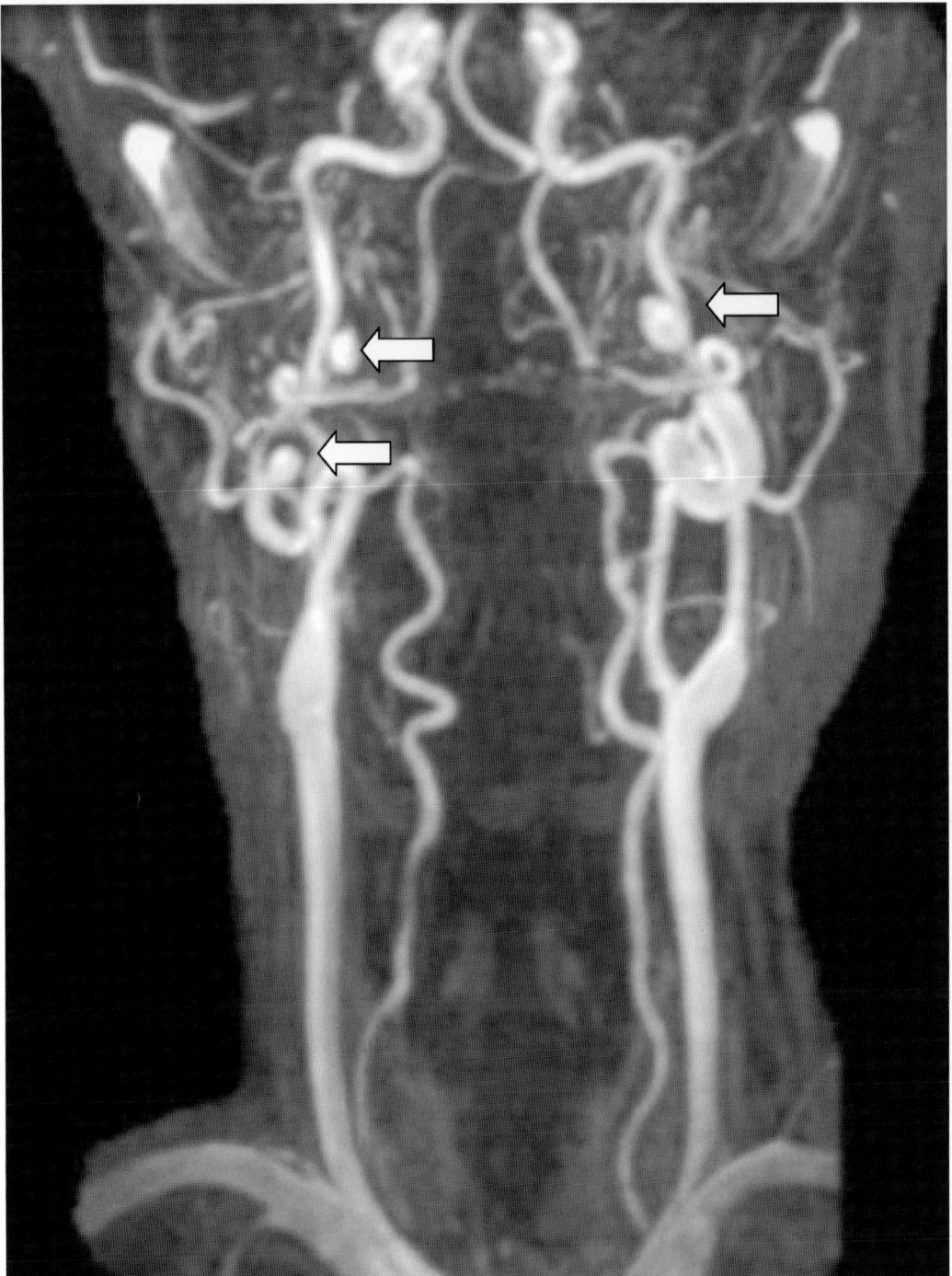

Fig. 6. MRA with gadolinium showing prominent tortuosity of both ICAs and presence of bilateral pseudoaneurysms (arrows).

pered that starts 2–3 cm above the bifurcation extending over several millimeters, often to the base of the skull ("string sign") (Fig. 11). Occasionally the dissection can extend to the cavernous portion of the carotid artery and sometimes involve the intracranial arteries. A carotid artery occlusion secondary to dis-

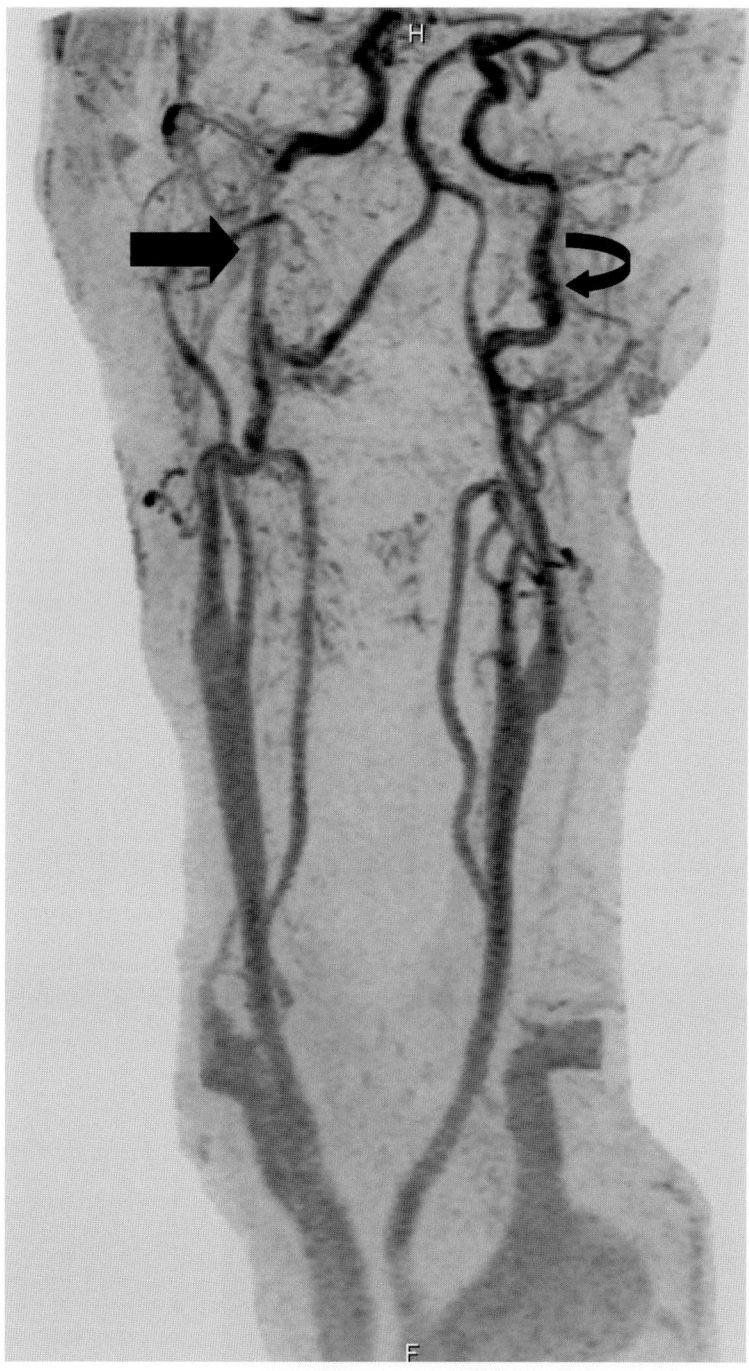

Fig. 7. MRA of the head and neck with gadolinium showing diffuse narrowing of the distal RICA (arrow) and mild iregularities of the distal LICA (curved arrow) compatible with bilateral ICA dissections.

section [6], [67], [15] also starts a few centimeters distal to the bifurcation and is characterized by a gradual tapering resembling a flame ("flame sign"). The incidence of dissecting aneurysms varies from 3% to 56% [76], [6], [67], [15], [32] and takes the appearance of an extraluminal pouch filled with contrast agent (Fig. 12). Occasionally the only abnormality seen in patients with carotid dissection is an irregularity of the vessel wall [15]. A combination of these different features may be observed as well.

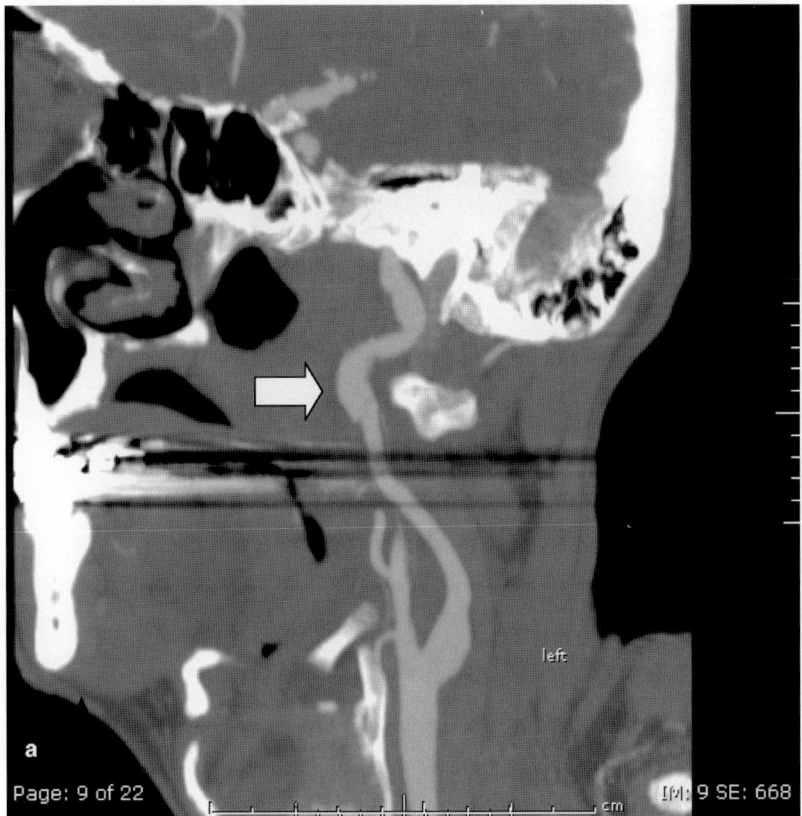

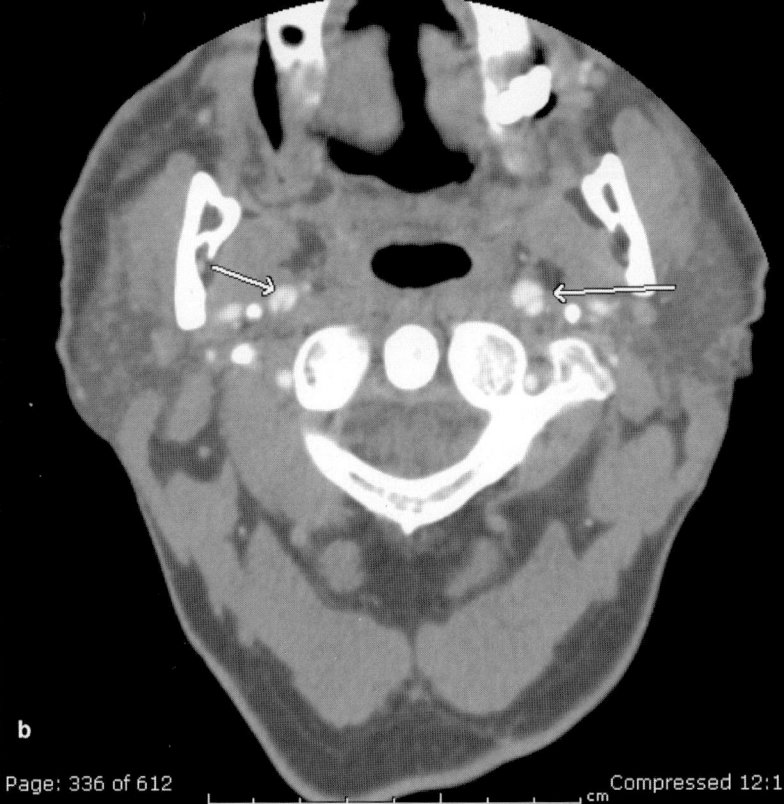

Fig. 8. a CTA of the neck from the same patient on Fig. 7 one week later showing a LICA pseudoaneurysm in the distal cervical segment; **b** CTA source images from the same patient showing bilateral ICA dissections.

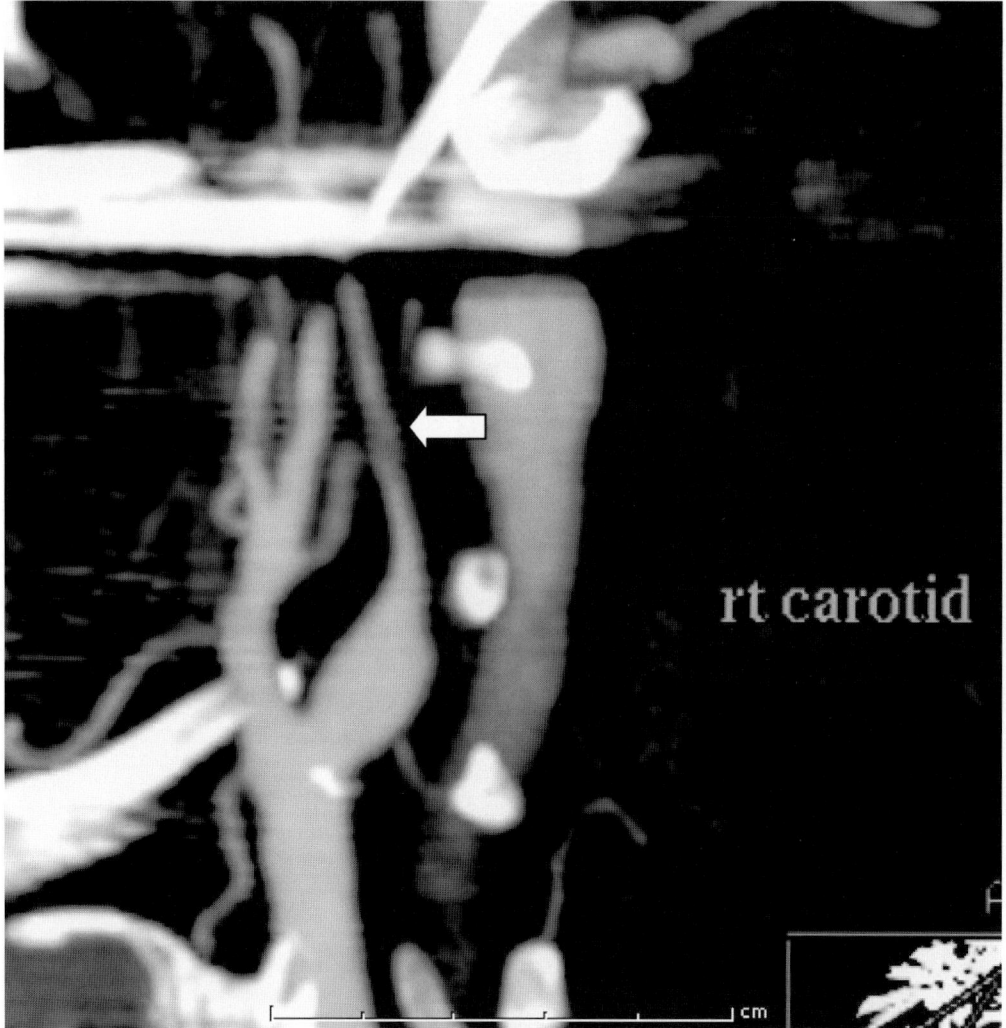

Fig. 9. CTA of the neck showing the presence of a luminal narrowing starting 2 cm above the RCA bifurcation and extending to the base of the skull (string sign).

Angiography can also document underlying abnormalities that can predispose to arterial dissections such as fibromuscular dysplasia and internal carotid artery redundancies (loops, coils and kinks).

Even though angiography is still considered the gold standard for diagnosis of carotid dissection, it carries an increased risk of complications [46] since it is an invasive technique. Also, a double lumen and intimal flaps are rarely visualized with this technique [6], [67], [16] and the external wall is also rarely visualized.

Differential diagnosis

Cluster headaches might be confounded with an ICA dissection since classically it presents as facial pain and an ipsilateral Horner's syndrome, however the episodes are usually brief and focal signs rarely occur [77].

Complicated migraine is also in the differential, even though most of the time, the patients recognize the attacks as their usual migraine. Changes in the characteristics of the headache should raise a red flag, since a possible association between mi-

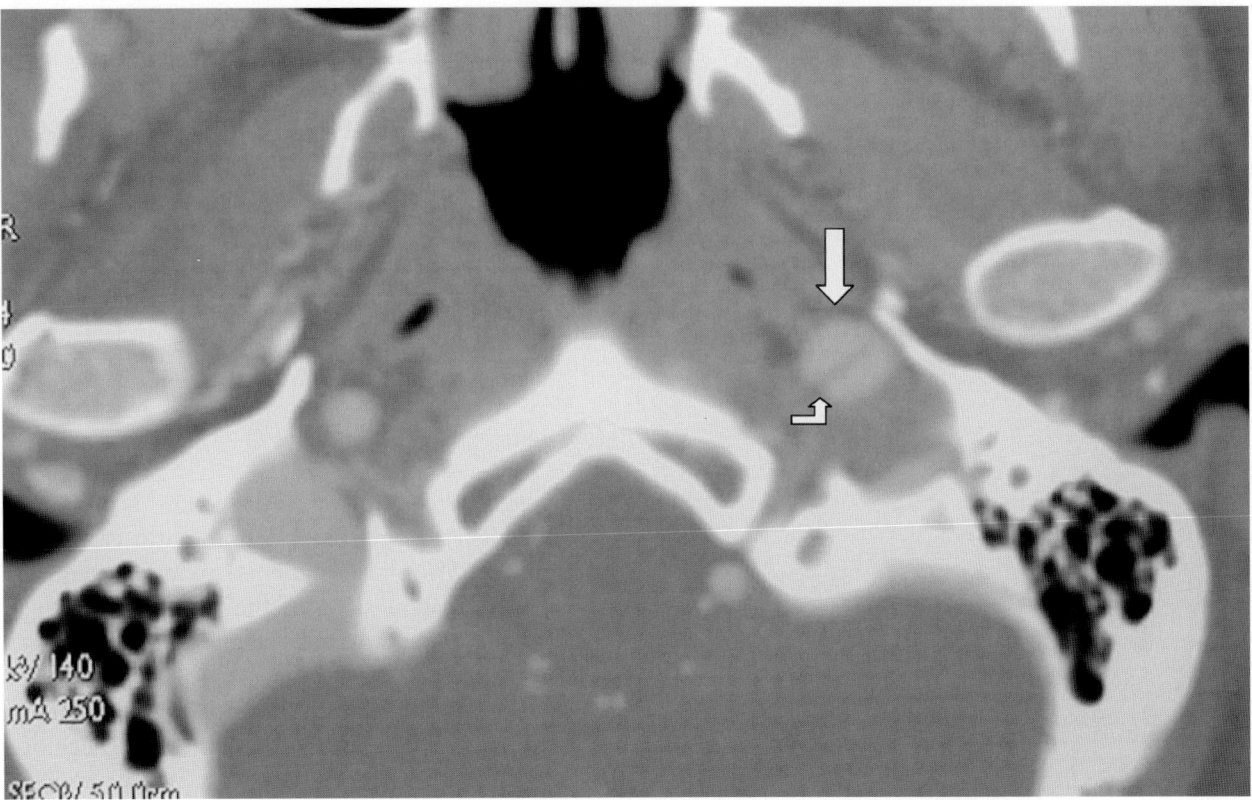

Fig. 10. CTA showing an increase in the diameter of the LICA (arrow) and the presence of an intimal flap (bent-up arrow).

graines and arterial dissections has been described [90], [37].

Herpes zoster involving the ophthalmic branch of the trigeminal nerve can also mimic dissection initially since it presents with unilateral facial pain and blurred vision before the typical rash develops [93].

Treatment

There have been no controlled trials of medical therapy for the treatment of ICA dissections. Some authors, with the goal of preventing intra-arterial embolism and further strokes, have advocated short-term anticoagulation with heparin followed by Coumadin [19], [79], [12], [58]. The long-term safety of antithrombotic therapy (anticoagulants or antiplatelets) has been shown in patients with carotid artery dissection [34] and the potential risk of a spread of mural hematoma, which has prevented some authors from using heparin, has never been demonstrated [40], [96]. The optimal duration of anticoagulation has not been established, but treatment for 3 to 6 months is usually advocated. Anticoagulation may be stopped earlier if complete recanalization is demonstrated or may be continued in cases of persistent stenosis of the artery. In patients with chronic occlusion of the artery, there is probably no benefit of continuing anticoagulation [19], [96].

The feasibility of IV TPA in patients with acute ischemic stroke secondary to carotid dissection has also been demonstrated [30], [5].

Fortunately in the vast majority of the cases there is complete recanalization and healing of the dissected arteries within the first few months of the initial event [90], [16], [87], [6], [67], [15]. However, in a subgroup of patients, the recanalization of the vessel fails to occur and patients are left with severely stenotic vessels, sometimes associated with

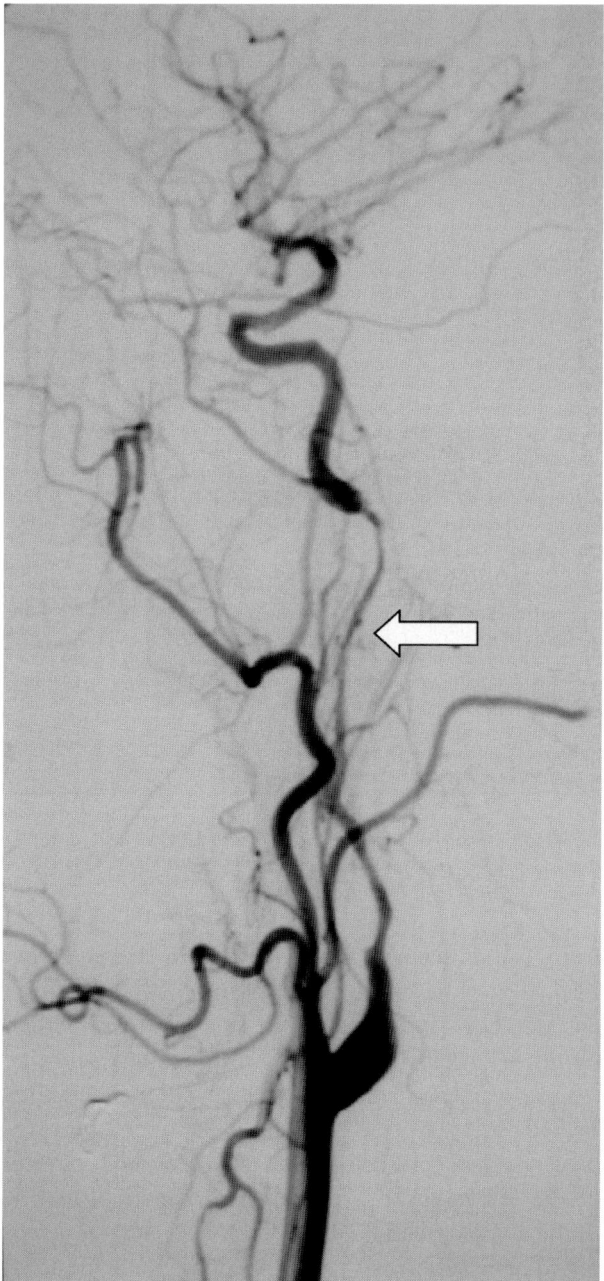

Fig. 11. Cerebral angiography showing a stenotic type of ICA dissection ("string sign").

pseudoaneurysm formation. In such cases anticoagulation will prevent further thromboembolic events, but not hemodynamic ones associated with low cerebral blood flow. Also, at times, anticoagulation may be contraindicated because of the risk of pseudoaneurysm rupture [3]. Occasionally, the false lumen can remain patent.

Surgeries including carotid ligation, resection with revascularization and bypass have been used when symptoms progress despite the best medical treatment or when a pseudoaneurysm is present. More recently, stents with and without coil placement have provided a new option for some of those patients with successful results [14], [23], [24], [59].

Prognosis

The prognosis of extracranial dissections is quite heterogeneous varying from asymptomatic cases (approximately 5% of the patients) to major sequelae and death in about 15% of the patients. However, most of the patients have excellent or good recovery [89], [87], [56].

Complete recanalization of the ICA occurs in approximately two thirds of patients with occluded vessels and 90% of patients with initial stenosis, usually within the first two months of symptom onset [90]. Rarely, recanalization is detected after 6 months of a dissection.

Recurrence rates for arterial dissection vary in different series from 3–8% [56], [11], [80] and are higher in younger patients, patients with positive family history or patients with an underlying arteriopathy [56], [11], [80], [81], [38].

Intracranial ICA dissection

Clinical presentation

Contrary to the patients with extracranial ICA dissection, patients with intracranial involvement usually present with a severe retro-orbital, frontal and/or temporal headache followed almost immediately by neurological signs [35], [22], [65], [95]. Fluctuation of the neurological signs during the first two weeks after symptom onset is common and likely secondary to cerebral hypoperfusion. The MCA territory is often involved [22].

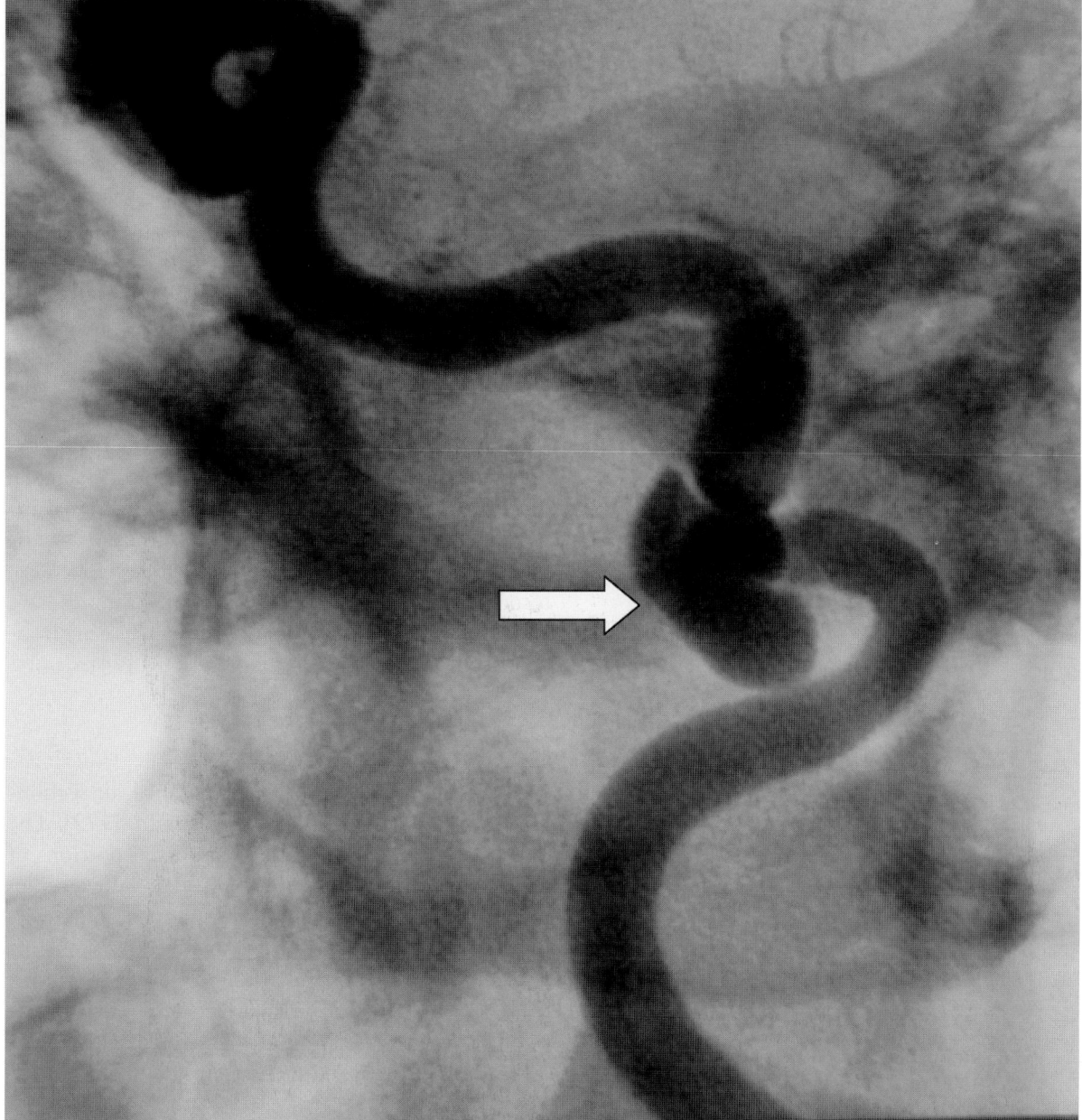

Fig. 12. Cerebral angiogram showing a saccular pseudoaneurysm (arrow) just below the skull base and immediately proximal to the carotid canal.

Even though more common in patients with vertebro-basilar dissection [60], [13], [2] subarachnoid hemorrhage due to rupture of a pseudoaneurysm has been reported in a few patients with intracranial carotid artery dissection [22], [62], [64], [43], [49].

Imaging studies

Most of the reports published so far have used angiography to diagnose those patients with intracranial dissection [22] (Figs. 13 and 14). Little is report-

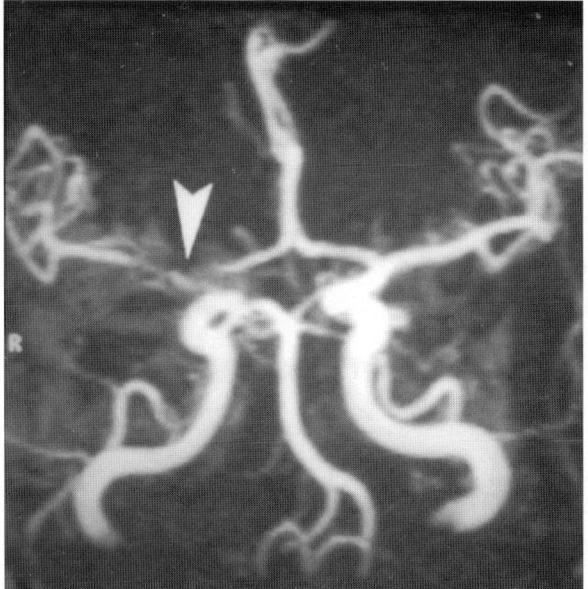
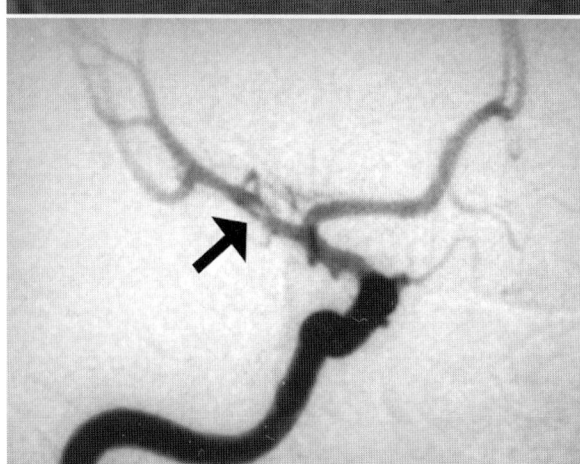
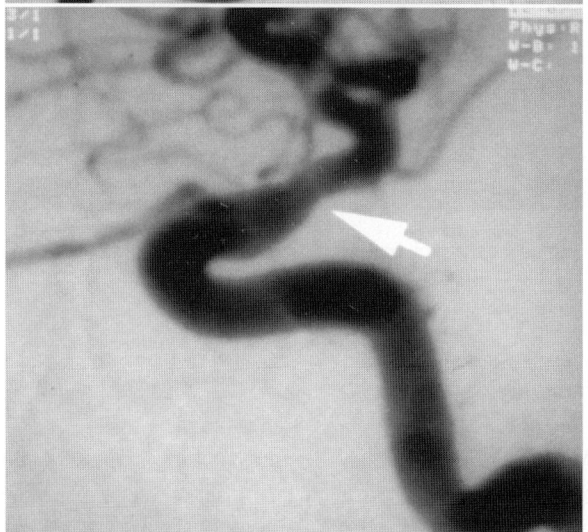

ed about the utility of other non-invasive imaging modalities, such as TCD, CTA and MRA, to diagnosis this condition.

The typical angiographic findings of intracranial ICA dissection are similar to those of its extracranial portion. String sign, double lumen (Fig. 13), irregular scalloped stenosis and vessel occlusion are usually seen when the dissection involves the subintimal and intramedial layers and aneurysm formation when the subadventitial layer is affected (Fig. 14) [10], [72], [73].

The most common intracranial site is the supraclinoid segment of the ICA with occasional extension to the MCA and/or ACA [72], [82].

Subarachnoid hemorrhage and aneurysm formation are common in patients with intracranial dissection, but rare in patients with extracranial involvement [13]. The presence of a thinner media and adventitial layers and lack of well-developed external elastica lamina in the intracranial arteries have been implicated as the main factors favoring subarachnoid hemorrhage in those patients [74].

Differential diagnosis

Occasionally patients with intracranial dissections have been diagnosed as having vasculitis [72]. The only vasculitis that can affect the distal portions of the ICA is giant cell arteritis [83]–[85]. However, in most of these patients, only the petrous and cavernous portions of the ICA are involved, without involvement of its supraclinoid portion [86]. Clinically, giant cell arteritis affects a much older population and is commonly associated with an increased erythrocyte sedimentation rate [87].

Treatment

The treatment of intracranial ICA dissection is controversial. The development of hemorrhagic trans-

Fig. 13. MRA of the head (left image) showing a filling defect (arrowhead) in the distal portion of the right ICA and proximal MCA. Cerebral angiography (right images) showing the presence of double lumen in the right MCA stem (black arrow) and a narrowing of the supraclinoid portion of the RICA (white arrow).

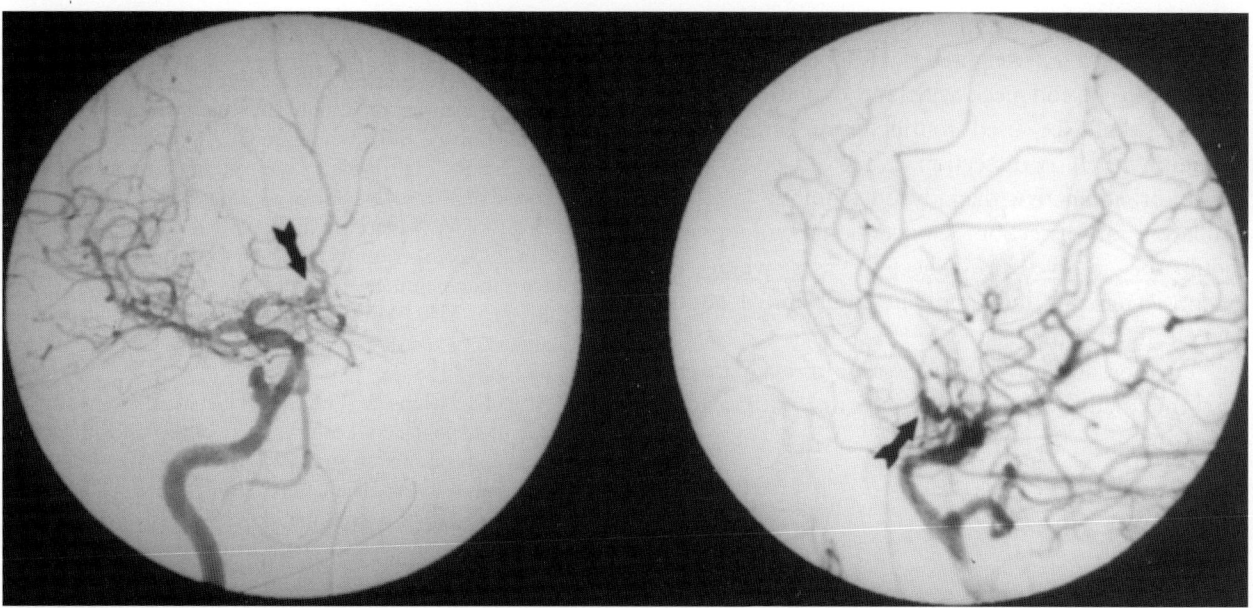

Fig. 14. Cerebral angiography showing an irregular aneurysm in the right A2 segment (left image, arrrow) with proximal narrowing of the right A1 segment and supraclinoid portion of the right ICA (right image, arrow).

formation and progression of the dissection during heparin treatment have prompted speculation that anticoagulation may be harmful in these patients [88], [89]. On the other hand, spontaneous progression in patients not anticoagulated has argued the opposite [90], [91].

Chaves et al. [72] reported no complication in patients with intracranial dissection treated with anticoagulation or antiplatelet treatment.

Surgical repair of intracranial dissections have been performed in patients with subarachnoid hemorrhage, but the incidence of spontaneous healing and recurrent bleeding is not known.

Prognosis

In contrast with most of the older literature [82], [92]–[94], in which massive stroke has been the rule with 75% mortality, most recent reports have shown better outcome probably due to a higher index of suspicion and improved diagnostic methods allowing antemortem diagnosis [72], [95], [96].

Aspects for the future

Further development of non-invasive imaging techniques will allow an easier detection of patients with intracranial dissection as well as of any associated underlying arteriopathy. High-field MRIs are currently being used primarily on an experimental basis and have shown to be a very promising technique allowing the identification of detailed morphologic changes in the brain and supplying vessels [97]–[99]. Perfusion MRI and CT have also been used recently in patients with cerebrovascular disease allowing the detection of areas of benign oligemia, penumbra and irreversibly infarcted tissue [100]–[102].

Hopefully, the advances in imaging techniques will translate into a better understanding of the stroke pathophysiology and a more rational therapeutic approach to those patients.

Take home message

Carotid artery dissections usually have a good prognosis and should be thought as a potential etiology of stroke and TIAs especially in young patients.

Non-invasive imaging techniques, in particular MRI (T1- and T2-weighted, fat-suppressed T1) and MRA of head and neck with and/or without gadolinium, should be used routinely for screening of patients with ICA dissection. CTA can be an alternative or adjunctive diagnostic technique used for evaluation of dissection. Conventional angiography should be reserved for selected cases where the diagnosis remains indeterminate after initial studies have been performed.

Further studies are necessary to evaluate the best therapeutic options for patients with arterial dissection.

References

[1] Adams C, Trevenen C: Middle cerebral artery dissection. Neuropediatrics 27: 331–332 (1996).
[2] Alom J, Matias-Guiu J, Padro L, Molins M, Romero F, Codina A: Spontaneous dissection of intracranial vertebral artery: clinical recovery with conservative treatment. J Neurol Neurosurg Psychiatry 49: 599–600 (1986).
[3] Anson J, Crowell RM: Cervicocranial arterial dissection. Neurosurgery 29: 89–96 (1991).
[4] Anzalone N, Strada L, Serra L et al.: Value of 3D contrast-enhanced MR: angiography in the diagnosis and follow-up of carotid and vertebral artery dissection. 2002 ASNR Annual Meeting Abstracts.
[5] Arnold M, Nedeltchev K, Sturzenegger M et al.: Thrombolysis in patients with acute stroke caused by cervical artery dissection: analysis of 9 patients and review of the literature. Arch Neurol 59: 549–553 (2002).
[6] Ast G, Woimant F, Georges B et al.: Spontaneous dissection of the internal carotid artery in 68 patients. Eur J Med 2: 466–472 (1993).
[7] Auer D, Karnath HO, Nagele T et al.: Noninvasive investigation of pericarotid syndrome: role of MR angiography in the diagnosis of internal carotid dissection [Review]. Headache 35: 163–168 (1995).
[8] Babikian VL, Forteza AM, Gavrilescu T, Samaraweera R: Cerebral microembolism and extracranial internal carotid artery dissection. J Ultrasound Med 15: 863–866 (1996).
[9] Bakke SJ, Smith HJ, Kerty E, Dahl A: Cervicocranial artery dissection. Detection by Doppler ultrasound and MR angiography. Acta Radiol 37: 529–534 (1996).
[10] Barbour PJ, Castaldo JE, Rae-Grant AD: Internal carotid artery redundancy is significantly associated with dissection. Angiographically based study comparing 13 patients with dissection and 108 without. Stroke 25: 1201–1206 (1994).
[11] Bassetti C, Carruzzo A, Sturzenegger M et al.: Recurrence of cervical artery dissection. A prospective study of 81 patients. Prospective study of cervical dissection recurrence. Dissections recur in 45 of cases during a mean follow-up period of 34 months. Stroke 27: 1804–1807 (1996).
[12] Beletsky V, Nadareishvili Z, Lynch J et al.: Canadian Stroke Consortium. Cervical arterial dissection: time for a therapeutic trial? Stroke 34: 2856–2860 (2003).
[13] Berger MS, Wilson CB: Intracranial dissecting aneurysms of the posterior circulation. J Neurosurg 61: 882–894 (1984).
[14] Biggs KL, Chiou AC, Hagino RT et al.: Endovascular repair of a spontaneous carotid artery dissection with carotid stent and coils. J Vasc Surg 40: 170–173 (2004).
[15] Biousse V, D'Anglejan-Chatillion J, Touboul PJ et al.: Time course of symptoms in extracranial carotid artery dissections. A series of 80 patients [Review]. Stroke 26: 235–239 (1995).
[16] Bogousslavsky J, Despland PA, Regli F: Spontaneous carotid dissection with acute stroke. Arch Neurol 44: 137–140 (1987).
[17] Brandt T, Hausser I, Orberk E et al.: Ultrastructural connective tissue abnormalities in patients with spontaneous cervicocerebral artery dissections. Ann Neurol 44: 281–285 (1998).
[18] Campeau NG, Huston J 3rd, Bernstein MA et al.: Magnetic resonance angiographic at 3.0 Tesla: initial clinical experience. Top Magn Reson Imaging 12: 183–204 (2001).
[19] Caplan LR, Biousse V: Cervicocranial arterial dissections. J Neuro-Ophthalmol 24: 299–305 (2004).
[20] Chakeres DW, Abduljalil AM, Novak P et al.: Comparison of 1.5 and 8 Tesla high-resolution magnetic resonance imaging of lacunar infarcts. J Comput Assist Tomogr 26: 628–632 (2002).
[21] Chang V, Rewcastle NB, Harwood-Nash DC et al.: Bilateral dissecting aneurysms of the intracranial internal carotid arteries in an 8 year-old boy. Neurology 25: 573–579 (1975).
[22] Chaves C, Estol C, Esnaola MM et al.: Spontaneous Intracranial Carotid Artery Dissection – Report of ten patients. Arch Neurol 59: 977–981 (2002).
[23] Cohen JE, Tamir B-H, Rajz G et al.: Endovascular Stent-Assisted angioplasty in the management of traumatic internal carotid artery dissections. Stroke 36: e45–e47 (2005).
[24] Cohen JE, Leker RR, Gotkine M et al.: Emergent Stenting to treat patients with carotid artery dissection. Stroke 34: e254–e257 (2003).
[25] Connett MC, Lansche JM: Fibromuscular hyperplasia of the internal carotid artery: Report of a case. Ann Surg 162: 59–62 (1965).

[26] Culebras A, Kase CS, Masdeu JC et al.: Practice guidelines for the use of imaging in transient ischemic attacks and acute stroke. A report of the Stroke Council, American Heart Association. Stroke 28: 1480–1497 (1997).

[27] Cull RE: Internal carotid artery occlusion caused by giant cell arteritis. J Neurol Neurosurg Psychiatry 42: 1066–1067 (1979).

[28] Dal Pozzo G, Mascalchi M, Fonda C et al.: Lower cranial nerve palsy due to dissection of the internal carotid artery: CT and MRI imaging. J Comput Assist Tomogr 13: 989–995 (1989).

[29] Davis SM, Donnan GA: Advances in penumbra imaging with MR. Cerebrovasc Dis 17: 23–27 (2004).

[30] Derex L, Nighoghossian N, Turjman F et al.: Intravenous tPA in acute ischemic stroke related to internal carotid artery dissection. Neurology 54: 2159–2161 (2000).

[31] Duyff RF, Snijders CJ, Vanneste JAL: Spontaneous bilateral internal carotid artery dissection and migraine: a potential diagnostic delay. Headache 37: 109–112 (1997).

[32] Ehrenfeld WK, Wylie EJ: Spontaneous dissection of the internal carotid artery. Arch Surg 111: 1294–1301 (1976).

[33] Elijovich L, Kazmi K, Law M: Diagnosis of carotid artery dissection: is multi-slice detector CT Angiography better than MR Angiography? [Abstract]

[34] Engelter ST, Lyrer PA, Kirsch EC et al.: Long-term follow-up after extracranial internal carotid artery dissection. Eur Neurol 44: 199–204 (2000).

[35] Fisher CM, Ojemann RG, Roberson GH: Spontaneous dissection of cervicocerebral arteries. Can J Neurol Sci 5: 9–19 (1978).

[36] Gelbert F, Assouline E, Hodes JE et al.: MRI in spontaneous dissection of vertebral and carotid arteries: 15 cases studied at 0.5 Tesla. Neuroradiology 33: 111–113 (1991).

[37] Goldberg HI, Grossman RI, Gomori JM, Asbury AK, Bilanuek LT, Zimmerman RA: Cervical internal carotid artery dissecting hemorrhage: diagnosis using MR. Radiology 158: 157–161 (1986).

[38] Goldstein LB, Gray L, Hulette CM: Stroke due to recurrent ipsilateral carotid artery dissection in a young adult. Case report of an ipsilaterally recurring ICA dissection. Microscopic examination of the resected pseudoaneurysm showed abnormalities consistent with fibromuscular dysplasia, while conventional angiography failed to demonstrate the usual features. Stroke 26: 480–483 (1995).

[39] Grosman H, Fomasier VL, Bonder D et al.: Dissecting aneurysm of the cerebral arteries. J Neurosurg 53: 693–697 (1980).

[40] Guillon B, Levy C, Bousser MG: Internal carotid artery dissection: an update. J Neurol Sci 153: 146–158 (1998).

[41] Hart RG, Easton JD: Dissection of cervical and cerebral arteries. Neurologic Clin 1: 155–182 (1983).

[42] Hausser I, Muller U, Engelter S et al.: Different types of connective tissue alterations associated with cervical artery dissections. Acta Neuropathol (Berlin) 107: 509–514 (2004).

[43] Hayashi N, Fukuda O, Endo S et al.: Intracerebral hemorrhage secondary to dissecting aneurysm of the anterior cerebral artery. No To Shinkei 48: 1053–1056 (1996).

[44] Hegedus K: Dissecting intracranial aneurysm. Arch Psychiatr Nervenkr 232: 25–32 (1982).

[45] Hennerici M, Steinke W, Rautenberg W: High-resistance Doppler flow pattern in extracranial carotid dissection. Arch Neurol 46: 670–672 (1989).

[46] Hessel SJ, Adams DF, Abrams HL: Complications of angiography. Radiology 138: 273–281 (1981).

[47] Hochberg FH, Bean C, Fisher CM et al.: Stroke in a 15 year-old girl secondary to terminal carotid dissection. Neurology 25: 725–729 (1975).

[48] Howard GF 3rd, Ho SU, Kim KS et al.: Bilateral carotid artery occlusion resulting from giant cell arteritis. Ann Neurol 15: 204–207 (1984).

[49] Kawaguchi T, Kawano T, Kazekawa K et al.: Dissecting aneurysm of the middle cerebral artery with subarachnoid hemorrhage and brain infarction: a case report. No Shinkei Geka 25: 1033–1037 (1997).

[50] Kidwell CS, Alger JR, Saver JL: Beyond mismatch: evolving paradigms in imaging the ischemic penumbra with multimodal magnetic resonance imaging. Stroke 34: 2729–2735 (2003).

[51] Koennecke HC, Trocio SH, Mast H et al.: Microemboli on transcranial Doppler in patients with spontaneous carotid artery dissection. J Neuroimag 7: 217–220 (1997).

[52] Koyama S, Kotani A, Sasaki J: Spontaneous dissecting aneurysm of the anterior cerebral artery: Report of two cases. Surg Neurol 46: 55–61 (1996).

[53] Leclerc X, Lucas C, Godefroy O et al.: Preliminary experience using contrast-enhanced MR angiography to assess vertebral artery structure for the follow-up of suspected dissection. AJNR 20: 1482–1490 (1999).

[54] Leclerc X, Godefroy O, Salhi A et al.: Helical CT for the diagnosis of extracranial internal carotid artery dissection. Stroke 27: 461–466 (1996).

[55] Levy C, Laissy JP, Raveau V et al.: Carotid and vertebral artery dissections: three-dimensional time-of-flight MR angiography and MR imaging versus conventional angiography. Radiology 190: 97–103 (1994).

[56] Leys D, Moulin T, Stojkovic T et al.: DONALD investigators. Follow-up of patients with history of cervical artery dissection. One of the largest series of cervical dissections with long-term follow-up assessment. Cerebrovasc Dis 5: 43–49 (1995).

[57] Long TD, Carter MP, Reynolds T: Spontaneous internal carotid artery dissection shown by magnetic resonance imaging. South Med J 84: 1140–1142 (1991).
[58] Lyrer P, Engelter S.: Antithrombotic drugs for carotid artery dissection. Cochrane Database Syst Rev 3: CD000255 (2003).
[59] Malek AM, Higashida RT, Phatouros CC et al.: Endovascular management of extracranial carotid artery dissection achieved using stent angioplasty. AJNR 21: 1280–1292 (2000).
[60] Manz HJ, Luessenhop AJ: Dissecting aneurysm of intracranial vertebral artery: a case report and review of literature. J Neurol 230: 25–35 (1983).
[61] Manz HJ, Vester J, Lavenstein B: Dissecting aneurysm of cerebral arteries in childhood and adolescence. Virchows Arch [Pathol Anat] 384: 325–335 (1979).
[62] Massoud TF, Anslow P, Molyneux AJ: Subarachnoid hemorrhage following spontaneous intracranial carotid artery dissection. Neuroradiology 34: 33–35 (1992).
[63] Meuli RA: Imaging viable brain tissue with CT scan during acute stroke. Cerebrovasc Dis 17 Suppl 3: 28–34 (2004).
[64] Miyahara K, Sakata K, Gondo G et al.: Spontaneous dissection of the anterior cerebral artery presenting subarachnoid hemorrhage and cerebral infarction: a case report. No Shinkei Geka 29: 335–339 (2001).
[65] Mizutani T, Golberg HI, Parr J et al.: Cerebral dissecting aneurysm and intimal fibroelastic thickening of cerebral arteries. J Neurosurg 56: 571–576 (1982).
[66] Mokri B, Houser W, Sandok BA et al.: Spontaneous dissections of the vertebral arteries. Neurology 38: 880–885 (1988).
[67] Mokri B, Sundt TM Jr, Houser OW et al.: Spontaneous dissection of the cervical internal carotid artery. Ann Neurol 19: 126–138 (1986).
[68] Moore P, Richardson B: Neurology of the vasculitides and connective tissue disease. J Neurol Neurosurg Psych 65: 10–22 (1998).
[69] Nguyen Bui, Brant-Zawadzki M, Verghese P et al.: Magnetic resonance angiography of cervicocranial dissection. Stroke 24: 126–131 (1993).
[70] Nunez DB Jr., Torres-Leon M, Munera F: Vascular injuries of the neck and thoracic inlet: Helical CT-angiographic correlation. RadioGraphics 24: 1087–1100 (2004).
[71] Oelerich M, Stogbauer F, Kurlemann G et al.: Craniocervical arterial dissection . MR imaging and MR angiographic findings. Eur Radiol 9: 1385–1391 (1999).
[72] Okamoto T, Miyachi S, Negoro M et al.: Experimental model of dissecting aneurysms. AJNR 23: 577–584.
[73] Ojemann RG, Fisher CM, Rich JC: Spontaneous dissecting aneurysms of the internal carotid artery. Stroke 3: 434–500 (1972).
[74] Ozdoba C, Sturzenegger M, Schroth G: Internal carotid artery dissection: MR imaging features and clinico-radiologic correlation. Radiology 199: 191–198 (1996).
[75] Pessin MS, Adelman LS, Barbas NR: Spontaneous intracranial carotid artery dissection. Stroke 20: 1100–1113 (1989).
[76] Petro GR, Witwer GA, Cacayorin ED et al.: Spontaneous dissection of the cervical internal carotid artery: correlation of arteriography, CT, and pathology. AJR Am Roentgenol 148: 393–398 (1987).
[77] Rosebraugh CJ, Griebel DJ, DiPette DJ: A case report of carotid artery dissection presenting with a cluster headache. Am J Med 102: 418–419 (1997).
[78] Schievink WI: Spontaneous dissection of the carotid and vertebral arteries. N Engl J Med 344: 898–906 (2001).
[79] Schievink WI: The treatment of spontaneous carotid and vertebral artery dissections. Curr Opin Cardiol 15: 316–321 (2000).
[80] Schievink WI, Mokri B, Piepgras DG et al.: Recurrent spontaneous arterial dissections. Risk in familial versus nonfamilial disease. Study of the risk recurrence among 200 patients with cervical dissection. Family history of arterial dissection is the main risk factor. Stroke 27: 622–624 (1996).
[81] Schievink WI, Mokri B, O'Fallon WM: Recurrent spontaneous cervical artery dissection. Long-term follow-up study of 200 patients with cervical dissection (163 involving the ICA), with emphasis on the risk of recurrence. N Engl J Med 330: 393–397 (1994).
[82] Schievink WI, Mokri B, Piepgras DG: Spontaneous dissections of cervicocephalic arteries in childhood and adolescence. Neurology 44: 1607–1612 (1994).
[83] Schmitt F, Grosu D, Mohr C et al.: 3 Tesla MRI: successful results with higher field strengths. Radiologe 44(1): 1–47 (2004).
[84] Sinclair W: Dissecting aneurysm of the middle cerebral artery associated with migraine syndrome. Am J Pathol 29: 1083 (1953).
[85] Srinivasan J, Newell DW, Sturzenegger M et al.: Transcranial Doppler in the evaluation of internal carotid artery dissection. Stroke 27: 1226–1230 (1996).
[86] Stapf C, Elkind MSV, Mohr JP: Carotid dissection. Annu Rev Med 51: 329–347 (2000).
[87] Steinke W, Rautenberg W, Schwartz A et al.: Non-invasive monitoring of internal carotid artery dissection. Assessment of ultrasound methods in 48 patients in the early stage and at follow-up. Demonstration of its accuracy in the recanalization process. Stroke 25: 998–1005 (1994).
[88] Stringaris K, Liberopoulos K, Giaka E et al.: Three-dimensional time-of-flight MR angiography and MR imaging versus conventional angiography in carotid artery dissections. Int Angiol 15: 20–25 (1996).
[89] Sturzenegger M, Mattle HP, Rivoir A: Baumgartner RW. Ultrasound findings in carotid artery dissection: analysis of 43 patients. Neurology 45: 691–698 (1995).

[90] Sturzenegger M: Spontaneous internal carotid artery dissection: early diagnosis and management in 44 patients. A large series of spontaneous ICA dissection. J Neurol 242: 231–238 (1995).
[91] Thielen KR, Wijdicks EF, Nichols DA: Giant cell (temporal) arteritis: involvement of the vertebral and internal carotid arteries. Mayo Clin Proc 73: 444–446 (1998).
[92] Tzourio C, Benslamia L, Guillon B et al.: Migraine and the risk of cervical artery dissection: a case-control study. Neurology 59: 435–437 (2002).
[93] Verghese J, Kachroo A, Sparr SA: Herpes zoster ophthalmicus mimicking carotid artery dissection: a case report. Headache 37: 663–664 (1997).
[94] Wilkinson IMS, Russell RWR: Arteries of the head and neck in giant cell arteritis. A pathological study to show the pattern of arterial involvement. Arch Neurol 27: 378–391 (1972).
[95] Yonas H, Agamanolis D, Takaoka Y et al.: Dissecting intracranial aneurysms. Surg Neurol 8: 407–415 (1977).
[96] Zetterling M, Carlstrom C, Konrad P: Internal carotid artery dissection. Review article. Acta Neurol Scand 101: 1–7 (2000).
[97] Zuber M, Meary E, Meder JF et al.: Magnetic resonance imaging and dynamic CT scan in cervical arterial dissections. Stroke 25: 576–581 (1994).

Chapter 2.3

HIGH SUITED CAROTID ARTERY STENOSIS AND IMAGING

B. Butz

Department of Radiology, University Hospital, Regensburg, Germany

Introduction

A stenosis of the internal carotid artery is typically irregular and approximately up to two centimeters distal the bifurcation. However, this is not what it is meant here. The so-called "high suited carotid artery stenoses" are different with respect to imaging procedure, more diagnosis, and particulary in treatment planning, and are a little bit complex than the stenoses just around the bifurcation. It is very important to understand the diagnostic techniques and therapy of traumatic or postsurgery carotid artery dissections and the complex intracranial stenosis. Furthermore, imaging and therapy of atherosclerotic extracranial brachiocephalic stenoses must also be considered. This chapter provides an overview of the various imaging options available, including a specific workflow in case of an emergency (traumatic lesions) and finally a discussion of the clinical, diagnostic and therapeutic knowledge based on the current literature.

Useful imaging techniques

Clinical and radiographic data should be combined for the selection of the most appropriate patients for surgical or interventional therapy.

Ultrasonographic assessment is often used as the initial diagnostic test. Abnormal flow pattern, stenoses, intramural hematoma or an intimal flap are seen as specific changes [20]. A combination of Doppler color-flow ultrasound and transcranial ultrasonography provides even more useful information. Unfortunately, limitations exist with this method due to the high variability of results depending on the physician, the device used and the measuring methods, e.g. the angle of measurement. For all types of carotid artery stenosis an overall sensitivity of 64–100% has been described [44].

Digital subtraction angiography is still the gold standard in imaging the carotid arteries. Transfemoral catheter arteriograms with aortic arch injection and selective catheterization of both carotid arteries and documentation of three different views (posterior–anterior, lateral and 45° oblique) of both internal carotid arteries are usually performed. Important information regarding intracranial circulation is obtained as well. Results are usually somewhat better in the skull base or petrous part of the carotid artery as are possible with computed or magnetic resonance tomography. Digital subtraction angiography methods are still indispensable for interventional procedures, but for diagnostic use, computed or magnetic resonance tomography methods are replacing digital subtraction angiography due to the non-invasive nature of the techniques and the fact, that the resolution now approaches that of the conventional angiography.

Computed tomography (CT) assessment of the carotid arteries has become increasingly important in recent years. Not only the single row CT scanners, but moreover the modern multislice CT scanners (e.g., 16-row, 64-row MSCT) is becoming more widely available for CT angiography. CT angiography has high diagnostic potential and provides information about vessel pathology, thrombus, intramural hematoma or aneurysmal dilatation as well as the surrounding tissue. Multislice scanners have excellent temporal and spatial resolution and multiplanar reformations can be done in each orientation to help visualize the extent of the dissection. Moreover, it is possible to image the entire supraaortic vessel system from the aortic arch to the circle of Willis, in about

10–15 sec. CT angiography shows low artifacts, e.g., low or no motion or pulsation artifacts, due to its high temporal resolution. CT angiography should be the preferred method in an emergency situation, combined with a cranial computed tomography. This combination not only provides critical information about the carotid arteries, but also cerebral perfusion can be evaluated and cerebral bleeding ruled out. To image the whole supraaortic vessel system a normalized pitch of 1 to 1.5 should be used. Normalized pitch and necessary table movement can be calculated as follows: normalized pitch = table movement/(collimation × rows). For a typical 16-row MSCT with a collimation of 0.75 mm and a necessary pitch of 1.0, the table movement must be 12 mm/sec (table movement = 1.0 × (0.75 mm × 16-row)). The voltage and ampere-second adjustments of the tube are set at 120 kV and 180–200 mAs, respectively. Using modulation of the radiation dose for the upper chest, results could be improved. For CT angiography, the use of an intravenous (cubital vein) contrast agent is imperative. Iodided contrast agent with 300 mg/ml iodide is usually used. A bolus of 100 ml contrast agent is delivered by a power injector at a flow rate of 3 ml/sec, followed by a saline flush at the same flow rate. To calculate the start delay, two methods are usually used; "bolus tracking" and "test bolus". Bolus tracking is an automatic or semiautomatic method, where a region of interest is set in the lumen of the target carotid artery or the aortic arch. During injection of the contrast agent, the Houndsfield Units are measured each second, and when a certain threshold value (e.g. 100 Houndsfield Units) is reached, the planned scan starts automatically. Obtaining a time-to-density diagram by preinjection of a small volume of contrast agent to obtain the right start delay is described as a "test bolus". Both methods can be recommended, but in the case of a suspected carotid artery dissection, it seems most effective to set the region of interest in the aortic arch and to add about 7–10 sec to the measured start delay. However, it may be that the region of interest was placed in the intramural hematoma or the low flow false lumen, thus resulting in a delayed start time. To avoid this, a reconstruction recruitment of 1–3 mm is necessary and rendering multiplanar reformations and maximum intensity projections are mandatory, especially when an interventional therapy is planned.

As described for the computed tomography, magnetic resonance (MR) methods are also becoming more and more important for carotid artery imaging. Before the era of contrast-enhanced MR angiography, two- and three-dimensional time of flight (TOF) or phase contrast techniques were used to image the supraaortic arteries. These bloodflow-based methods are limited, however, by intravoxel dephasing due to complex flow, rising peak systolic velocity, low flow, and disturbances, caused by vascular lesions in stenotic areas. Methemoglobin in thrombus can imitate a perfused lumen. TOF is most important for imaging the intracranial vessel. 2D TOF and 3D TOF each have certain strengths and weaknesses. 3D TOF shows a higher spatial resolution and a higher signal to noise relationship, whereas 2D TOF does not show significant saturation effects, but does have a lower spatial resolution. For optimal results, a hybrid technique with multiple overlapping thin slab acquisitions (MOTSA) can be used. The use of contrast agent has reduced this signal loss substantially due to the reduction of echo time and the diminution of saturation effects, resulting in more accurate imaging of the stenoses. The vessel signal is related to the contrast agent enhanced T1 shortening effect in the vessel lumen. Spin saturation effects, from in-plane flow or slow flow are reduced and short echo times reduce intravoxel spin-dephasing in turbulence flow caused by vascular lesions. Contrast enhanced MR angiography has been shown to reliably produce high-quality images of the carotid arteries with conventional angiography analogous lumen filling characteristics. Unenhanced and enhanced images of the carotid arteries are obtained with 3D field gradient echo techniques. A dedicated head and neck coil plus at least a 1.5 Tesla whole body superconducting scanner is mandatory for excellent image quality. Contrast agent (e.g., gadopentate dimeglumine) is injected into a cubital vein at a dose of 0.2 mmol/kg body weight of gadolinium. The bolus must be delivered by a power injector at a flow rate of 2–3 ml/sec, and followed by a saline flush at the same flow rate. Patients are instructed to breath quietly throughout the entire acquisition phase or breath-holding techniques can also be used. Unenhanced and contrast enhanced images are subtracted, similar to digital subtraction. The source coronal images are post-processed with a standard maximum intensity projection algorithm. In addition, fat-suppressed T1 weighted coronal and axial images must to be acquired to differentiate an intramural hematoma from the surrounding soft tissue [73], [32]. For all types of carotid artery stenoses, the overall sensitivity and specifity for CT and MRA in the literature is 82%–100%.

For an acutely occurring carotid artery stenosis with neurological symptoms, e.g., a dissection, it may be necessary to obtain information, regarding critically hypoperfused brain tissue, to aid in the decision-making process for therapy. The definition of ischemic penumbra, a critically hypoperfused and functionally impaired and viable brain around the infarct core, was introduced in the late 1990s. This area is potentially resolvable and could be salvaged by restituting the perfusion. In order to perform MR diffusion studies, field gradients have to be applied in addition to radio frequency and gradient pulses. During the time evolution, diffusion-encoding is performed by a pair of field gradients. The gradient factor is called the b-factor. Diffusion results from the Brownian motion of the water molecules. When the spins move excessively inside the field gradient, they dephase each other destroying the alignment of the spins, thus resulting in a low measured signal. If they do not move, no or less early dephasing is seen and thus a high signal is obtained. Hyperintense diffusion weighted imaging lesions have to be correlated with severely depressed apparent diffusion coefficient values (ADC). Calculated ADC maps reflect the strength of diffusion in the pixels by obtaining diffusion weighted images (DWI) with different b-values (increasing magnitude, e.g., 1000 s/mm). DW images are T2 weighted and the effect of T2 prolongation is a well known artifact called "T2 shine-through". Exponential image processing eliminates this effect. For DWI, a reasonably short TE (120 ms) and an adequate diffusion sensitivity is required. Images must be obtained in the x, y, and z-axis plus two b-factors for best results. Single shot echo-planar imaging techniques are most performed in clinical practices [19], [64]. Perfusion weighted imaging (PWI) is usually obtained with an echo-planar gradient-echo sequence, measuring several time points per slice and centered on the DWI lesion. A bolus of gadolinium contrast agent is injected at the beginning of the measurement. Subsequently, the relative mean transit time (rMTT), time to peak (TTP), relative cerebral blood flow (rCBF) and relative cerebral blood volume is calculated and displayed as color-coded maps. The penumbra is the area with no reduced diffusion, but changes in PWI (reduced rCBF and increased rMTT), the so-called PWI > DWI mismatch [70].

Carotid artery dissections (traumatic, spontaneous, iatrogenic)

Clinical knowledge

Studies describe an annual incidence of spontaneous carotid artery dissection of about 2.5 to 3 per 100,000 people [73], [78]. These spontaneous dissections account for only about two percent of all ischemic strokes [75], [52], [26]. However, carotid artery dissection is a very common cause of stroke in children and in young or middle-aged patients [26]. There, it occurs in 10 to 25 percent of ischemic strokes. Most dissections are observed after trauma, particulary motor vehicle accidents, although they may also occur spontaneously. Typical common risk factors for vascular disease and atherosclerosis, like smoking, hypertension and hypercholesterolemia, may play a minor role, but are not the main reasons for vessel wall pathology. Generally, atherosclerotic changes are not seen in the average patient, but carotid artery dissection can be found in apparently healthy vessels or vessels weakened by inherited connective-tissue disorders. Well-known collagen abnormalities show an increased risk of spontaneous carotid artery dissection and have been identified in most young patients with spontaneously dissections. In all vessels, dissections arise from an intimal tear (entry), which allows blood to enter the artery wall and split its layers. An intramural hematoma is formed which is located within the layers of the tunica media towards the intima. This hematoma can cause high-grade carotid stenosis. The so-called false lumen (subintimal dissection) can disrupt twice causing a reentry into the true arterial lumen leading to what is known as a perfused false lumen. This false lumen is normally wider than the true lumen, due to a lower blood flow and a thinner vessel wall. Simultaneously the true lumen can be tightened. Furthermore, the subintimal dissection can cause an intimal layer, floating in the perfused artery lumen and causing a high-grade stenosis or thrombembolic events. Based on this pathogenic mechanism, stroke as a complication of carotid artery dissection is caused by critical stenosis of the true arterial lumen with a resulting hemodynamic insufficiency. Moreover, embolization of thrombi that develop on the intimal layer may occur [47]. Young patients with spontaneous carotid artery dissections are thought to have an underlying structural defect of the vessel wall, although the exact type of arteriopathy remains obscure in most cases [73]. In some families, a history of a dissection of the aorta or its branches is known. Schievink WI [73] gives an excellent overview of the most common inherited connective-tissue disorders or collagen abnormalities with an increased risk of spontaneous carotid artery dissections. Foremost is Ehlers-Danlos-Syndrome type IV [75], but others like Marfan's-Syndrome, autosomal-dominant polycystic kidney-disease and osteogenesis imperfecta are important as well. These inherited abnormalities have been identified in about one to five percent of all patients with spontaneous dissections. Twenty percent of all patients have clinically apparent, but as yet unnamed connective-tissue disorders. In addition, it seems that fibromuscular dysplasia is found in up to 15 percent of patients with carotid artery dissections [75], and ultrastructural abnormalities of dermal connective-tissue components have been detected in 66 percent of all spontaneous carotid artery dissections [73].

For serious head or cervical spine trauma, for example a hyperflexion-hyperextension (whip-lash trauma) or rotation trauma of the cervical spine from a motor vehicle accident, as well as a spontaneous carotid artery dissection, mechanical stress, like stretching of the carotid artery wall is mandatory. Even minor precipitating events like sudden neck movements, sports, working over head, painting a ceiling, less forceful focal trauma, chiropractor manipulation, a history of respiratory tract infection, in addition to coughing, sneezing or heavy vomiting may injure the vessel mural, which has been weakened by inherited connective-tissue disorders. It should also be mentioned, that acute carotid artery occlusion or dissection following carotid endarterectomy is often accompanied by a sudden deterioration in clinical status, e.g., hemiparesia and somnolence, where emergency stent replacement as an alternative method of treatment should be considered [45]. The extracranial part of the internal carotid artery and the external carotid artery undergo more dissections than the intracranial part. This is due to the fact that there is a greater mobility of the extracranial part between its origin and its entry into the skull, while the intracranial part is fixed. This mobility and the proximity to bone structures like the cervical spine or the styloid process increases the potential for vessel wall injuries. Nevertheless, despite the reduced mobility of the intracranial portion, dissections were also observed in this area.

Due to modern non-invasive imaging methods, carotid artery dissection is often diagnosed more often than at later times and the number of diagnosed dissections has increased over the last several years. Patients present either no signs at all, only subtle signs or obvious manifestations of acute carotid artery dissection [84]. Before cerebral ischemia actually occurs, patients often undergo diagnosis and therapy due to some other localized warning sign. The typical symptoms are pain on one side of the face, partial oculosympathetic palsy (Horners syndrome) or severe ipsilateral headache miming a subarachnoid hemorrhage, migraine or a cluster headache. Pain is usually the initial manifestation of carotid artery dissection before cerebral or retinal ischemia occurs. This classic triad (pain, Horners syndrome and cerebral ischemia) is observed in only one third of all patients [73], [84]. Patients with symptoms develop cerebral or retinal ischemia in about 50 to 95 percent of the cases. One fifth of them show cerebral ischemia without any warning signs

[73]. Related to atherosclerotic high-grade carotid artery stenoses, are hemispheric neurological symptoms like transient ischemic attacks or recurrent episodes of transient monocular blindness (amaurosis fugax) and cranial-nerve palsies. In the worst case scenario, it progresses to ischemic stroke and permanent loss of vision. The average time from the initial manifestation and the appearance of more severe symptoms is about four days [73], [84].

Imaging knowledge

In the detection and follow-up of carotid artery dissections, a combination of Doppler color-flow ultrasound and transcranial ultrasonography may some merit [3], but it is not very useful for decision-making. In diagnosing carotid artery dissections, magnetic resonance imaging and computed tomography is superior to digital subtraction angiography [73]. It provides more information about the extent of the dissection, and shows the intramural hematoma with its characteristically crescent-shape, the intimal flap and the true and false lumen. Intracranial bleeding can be ruled out before intervention, and as an aid to the decision-making for planning therapy, diffusion- and perfusion-weighted magnetic resonance images can indicate the presence of ischemic areas as well as identify the brain tissue at risk by finding a diffusion-perfusion mismatch. In dissected vessels, conventional angiography usually only shows a narrowing or an occlusion of the lumen, although sometimes the intimal flap can be seen. In an emergency, we prefer to perform a native cranial computed tomography and a contrast-enhanced CT angiography from the aortic arch to the circle of Willis. The presence of objective cerebral ischemia and an available magnetic resonance tomography scanner, contrast-enhanced MR angiography should be performed in the same way as described for the CT angiography. Additional axial and coronal views must also be obtained with fat-suppressed T1 weighted images to help identify an intramural hematoma. Furthermore, diffusion- and perfusion-weighted images of the brain are mandatory in the presence of objective neurological symptoms. By finding a larger perfusion deficit than diffusion deficit, the area of the salvageable brain tissue can be shown (penumbra). This can help to identify patients requiring emergency stent replacement, since penumbra tissue only survives about 6 hours, or perhaps a bit longer [46], [27]. Studies have shown that patients with radiological evidence of viable penumbra tissue benefit from emergent interventional therapy and show a resolution of neurological symptoms [15]. Magnetic resonance imaging is also very important for follow-up series during the healing process, especially under conservative treatment.

Treatment knowledge

Carotid artery dissection (extracranial) is an acute (spontaneous, traumatic) disease in which most dissections heal spontaneously. However emergency treatment is necessary in patients with severe or persistent symptoms of ischemia to prevent cerebral or retinal ischemia which can lead to significant disabilities. Blood clots formed in the false lumen or on the intimal flap give rise to distal emboli, e.g., in the middle cerebral arteries, and the mural hematoma may induce a critical stenosis or even occlude the true lumen. It is thus recommended that anticoagulation therapy be the first step in treatment. In fact, this has been advocated since the 1970s and is widely accepted, but no controlled studies of anticoagulation have been performed to assess the benefits and risks of anticoagulation in carotid artery dissections and the actual validity of such treatment has never been truly evaluated. Furthermore, it is not known which patients will respond to anticoagulation, which will show persistent symptoms or an exacerbation of ischemia despite anticoagulation therapy, and how many patients might even show spontaneous improvement [15]. To prevent these thromboembolic complications, anticoagulation with intravenous administration of heparin, followed by oral marcumar or warfarin is used in most institutions. No specific parameters have yet been identified for predicting the clinical history, although anticoagulation has to be recommended for all patients, regardless of the type of symptoms (except contraindication for anticoagulation, e.g. intracerebral bleeding). The target international normalized ratio of 2.0–3.0 (INR) should generally be used for three to six months [57],

[74]. A high rate of recanalization within the first three months after the event is observed. Schievink et al. [74] describe an approach to obtaining the appropriate level of anticoagulation, and recommend performing a magnetic resonance angiogram after three months. Anticoagulation therapy should be subsequently continued for three or more months if luminal irregularities are found, and then repeat the imaging and change to antiplatelet therapy (e.g., clopidogrel) if the luminal irregularities still persist.

The most common mechanism of cerebral ischemia is the embolization of thrombi or microemboli from the dissected vessel [47]. Hemodynamic insufficiency (i.e., caused by insufficient flow) due to a critical high-grade stenosis of the origin true lumen, caused by the mural hematoma or a moving intimal flap, is another mechanism for cerebral ischemia or stroke. Over the past decade, endovascular stent therapy of vessel lesions has become increasingly important in modern interventional therapy. Recently, stent therapy has been proposed as an alternative method for the treatment of patients with carotid artery lesions such as traumatic and spontaneous dissections. Most data are based on emergency settings and long-term results are limited [4]. As mentioned above, most dissections of the carotid artery heal spontaneously under anticoagulation/antiplatelet treatment [73]. Thus, open surgery [67], [69] or percutaneous interventional repair should be reserved for patients with persistent symptoms, recurrent neurological episodes, persistent high-grade stenosis or failed anticoagulation treatment. The major advantage is that stent repair achieves immediate restoration of vessel caliber thereby preventing formation of emboli, plus coverage of the arterial defect and restoration of a normal circulation.

All surgical methods, including ligature of the carotid artery combined with an in situ extracranial-to-intracranial bypass or vein-graft replacement are quite challenging in carotid artery surgery. In contrast, percutaneous interventional methods are very beneficial and are easier to perform. Percutaneous endovascular treatment consists of percutaneous balloon angioplasty and placement of one or more naked or covered metallic stents. In iatrogenic, traumatic or spontaneous carotid artery dissections, non-covered metallic stents are common, whereas in carotid artery aneurysm, covered stents are often used. The major limitation of endovascular stenting in carotid artery dissections is related to technical difficulties. Malek et al. [58] have demonstrated that it is often difficult, although possible to navigate a microcatheter through a dissection to reconstruct the true lumen, even in the case of complete carotid occlusion [58]. The arterial segment is usually extensive and frequently requires a long stent or several combined stents, in which the combined stents have to be exactly overlapped (telescoping). In our opinion, self-expanding stents should be given precedence. Self-expanding stents open with different diameters over their entire length according to the actual vessel diameter are thus more adaptable than balloon-expandable stents. Most often, an emergency stenting procedure is necessary, and recent studies have shown that emergency endovascular stenting may be a feasible and effective treatment for symptomatic patients [45], [15], [29]. During the interventional procedure, heparinization with up to 10,000 IU (acquired coagulation time ACT about 200–300 sec) is recommended. If the stenting procedure is elective, 75 mg clopidogrel daily or 250 mg ticlopidine daily should be administered for five days. Additionally, 100–300 mg acetylsalicylic acid daily should be administered five days prior to the procedure. Intraarterial papaverine or nitrogylcerin may sometimes be necessary in cases of arterial spasm during the procedure. Some physicians use abciximab or eptifibatide (platelet glycoprotein IIb/IIIa inhibitors) before the first angioplasty, but this is not a general practice. The intervention should be followed by a daily dose of clopidogrel or ticlopidine for at least three to six weeks and acetylsalicylic acid should be continued for at least half a year.

Prognosis

As shown above, the incidence of detected carotid artery dissections is reported to be 2.5 to 3 per 100,000 people [73], [78]. Due to the fact that most ischemic events after dissection are thrombembolic arising from the intimal flaps, the reported recurrence rate of thrombembolic events varies from 0.6% to 10.4% a year [47], [6]. Most observers describe an annual recurrent stroke rate in patients of < 1% [77], [54]. These dissections account for only two percent of all ischemic strokes [77], [52], [26], but are the cause of ischemic stroke in up to 25% of younger adults [26]. Within the first two to three months, spontaneous recanalization was described in 47% to 90% of all cases, whereas two thirds of occlusions and up to 90% of all stenosis are recanalized [73], [4], [42], [25]. It seems that adequate anticoagulation therapy supports this process, in particular by reducing the number of complications. After six months changes are rare.

Surgical techniques are demanding and are associated with a high morbidity rate. Perioperative stroke occurs in up to 10%, and peripheral cranial nerve injury rates of 58% and mortality rates of 2% are observed [4], [67]. Perhaps the use of the hybrid technique (open surgical implantation of a covered stent) may reduce this substantial complication rate [4]. The occurrence of microembolic shower in intracranial circulation during carotid artery angioplasty or stenting is well known, but recent studies showed neurological events after carotid artery stenting (without protection devices) in 5.4% of all cases. Major strokes were seen in 0.7% and minor complications (e.g., transient ischemic attacks, minor stroke) in 4.7% [86]. 64.3% of all neurological symptoms occurred postprocedurally. The basic complication rate for angiography is known to be about 4% for minor complications (e.g., puncture site hematoma) and < 0.01% for major complications. Reports on the long-term results of carotid artery dissection stent repair are rare, but they seem to be positive and indicate that recovery will ultimately be achieved [4], [53]. The prognosis of stroke is related to the initial ischemic insult and the collateral circulation. Once stroke has occurred, the prognosis is generally poor and anticoagulation does not really affect any significant change [7]. Therefore, diffusion- and perfusion-weighted magnetic resonance images could help to identify those patients which did not respond to anticoagulation and therefore are very good candidates for endovascular stent repair. Diffusion- and perfusion-weighted images identify potentially salvageable, but at-risk cerebral tissue by showing the hypoperfused ischemic penumbra (brain tissue at-risk). Less than five percent of all patients with carotid artery dissections die from the dissection or its complications.

Take home points

The spontaneous, traumatic or iatrogenic (post-surgery) dissection of the carotid artery is a dynamic process associated with a potentially poor clinical outcome and significant disabilities. It affects predominantly younger adults. The main reasons for cerebral ischemia complicating a carotid artery dissection are microembolic events. To date, primary treatment of acute carotid dissection is nonsurgical or noninterventional. Despite the lack of evaluative studies, primary therapy should include anticoagulant or antiplatelet agents over at least three to six months, since most dissections of the carotid artery heal spontaneously under anticoagulation/antiplatelet treatment. Open surgery or percutaneous interventional repair should be reserved for patients with persistent symptoms, recurrent neurological episodes, persistent high-grade stenosis and a failed anticoagulation treatment. To identify potential patients, urgent magnetic resonance imaging of the brain, including diffusion- and perfusion-weighted images and a magnetic resonance angiography should be performed. Cohen et al. [15] stated "The presence of objective evidence of cerebral ischemia and salvageable tissue on magnetic resonance imaging studies could help in the selection of the most appropriate patients for stenting". Due to a lower complication rate and an excellent success rate, percutaneous interventional therapy by stenting the dissection should be preferred. After stenting, an antiplatelet therapy with clopidogrel or ticlopidine and acetylsalicylic acid is mandatory. Although long-term studies are rare, endovascular stent repair seems to achieve good results and should be considered as more than just an option to open surgery. Normally, the procedure is easy to perform, but it should only be reserved for patients with ongoing clinical symptoms, despite adequate anticoagulations. Endovascular stent repair allows immediate recanalization of

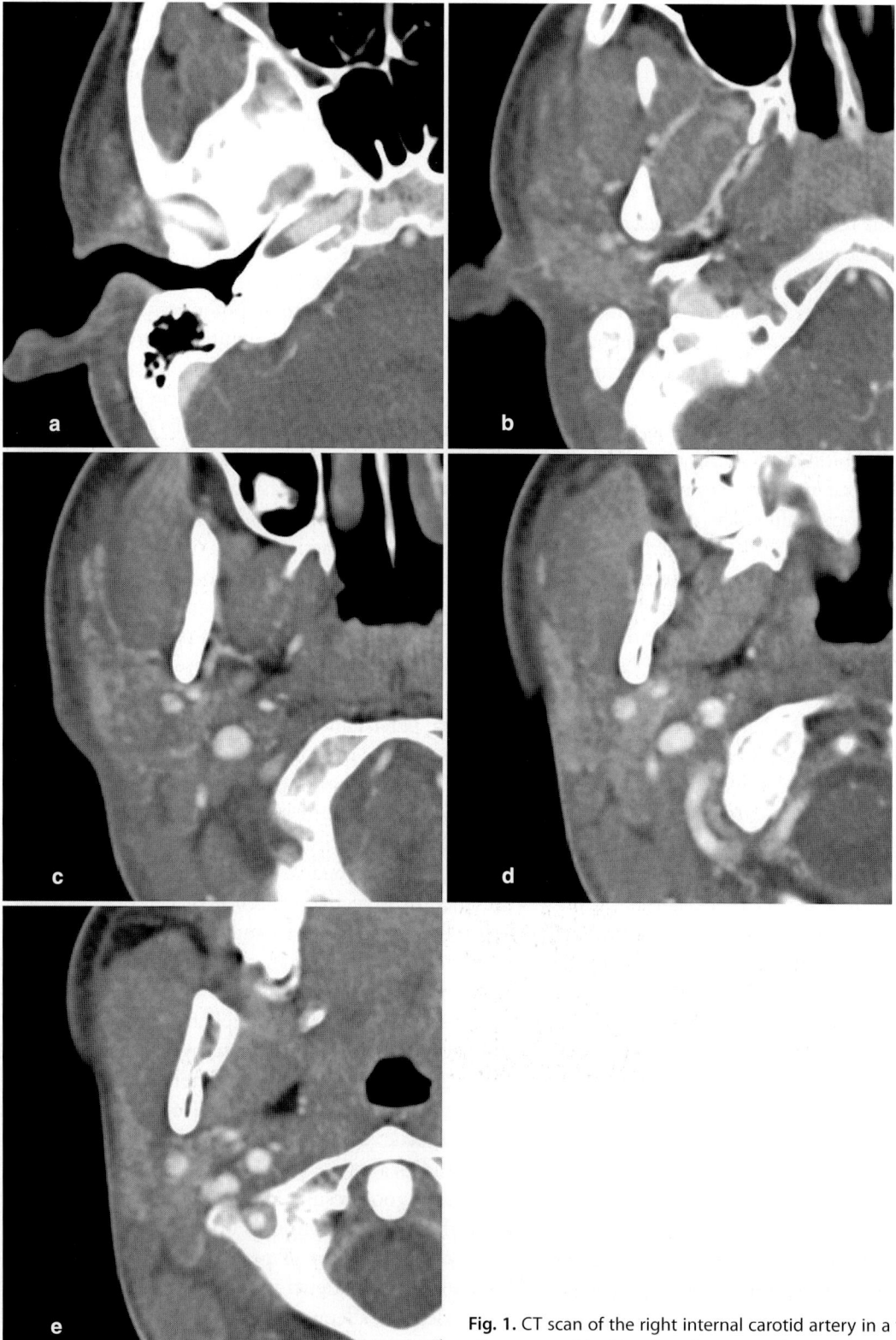

Fig. 1. CT scan of the right internal carotid artery in a young female patient after a car accident (explanation see text).

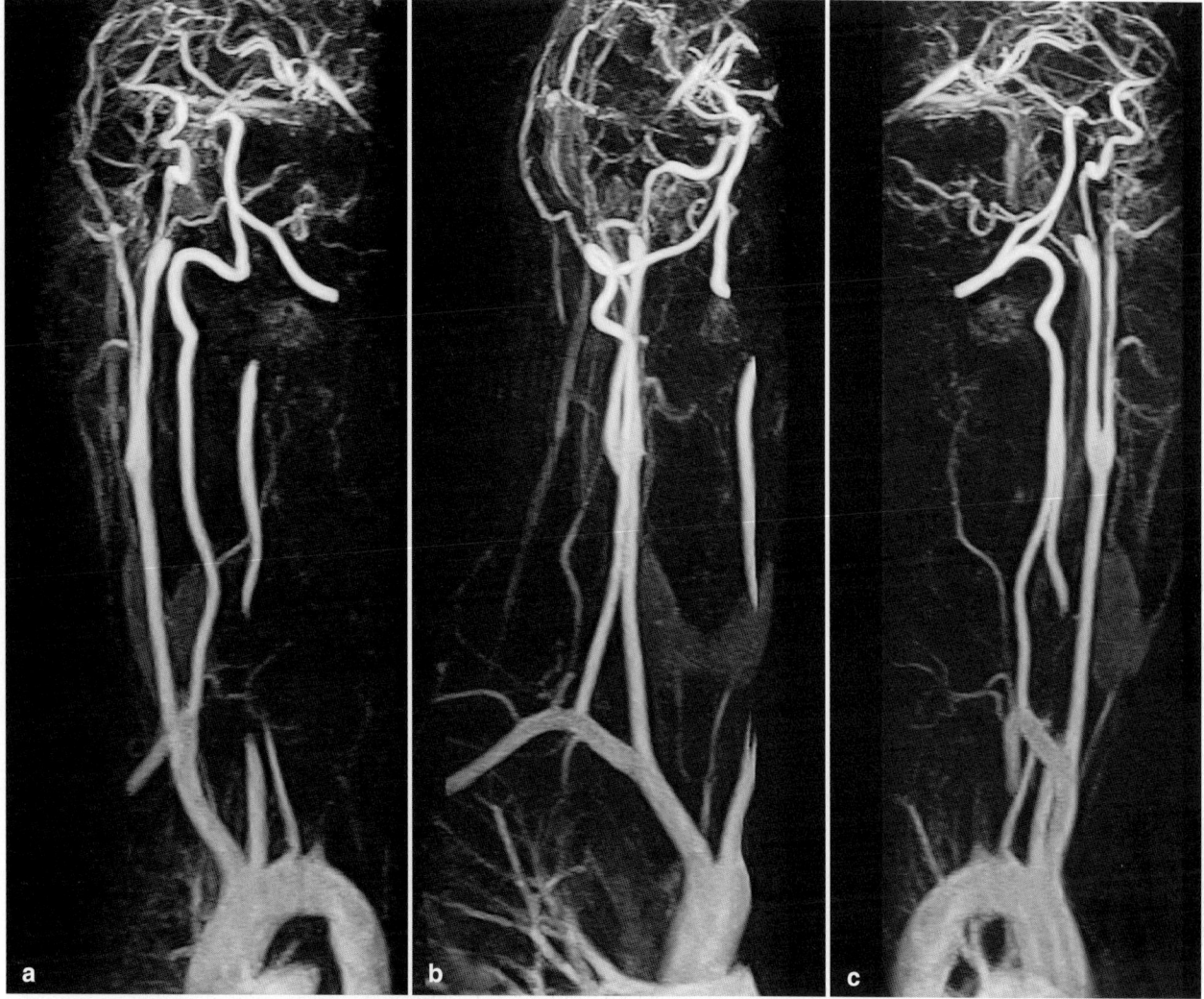

Fig. 2. MRA of the right internal carotid artery in a young female patient after a car accident (same patient as in Fig. 1; explanation see text).

the dissected vessel with immediate reperfusion of the brain, and is therefore also suitable for emergency treatment [15].

Clinical examples

Fig. 1 shows a CT scan of the right internal carotid artery in a young female patient after a car accident. The traumatic dissections typically begins before entry into the skull base (see arrow Fig. 1d; Fig. 1e shows a normal internal carotid artery). Due to the intramural hematoma, the perfused true lumen of the petrous part shows a high-grade stenosis of a short distance (see arrows Fig. 1b, c). After passing through the skull base, the cavernous part of the internal carotid artery shows a regular caliber (see arrow Fig. 1a). The same findings were depicted on MRA (see arrows Fig. 2a–c). The patient showed no symptoms and no signs of ischemia in cranial MRI and was treated long-term with acetylsalicylic acid. More than one year later, the stenosis had not significantly changed on MRA follow-up, and no symptoms had occurred.

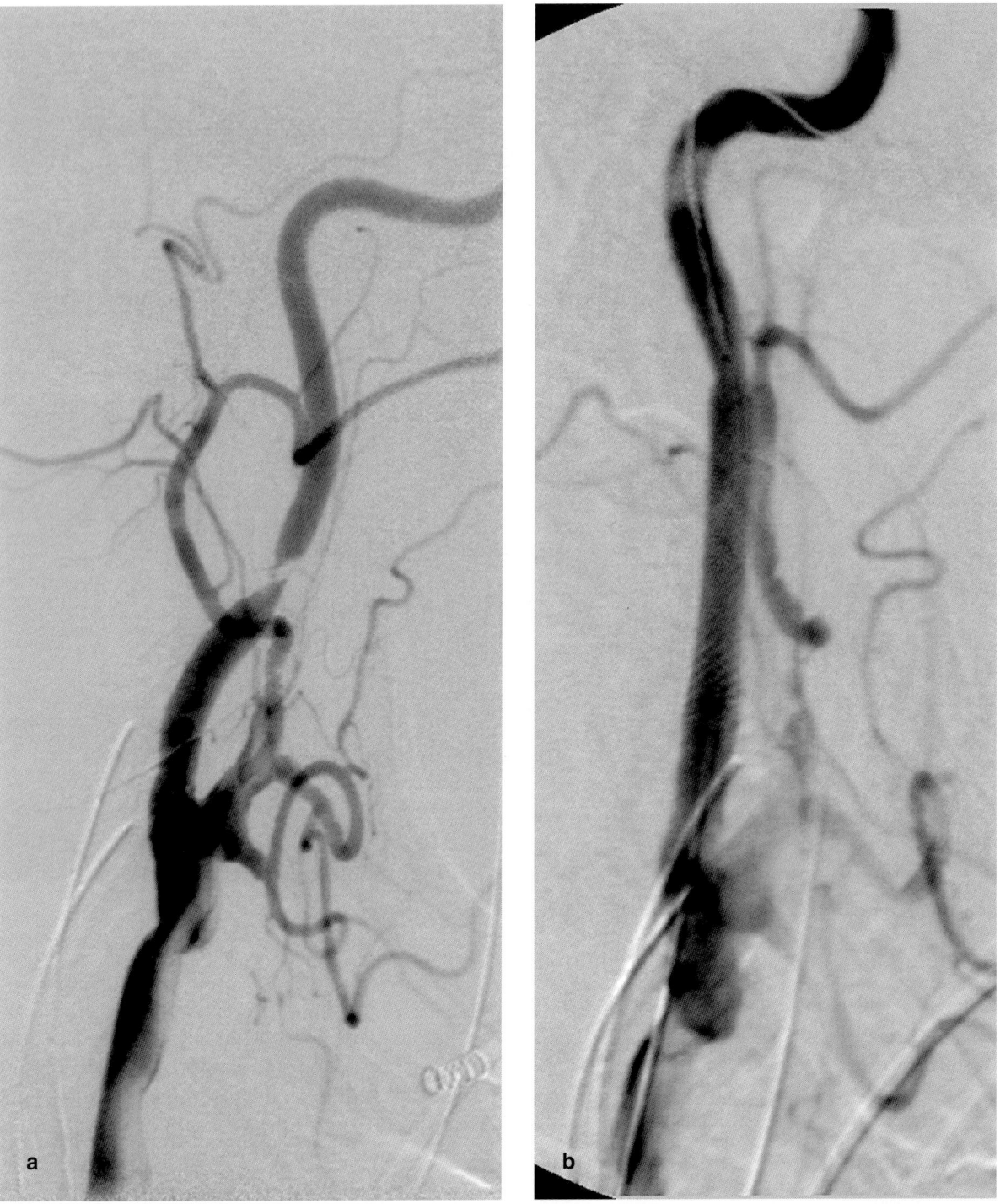

Fig. 3. Carotid artery angiogram after endarterectomy due to a high-grade stenosis of the carotid artery bifurcation (explanation see text).

Fig. 3 shows the carotid artery angiogram of a patient who underwent endarterectomy due to a high-grade stenosis of the carotid artery bifurcation. After surgery, a new weakness in the left arm occurred although the cranial MRI did not show any signs of acute ischemia or bleeding. However, the MRA depicted a high-grade stenosis of the internal carotid artery and consequently a DSA was performed. Fig. 3a shows an iatrogenic dissection (see arrow) of the right internal carotid artery. As shown in Fig. 3b, it could be successfully treated with a 6 mm diameter and 22 mm long Carotid-Wall-Stent. Clinical symptoms resolved and the patient was subsequently treated with clopidogrel and acetylsalicylic acid.

Intracranial carotid artery stenosis

Clinical knowledge

Atherosclerotic lesions and dissections of the main intracranial carotid artery stenosis cause stroke in 8–29% of patients per year [88], [14], [72], [90], [89]. Intracranial atherosclerotic lesions are present in 8–12% [72], [90], [16], [55] of all patients with cerebrovascular symptoms. The typical risk factors for atherosclerotic lesions in intracranial and peripheral vessels are well known and need not be mentioned here. A high risk of death from ischemic heart disease correlates with symptomatic intracranial atherosclerotic lesions. The incidence of intracranial carotid artery stenosis is higher in certain ethnic groups, like Hispanics, African Americans and Asians [72], [90]. Novel magnetic resonance imaging techniques, such as MRA, diffusion- and perfusion-imaging, can increasingly detect intracranial stenoses, even in clinically asymptomatic patients, and give an acute evaluation of stroke patients. Most patients with an intracranial artery stenosis have recurrent cerebral ischemic events despite antiplatelet or anticoagulation regimens. The risk of suffering a stroke is dependent on the one hand on the general hemodynamic situation and thrombembolic events, and on the other hand on the severity of the intracranial stenosis [14], [13]. Patients with a high-grade stenosis run a more than 80% higher risk of stroke. The yearly risk of stroke in patients with an intracranial carotid artery stenosis is listed above and, for patients with a history of stroke, suffering a stroke again in the same vessel territory carries a risk of about 25% [88].

Intracranial stenoses are mostly found in the petrous and cavernous siphon parts of the internal carotid artery and the M1-segment of the middle cerebral artery. Intracranial stenoses may be either stenotic or dilatative. A symptomatic stenosis occurring under a reduced hemodynamic situation manifests itself in transient ischemic attacks, minor and major strokes. In contrast to extracranial carotid artery stenosis, intracranial carotid artery stenosis can cause stroke due to thrombembolic events or local thrombosis. Microembolic events can cause small vessel cerebrovascular disease with leukoaraiosis, patchy lesions and lacunes [21], [22], [91], [92]. The same pathological patterns are found in vessels with atherosclerotic plaques occluding the small penetrating vessels, like the important lenticulostriate arteries. Due to similar pathological image patterns, a differentiation of the cause is usually not possible [21], [22], [91], [92]. Stenosis in more peripheral parts of the intracranial vessels, e.g. the peripheral middle cerebral artery, cause perfusion deficits as a results of hemodynamic insufficiency, whereas stenosis in the major intracranial arteries can be asymptomatic due to better collateral perfusion. Thus, in addition to the grade of stenosis and its localization, the presence of collateral circulation is decisive for possible perfusion deficits which lead to actual clinical symptoms [21], [22]. The circle of Willis, and the leptomeningeal and extracranial anastomoses are the main arteries responsible for sufficient collateral circulation. Particulary the internal carotid artery can be well perfused via the circle of Willis. Once detected, intracranial atherosclerosis usually has a progressive course, but when dynamic behavior of the intracranial stenoses is observed, stabilization or even a regression may be possible.

Imaging knowledge

Before performing therapy, the clinical symptoms and neurological history, obtained by a neurologist or neurosurgeon, have to be compared with the neuroimaging findings. This is mandatory for planning a successful interventional treatment or an optimal medical treatment program alone. Currently imaging diagnostics is mostly based on MRI and MRA. To assist in decision-making for therapy planning, diffusion- and perfusion-weighted magnetic resonance images are necessary since they can image the presence of ischemic areas and identify the brain tissue at risk by finding a diffusion-perfusion mismatch, thus providing critical information about the extent of ischemic brain damage. Additional positron emission tomography with an oxygen 15-labeled radiotracer can be performed to obtain information about impaired cerebrovascular reserve as an indicator of perfusion failure distal to the stenosis [80]. Intracranial bleeding must be excluded before intervention (e.g. with CT). For diagnostic purposes, an MRA is usually performed from the aortic arch to the circle of Willis (usually with a contrast-enhanced technique) and additionally thin slabs of the circle of Willis (usually with time-of-flight techniques) should be obtained to give clear information about the localization and extent of the intracranial stenosis. CT and CT angiography are somewhat limited due to the beam-hardening artifacts at the skull base and after stent implantation due to the metal of the stents. Accurate depiction is not ensured in these cases. Collateral blood flow is of tremendous importance for adequate brain tissue perfusion, since insufficient collateral blood flow and stenosis of the supplying vessel are both responsible for the perfusion failure. This collateral blood flow has to be carefully evaluated on conventional DSA images and is indicated by a delayed flow or a border-zone shift [80]. Transcranial ultrasound does not play an important role in the detection of intracranial artery stenosis, but transcranial Doppler ultrasound is a useful method for the detection of microembolic signals as a marker for a soft, local unstable plaque. This method can not only be performed before intervention, but gives critical information about plaque stability, especially when performed during crossing of the lesions [82], [91], [92]. Ultrasound allows differentiation between the white stable plaques and the yellow unstable plaques. In the case of unstable plaques with evident microembolic showering, the primary strategy should focus on plaque stabilization and anticoagulation, whereas angioplasty or stenting is secondary and should be considered carefully [80].

The primary aim of imaging techniques is to identify those patients with a high risk of stroke. Furthermore, it is to detect the stenosis, determine whether it is accessible and suitable for angioplasty or stenting, or to exclude patients with other possible differential diagnoses like cerebral vasculitis, intracranial bleeding or a tumor, which are clearly not treated with interventional techniques. Imaging should help to detect patients with acute ischemic events which run a much higher risk of complications under intervention, predominantly intracerebral hemorrhage by reperfusion or stroke, based on an unstable plaque. Posttreatment imaging follow-up must detect subacute to late restenosis and must depict ischemic events. MRI and MRA are the best methods to accomplish this. Follow-up with extra- and intracranial Doppler ultrasound can easily be performed and provides important information about a significant restenosis. A peak systolic velocity of over 220 cm/sec in the carotid artery or middle cerebral artery indicates a > 50% restenosis [5].

Treatment knowledge

Patients with stenoses of the intracranial arteries frequently show cerebral ischemic events while being traditionally treated with an antiplatelet agent or oral anticoagulant and general management of vascular risk factors [88]. Despite the dynamic course, prognosis is poor with significant morbidity and death rates. These limitations and the high current stroke rates require a more aggressive treatment regimen in patients with symptomatic intracranial artery stenosis. The treatment of these patients is still controversial and several questions have to be answered. For example, whether only antiplatelet/anticoagulation therapy or angioplasty/stenting is the best first-line therapy [13], or what is the best or maximal medical therapy? Furthermore, what is the risk of stroke with medical therapy or with interventional therapy or, what is the risk of complications from interventional therapy? Is stenting necessary or is angioplasty alone sufficient? Do the interventionalists have sufficient experience and routine clinical use. Are there any contraindications against a sufficient peri- and postprocedural anticoagulation/antiplatelet therapy? [13]. All of these questions have not yet been clearly answered and must be considered for each patient on an individual basis.

The so-called best medical treatment plan is based on the control of vascular risk factors and the application of antiplatelet/anticoagulation drugs, statins (HMG-CoA reductase inhibitors) and angiotensin-converting enzyme inhibitors. Maximal medical treatment can be defined as receiving daily doses of >81 mg acetylsalicylic acid, 500 mg ticlopidine, 75 mg clopidogrel, or comparable doses of marcumar/warfarin or heparin [80]. A more aggressive treatment regimen like angioplasty should be considered in cases where maximal medical therapy fails to prevent massive ischemic stroke. Medical therapy failure is not clearly defined, but should be assumed when recurrent cerebral symptoms occur under maximal medical treatment [80].

Despite unsatisfactory experiences during the 1980s involving high rates of stroke or death, advances in micro-guidewires, microcatheters, balloon technology and stent technology have been made as a result of positive in coronary angioplasty and stenting. Angioplasty or stenting methods have emerged as a potential therapeutic option over the last decade. Stent placement has proven to be as technically feasible as for angioplasty or stenting of the extracranial carotid artery [56].

Angioplasty or stent treatment can be performed using the typical transfemoral access. Some physicians perform the interventional procedure without general anesthetic or sedative, in order to recognize slight changes in clinical neurological status such as motor activity or speech. But for quiet examination conditions and reduced patient movement, a general anesthetic is recommended. During all examinations, the continuous measurement of blood pressure, electrocardiogram and transcutaneous oximetry is mandatory during the entire interventional procedure. Despite preexisting imaging modalities, like a MRA of the circle of Willis or the carotid arteries, a four-vessel cerebral DSA must be performed to verify the stenosis and to provide a description of the existing collateral circulation. Three-dimensional rotational angiography can be a very helpful method for the imaging and evaluation of the stenosis. The diameter of the stenosis, referring to the next normal sized vessel part and the stenosis length have to be measured based on the standardized criteria [68]. The choice of the appropriate micro-guidewire to be used for probing the stenosis is also of considerable importance. Intracranial vessels are located in the subarachnoid space surrounded by the cerebrospinal fluid and follow quite a convoluted course. Additional, small penetrating vessels extend from the major intracranial arteries supplying the brain tissue with blood. These small penetrating vessel are invisible in neuroimaging. Particular care must be taken with the lateral lenticulostriate arteries arising from the M1-segment of the middle cerebral artery. The use of stiff micro-guidewires, involves the risk of injuring (e.g., dissection) or penetrating the vessel and tearing off the small penetrating vessels. Subsequent severe intracranial bleeding or infarction may occur. Occlusion caused by a stent or a dissection or microtrauma to the vessel wall as a result of angioplasty may lead to subsequent ischemic stroke. Hydrophilic micro-guidewires (usually 0.010–0.014 inches) with a soft or floppy tip should thus be used. These wires must be placed more peripherally, so that the system can be well stabilized [21], [22]. In case of an M1 medial cerebral artery stenosis, this requires the positioning of the tip in the M2 insular branches. All manipulations with the micro-guidewire – microcatheter-system have to be performed very carefully since each step runs the risk of vessel rupture, vasospasm or dissection. After positioning a 6 French guiding catheter in the upper cervical part of the internal carotid artery and crossing of the intracranial lesion by the micro-guidewire or micro-guidewire – microcatheter-system, a predilation of a high-grade stenosis is often necessary, since the stent delivery system might not cross the lesion or can cause a dissection or shearing off of atherosclerotic plaques. Otherwise, primary stenting is normally preferred. Some authors are of the opinion that a predilation should always be performed if the diameter of the stent delivery system is smaller than that of the lesion [21], [22]. Small-profile balloon-catheter-systems should be given preference and, in order to reduce the risk of rupture or dissection, a balloon diameter size smaller than the normal adjacent vessel diameter should be used. Balloon-dilation should be performed very slowly lasting several seconds or even minutes [80]. As mentioned above, intracranial vessels follow a quite tortuous course, thus the matched stent and the stent delivery catheter system have to be soft, flexible and must offer a low profile with excellent trackability and pushability. Balloon-expandable stents derived from coronary angioplasty are very suitable stents and, based on experience in this area, special stents for intracranial angioplasty were developed [85]. In general, the stent size should be matched to the vessel diameter proximal or distal to the stenosis or slightly undersized, and in case of a less than optimally deployed stent, a further expansion with a balloon catheter can be performed [85].

Clearly, postprocedural angiograms have to be carried out immediately in order to evaluate cerebral blood flow. The main risks of intracranial intervention remain the possibility of vessel rupture, vasospasm, dissection, stroke, severe intracranial bleeding or even death. These risks can be reduced by increased experience and the use of novel, improved materials, as described above. Crossing and dilating the lesion carry the greatest risks in intracranial intervention. Careless pushing of the stent delivery system leads to the danger of a shear stress to these small vessels with associated disruption or dissection. It is well known from coronary or peripheral angioplasty, that abrupt inflation of the balloon produces severe stress on the vessel wall causing the vessel to dissect. Slow inflation and deflation of the balloon is mandatory and can reduce the dissection rate for angioplasty from 75% to 14% [66]. After predilation, the stent should be positioned and deployed quickly but carefully in order to diminish the vessel recoil.

Initial positive experiences with undersized stents have been reported in the literature [21], [22]. These studies showed a good balance between efficacy and safe procedure, where the risk of vessel rupture could be reduced, without affecting the clinical outcome. If the predilated lesion can not be easily reached with the stent delivery catheter, prolonged attempts should be abandoned to reduce procedural risks. In such cases, angioplasty alone can sometimes be safer than stent placement [66]. The aim being to just slightly stretch the vessel, since a small increase in vessel diameter results in a large increase in perfusion [80].

After the recanalization of a major intracranial artery, intracerebral reperfusion hemorrhage within a preexistent hemodynamic stroke can occur. In case of acute thrombosis, the application of urokinase or tissue plasminogen activator during intervention is necessary. It should be clear that this thrombolytic treatment increases the risk of intracerebal hemorrhage. Intraarterial papaverine or nitroglycerin may sometimes be necessary in case of arterial spasm during the procedure.

To reduce the risk of acute vessel occlusion due to acute thrombosis, a rigorous periinterventional anticoagulation/antiplatelet therapy is mandatory. As mentioned above, the best medical treatment in patients with intracranial atherosclerotic lesions is still unknown. Similarly, the best periinterventional medical treatment is also not known [14], [13], [21], [22]. Despite the increased risk of intracerebral hemorrhage, the risk of thrombembolic events during and after intervention has to be reduced. The anticoagulation and antiplatelet regimen should be performed as known from interventions for the extracranial internal carotid artery. Before intervention, 75 mg clopidogrel daily or 250 mg ticlopidine daily should be administered for three to five days. Additionally, 100–300 mg acetylsalicylic acid daily should be administered three to five days prior to the procedure. During the interventional procedure, heparinization with up to 10,000 IU (acquired coagulation time ACT about 200–300 sec) is recommended. In addition to heparin, glycoprotein IIb/IIIa inhibitors can be used as well with similar results [56], but with a possibly higher risk of intracerebral hemorrhage. A burst suppression-inducing dose of etomidate may help to protect the brain from ischemic events, especially while the treatment device transverses the stenosis [80]. The intervention should be followed by a daily dose of clopido-

Table 1. Classification of intracranial stenotic lesions modified from a scheme for coronary arteries for intracranial angioplasty alone [63]

Lesion Type A	Lesion Type B	Lesion Type C
Concentric or moderate eccentric	Eccentric	Eccentric
Angulation < 45°	Angulation 45°–90°	Severe tortuosity
Smooth contours	Irregular contours	
No prominent calcifications	Heavy calcifications	
Non ostial	Ostial	
Non occlusive	Total occlusion < 3 months old	Total Occlusion > 3 months old
No thrombus present	Some thrombus present	
No major branch involvement	Major branch involvement possible	
Lesion length < 5mm	Lesion length 5–10mm	Lesion length > 10 mm

grel or ticlopidine and acetylsalicylic acid for up to six months and acetylsalicylic acid monotherapy (or clopidogrel/ticlopidine monotherapy if necessary) should be continued for life.

Prognosis

The risk of stroke per year is about 3.9–28.7% in patients with atherosclerosis of the internal carotid artery and about 2.8–12% in patients with atherosclerosis affecting the middle cerebral artery [88], [14], [72], [90], [89], [18], [30], [8]. The prognosis depends on the localization and extent of the stenosis, as well as the plaque morphology, the collateral circulation and the general hemodynamic situation. Intracranial stenoses are dynamic lesions. They can show progression, can remain stable or even undergo regression. Predicting these changes is impossible and the dynamic process is not really completely understood. Several studies have suggested that intracranial stenoses have the potential to regress with medical treatment alone [80], [82], [91], [93], [1]. The annual risk of stroke in patients with symptomatic intracranial atherosclerosis where anticoagulation/antiplatelet therapy failed is about 4–12% (−45%) [88]. Patients who show symptoms despite best medical treatment have an annual risk of stroke of up to 25% [88]. Surgical methods like an extracranial-intracranial bypass do not reduce the risk of stroke [87]. Several attempts were made to evaluate the effectiveness of medical treatment alone. All of these studies (WASID, TASS, ESPS, CAPRIE [89], [39], [24], [10] showed the potential to reduce the risk of suffering from stroke. Anticoagulation or antiplatelet therapy positively influences thrombembolic induced events, but may only have a reduced effect on events induced by hemodynamic insufficiency. Nevertheless, best medical treatment is always mandatory. Despite best medical treatment and the potential of a regressive course, prognosis is generally poor. In case of maximal medical treatment failure, angioplasty or stenting must then be considered. Experienced physicians are able to perform most lesions and the technical success rate is high (up to 95%). To reduce the complication rate, recent technological advances in microcatheter – microwire-systems, balloons and stents should be taken advantage of.

The short-term patency rate in cases of primary intracranial stent placement seems to be slightly favorable compared with angioplasty alone, but the long-term results have yet to be determined. The intracranial complication rates of intracranial angioplasty or stent placement are as high as 20% (general angiographical complication rate not included). During treatment, ischemic stroke has been reported in 0–20%, intracranial hemorrhage in 0–4%, vessel dissection in 0–10%, vessel rupture in 0–4%, vessel occlusion/thrombosis in 0–4% and death in 0–8% [80], [56], [61], [62], [2], [33], [34], [65], [35], [17], [49]. In neurologically unstable patients, e.g. with a recent ischemic stroke, an intracranial complication rate of up to 50% [36] was observed. As mentioned above, for patients with acute stroke or after thrombolysis, the risk of intracranial hemorrhage after angioplasty or stenting is very high. But sometimes recanalization is the only option in order to prevent the extension of the stroke or vessel reocclusion. The risk of intracranial hemorrhage versus the benefit of brain tissue salvage has to be weighed very carefully. Mori et al. [60]–[62] developed an angiographic classification system modified from a scheme for coronary arteries to predict the outcome of cerebral intervention with angioplasty alone. Lesions were categorized as shown in Table 1. Corresponding to this classification system, procedural success and short- and long-term outcome was either more or less satisfactory based on the type of lesion. Type A lesions show the best results, type B lesions have an intermediate risk and type C lesions have the poorest outcome and do not respond sufficiently to angioplasty alone. Mori reported procedural success for a type A lesion as 42% and for a type C lesion as 33%. In type C lesions, the short-term patency rate can even be totally unsatisfactory 0%. This classification system is developed for angioplasty alone, and the typical limitations of angioplasty (see above) can be reduced by primary stenting. The 30-day stroke and death rates after angioplasty or stenting are about 10% (maximal 36% in earlier studies) in the literature. Subacute or late restenosis is mostly related to neointimal hyperplasia and vascular remodeling. Neointimal hyperplasia seems to carry a lower risk

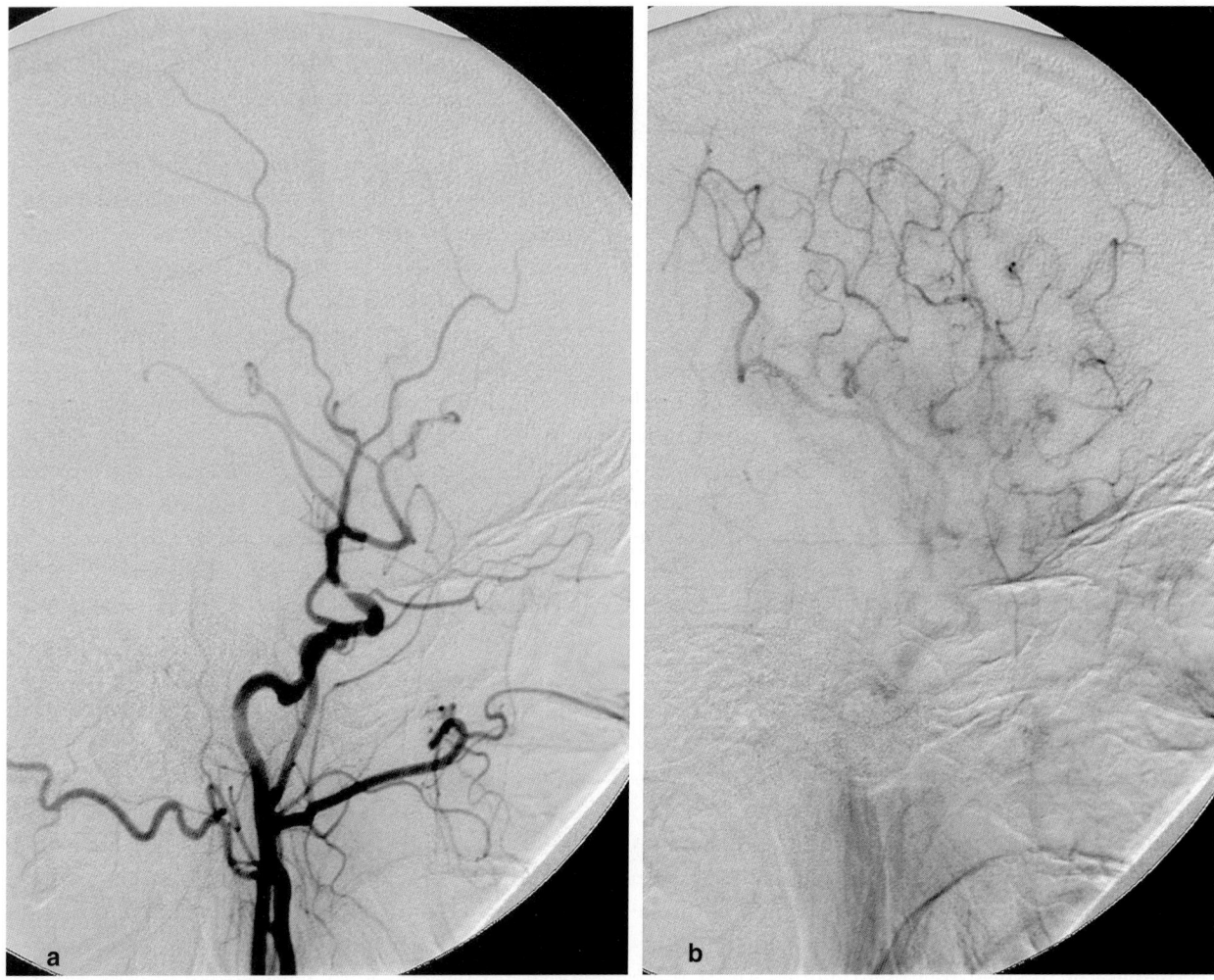

Fig. 4. Carotid artery angiogram of a high-grade intracranial internal carotid stenosis of the supraclinoid portion (explanation see text).

of thrombembolic events than does atheroselcerosis. In recent studies, about 60% of patients remain asymptomatic at the six month follow-up after interventional treatment. In stented lesions, restenosis > 50% occurred in about 11% after one year (0–30%) [56], [85], [21], [22], [33], [34], [65], [17], [60], [50], [51]. Nevertheless, the long-term patency rate of angioplasty or stent placement needs to be evaluated in further studies. It seems that patients with one event in their clinical history do not benefit from stenting, but for patients with recurrent events, interventional therapy is a good treatment option. The risk-to-benefit ratio has to be considered individually for each patient.

Take home points

In patients with intracranial atherosclerotic disease, angioplasty or stent placement should not be the first-line therapy. Instead, initial treatment should include the standard control of vascular risk factors and application of antiplatelet/anticoagulation drugs, statins and angiotensin-converting enzyme inhibitors. Unfortunately, best-medical treatment, intracranial atherosclerosis is associated with a poor prognosis. However, only in the case of maximal medical therapy failure, should interventional treatment be considered. Elective stenting of intracranial atherosclerotic lesions of the major intracranial arteries is technically feasible

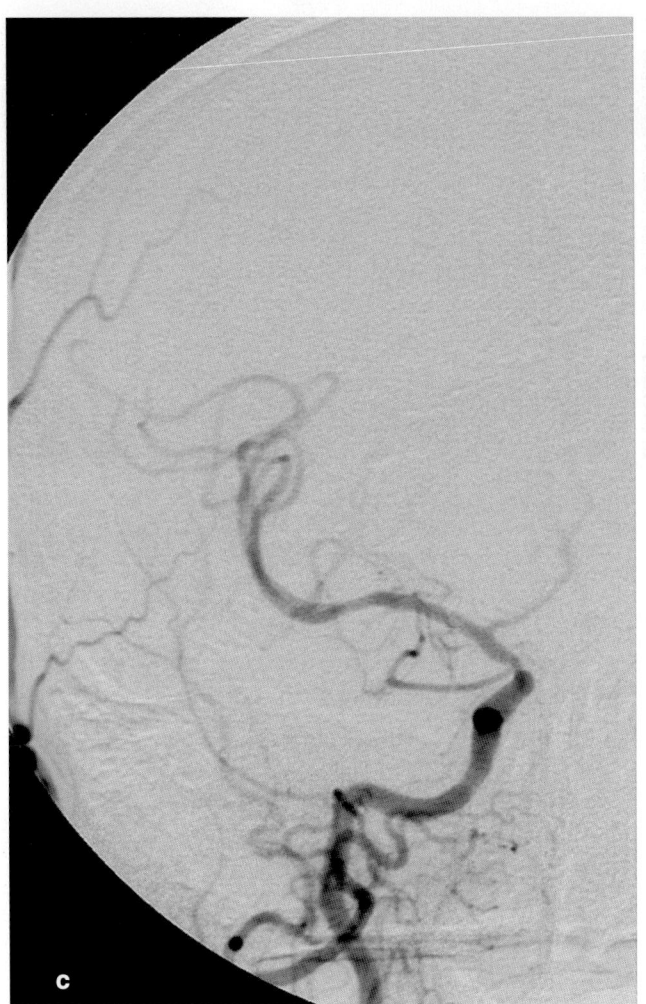
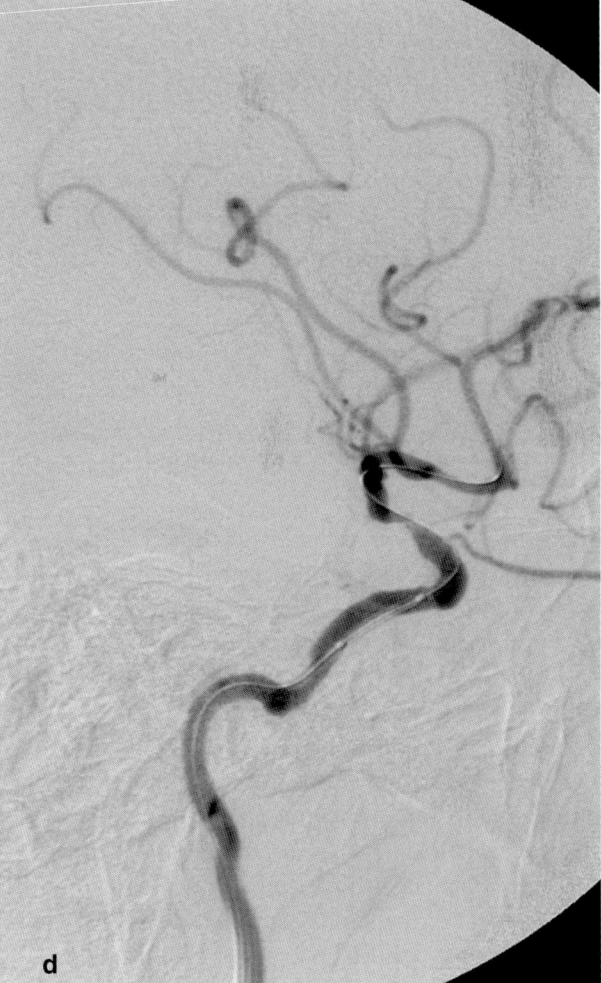

Fig. 4. (Continued)

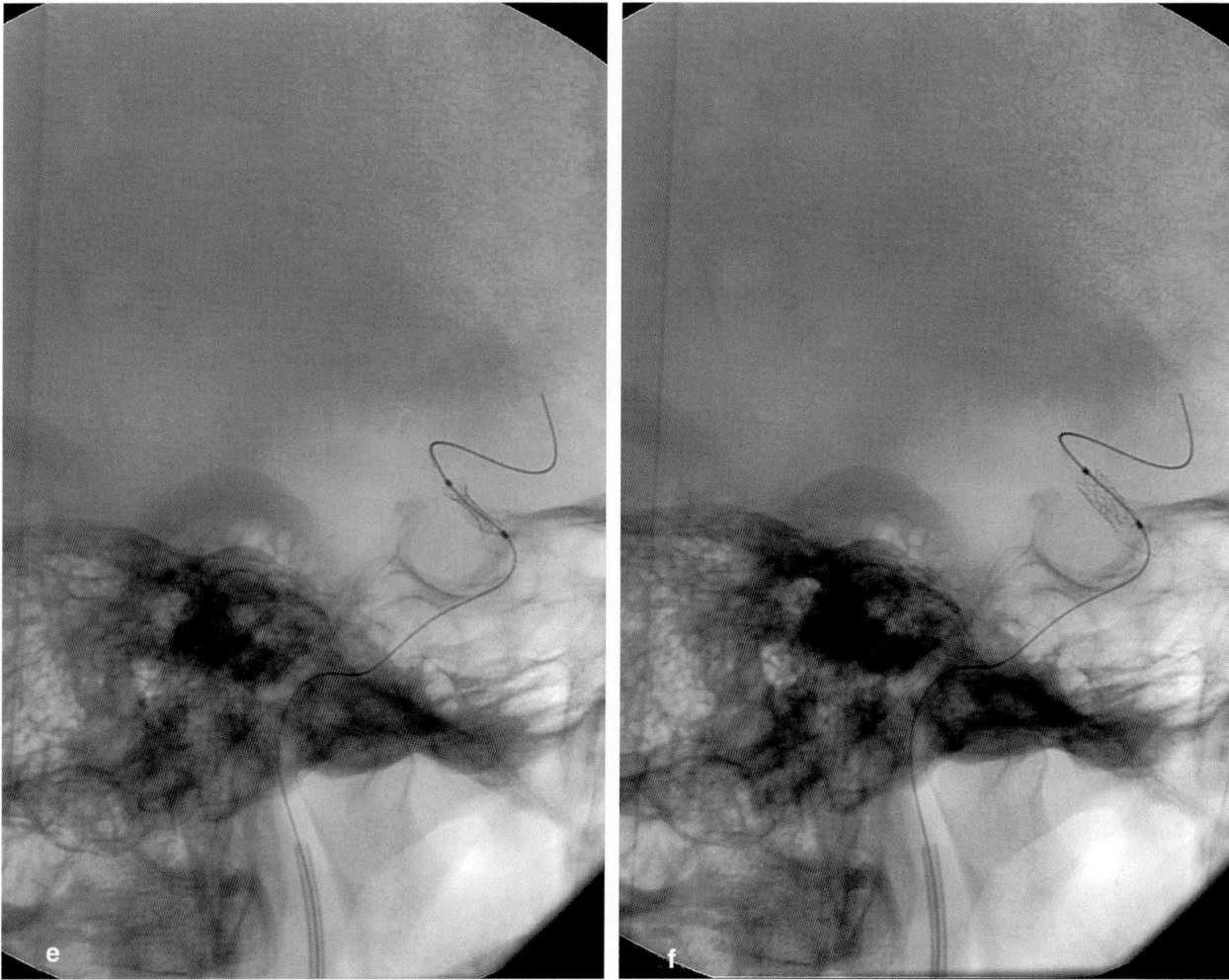

Fig. 4. (Continued)

and shows a good procedural and clinical success rate. Angioplasty and stent placement have to be done very carefully because, unlike extracranial arteries, the wall layers of intracranial arteries are very vulnerable. Using an oversized the balloon or stent could lead to vessel rupture with subarachnoid bleeding and the resulting devastating consequences. The small penetrating vessels can be covered by the stent or angioplasty, thus inducing dissection or microtrauma to the vessel walls resulting in stroke. Special attention has to be paid to the lateral lenticulostriate arteries arising from the M1-segment of the middle cerebral artery. Here, stent placement can produce better angiographic and short-term clinical results than balloon angioplasty alone due to the prevention of vessel dissection or vessel recoil. Therefore, the safety of interventional treatement can be increased by using stents versus angioplasty alone.

Angioplasty or stent therapy remains technically difficulty, and application of the interventional approach should always take into account multidisciplinary factors to ensure careful selection of the right patient and to reduce periprocedural complications. Up-to-date techniques using flexible and soft catheter and stent-delivery systems should be used and an experienced team of physicians is mandatory. It must always be kept in mind that interventional therapy of intracranial artery stenosis has a high periprocedural complication rate of up to 20% including stroke, intracranial hemorrhage and death. This com-

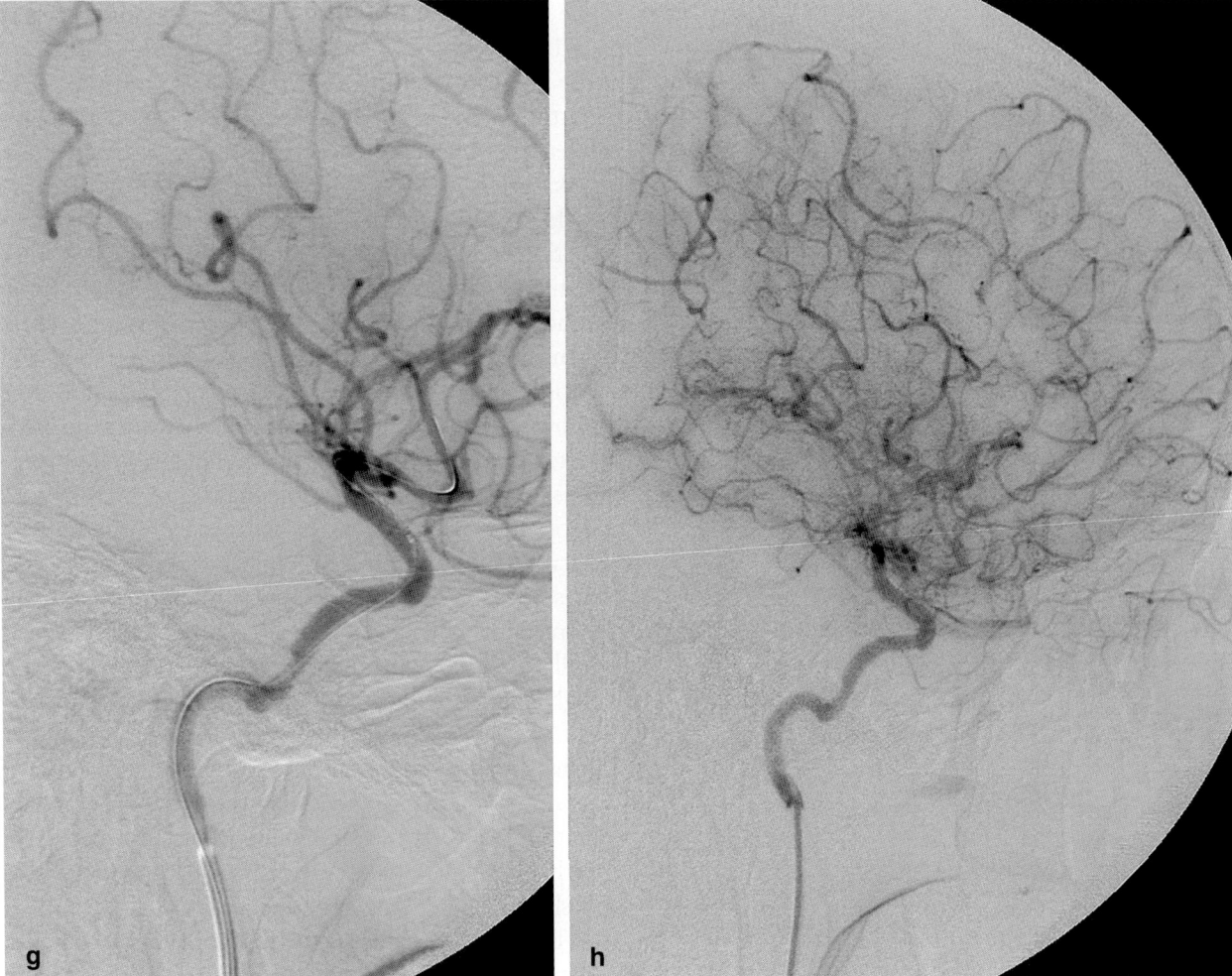

Fig. 4. (Continued)

plication rate will be even higher in neurologically unstable patients or in emergency situations. The goal of preprocedural imaging, in conjunction with a complete neurological history obtained by a neurologist, is to exclude patients with acute ischemic symptoms or exclude other potential differential diagnoses like cerebral vasculitis. The effectiveness of stroke prevention is not really known yet and the long-term results have to be further evaluated in the future. It seems that patients with recurrent events benefit more from interventional treatment than from medical treatment alone, whereas the benefit in patients with only one event in their clinical history has to be carefully considered. As with interventional therapy performed in other vessel territories, a periprocedural and a life-long post-procedural anticoagulation/antiplatelet treatment is mandatory.

Clinical examples

Fig. 4 shows a high-grade intracranial internal carotid stenosis of the supraclinoid portion (see arrows Fig. 4a for lateral view and Fig. 4c for anterior-posterior view) in a symptomatic patient. A concurrent reduced blood flow in the anterior and middle cerebral artery branches is well demonstrated (Fig. 4b). The stenosis could be easily crossed with a 0.014 inch microcatheter (Fig. 4d). Fig. 4e and f depict the opening of a balloon-

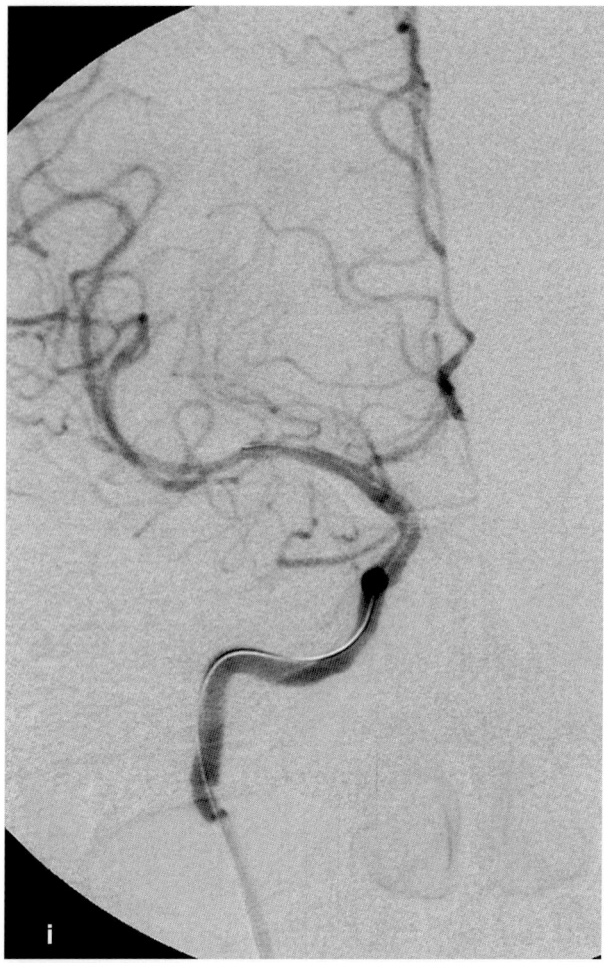

Fig. 4. (Continued)

expandable stent with of 2.5 mm in diameter and 20 mm in length. This stent is usually used in the coronary arteries. Fig. 4g and i depict the excellent result, with no restenosis or any vascular complications. In comparison to Fig. 4b, the anterior and middle cerebral arteries are again well perfused (Fig. 4h).

Extracranial brachiocephalic and common carotid artery stenosis

Clinical knowledge

Not only are the internal carotid arteries or major intracranial vessels affected by atherosclerosis, but also the common carotid arteries, the innominate artery and the subclavian arteries. Vasoocclusive disease of the upper extremities is much less common than in the lower extremities. Usually, lesions are atherosclerotic, whereas non-atherosclerotic changes like Takayasu's arteritis, connective-tissue disorders or collagen abnormalities, fibromuscular dysplasia and radiation-induced fibrosis are quite rare [83], [3]. Symptomatic lesions show a prevalence of 1.9% to 7.1% in cohort studies [83], [28]. As for internal carotid artery stenosis and stenosis of the major intracerebral and peripheral vessels, the typical risk factors are well known. Extracranial brachiocephalic stenoses are associated, e.g., with a history of smoking, systolic hypertension and hypercholesterolemia or low high-density lipoprotein cholesterol. A coexistence with atherosclerotic lesions in the intracranial vessels, lower extremities [37], in the cardiovascular system or in other extracranial brachiocephalic arteries can be observed as well. Unlike intracranial atherosclerotic lesions, no higher risk is found to be associated with certain ethnic groups like Hispanics, African Americans or Asians [83]. Whereas a male predominance is known for other atherosclerotic lesions, lesions in the innominate artery occur with no significant differences in both sexes [43]. Stenoses of the subclavian artery tend to show a higher incidence on the left side [28], and in up to a third of patients, the innominate artery is also affected [83], [94]. Furthermore, it has been observed that stenoses are more common in the proximal vessel segments or proximal to the origin of the vertebral artery. This can be attributed to the fact that a more turbulent flow in the aortic arch, nearer the origin, induces more extensive plaque deposits [79].

Major symptoms of stenosis or occlusion of the subclavian artery include upper limb ischemia/claudicatio (palor, finger coldness, functional raynaud disease), peripheral emboli to the brachial-, forearm-, hand- and finger-arteries, sensory- and motor deficit, considerable interarm blood pressure difference and vertebrobasilary insufficiency (subclavian steal syndrome). Patients with a high grade stenosis of the subclavian or innominate artery show a reversal of blood flow in the ipsilateral vertebral artery. This steal phenomenon leads to the typical symptoms of a hemodynamic insufficiency in the posterior brain circulation

[40], e.g., vertigo or collapsing after arm exercises. The same phenomenon is observed in patients with an arterial thoracic outlet syndrome, but there the stenosis is caused by compressive fibrous, muscle or bone structures, and is usually treated by transaxillary or supraclavicular surgery. Subclavian stenosis in patients with an internal mammary interventricular anterior artery bypass or a Blalock-Taussig shunt can lead to a coronary-subclavian steal with myocardial ischemia [31]. An interarm difference of > 15 mm Hg of the systolic blood pressure is considered clinically significant [48]. for patients with subclavian or innominate artery stenosis, a sensitivity of about 50% and a specifity of 90% is described, with an interarm systolic blood pressure difference of > 15 mm Hg [28]. This relatively low sensitivity is a result of a low or moderate grade stenosis, whereas a high grade stenosis or an obstruction shows a more significant sensitivity [83], [28]. Stenoses or occlusions of the common carotid artery cause symptoms similar to that of the internal carotid artery, e.g., cerebral or ocular ischemia, like transient ischemic attacks or amarousis fugax and are a source for thrombembolic events. The risk of ischemia is not only dependent on the grade of stenosis, but also on the plaque morphology, especially in incomplete occlusions or ulcerations. Stenoses or occlusions of the innominate are markedly different than a single subclavian or carotid artery stenosis. They are symptomatic as a result of the reduced blood flow in the subclavian and carotid artery, and can thereby result in upper limb ischemia and ocular or cerebral ischemia.

Clinical examination includes comparative blood pressure measurements on both arms, pulse palpation and a subclavian, carotid and vertebral Doppler color-flow ultrasound to verify suspected stenosis or a steal phenomenon. Examination by a neurologist is mandatory in the case of common carotid artery lesions, but should also be performed as well in lesions affecting the other supraaortic vessel.

Imaging knowledge

In the detection of extracranial brachiocephalic and the common carotid artery stenosis, Doppler color-flow ultrasound is routinely used. It should always include an examination of both common carotid arteries, both subclavian arteries and both vertebral arteries. The duplex of the vertebral arteries provides evidence for the reversed blood flow in the ipsilateral vertebral artery in case of a subclavian stenosis. Ultrasound can also be useful in evaluating plaque morphology. DSA is still the gold-standard and must be performed before any intervention. Every DSA should start with an overall view from the aortic arch to the circle of Willis, usually with a left-anterior-oblique projection of 30°. After that, the affected vessel can be depicted selectively. In case of a common carotid artery stenosis, a four-vessel angiography is recommended to obtain detailed information about intracranial blood flow, performed as well in internal carotid artery lesions. In patients with subclavian artery stenosis, it can be necessary to perform semiselective angiography of the contralateral vertebral artery to depict the reversed blood flow in the ipsilateral vertebral artery. For diagnostic use or interventional or surgery planning, non-invasive imaging methods can be used. Magnetic resonance angiography is the most preferred non-invasive method. However, with new CT technologies (multirow scanner), an excellent depiction of the supraaortic vessel is possible as well. In addition, the extent of calcification can also be clearly visualized. For patients with a history of cerebral or ocular ischemic events, a supplemental image of the brain is obligatory. Diffusion- and perfusion-weighted magnetic resonance images are optional, but should be performed to determine the presence of possible ischemic areas. Non-invasive imaging techniques are sufficient, if only surgery treatment is planned, but naturally, DSA must be performed if interventional treatment is the chosen course of action.

Treatment knowledge

Traditionally, surgical revascularization of extracranial brachiocephalic and common carotid artery lesions using a transthoracic or extrathoracic route has procedural good technical success rates and acceptable long-term results. More recently, angioplasty of the extracranial brachiocephalic and the common carotid artery, which began in the 1980s, has become increasingly important. Surgical treatment is associated with a considerable morbidity and mortality rate [43], [12], [59], [9], resulting in potential lung atelectasis, pneumothorax, chylothorax, pleural effusion, stroke, phrenic nerve palsy or Horner's syndrome. In contrast, angioplasty is very effective, shows a low incidence of complications and produces excellent short- and midterm results [38].

DSA, angioplasty or stent treatment is generally performed using the transfemoral access and local anesthesia. Sometimes, an additional transbrachial approach can be very helpful if a subclavian occlusion can not be crossed via the transfemoral route and the aortic arch. Often the lesion can be crossed via the transbrachial route, and then grasped with a lassocatheter and drawn out transfemorally. Further operations can be performed via the femoral access. Using small delivery systems, all operations can also be performed via the transbrachial access and recanalization can also be attempted from this point. For the transfemoral access, usually a short sheath in combination with a guiding catheter or a long sheath alone are used. If a lesion is suspected in the common carotid artery, a four-vessel angiography should be performed to obtain additional information about the intracranial circulation and collaterals. In case of a subclavian or innominate artery stenosis, the aortic arch must be depicted and the reversed blood flow of the ipsilateral vertebral artery documented to provide evidence of the steal phenomenon. After the lesion was crossed, angioplasty can be performed as usual. Common carotid artery stenosis should be primary stented, similar to the internal carotid artery stenosis. Self-expanding stents, e.g., Wallstents are highly recommended.

In the literature, no consensus has been reached as to whether angioplasty alone or primary stenting is more favorable in the treatment of the subclavian and the innominate artery. Several authors did not report any differences between primary stented lesions or nonstented lesions as far as the recurrent stenosis rate was concerned [23], [41]. Often, additional stent placement is necessary in the case of a dissection after angioplasty or if a residual stenosis of > 20% persists, as well in cases of a persisting pressure gradient of > 5 mm Hg. Residual stenoses are mostly seen in highly calcified lesions. To avoid dissection or covering up of the vertebral origin after angioplasty or stenting, the subclavian lesions must be proximal and at a safe distance from the origin of the vertebral artery. Balloon-expandable stents should be preferred due to the high accuracy of placement with respect to the origin of the vertebral artery and the aortic arch. The anticoagulation and antiplatelet regimen should be performed according to standard procedure. Before intervention, 75 mg clopidogrel daily or 250 mg ticlopidine daily should be administered for at least three days. During the interventional procedure, heparinization with up to 10,000 IU (acquired coagulation time ACT about 200–300 sec) is recommended. After the intervention, a daily dose of clopidogrel or ticlopidine and acetylsalicylic acid (100–300 mg) for up to six months is necessary and acetylsalicylic acid monotherapy (or clopidogrel/ticlopidine monotherapy) should be continued for at least an additional six months. As opposed to surgery, patients can usually be discharged within two days after the interventional procedure.

Angioplasty or stenting should be preferred in the treatment of extracranial brachiocephalic and common carotid artery stenosis. However, surgery is still indicated after unsuccessful interventional treatment or long segment occlusions, heavy calcification or in lesions located very close to the vertebral origin. Furthermore, a history of embolization from incomplete occlusions or ulcerative plaques in the innominate or common carotid artery is also an indication for surgery. Innominate artery stenosis can be responsible for both cerebral and upper limb ischemia, therefore the indication for interventional therapy has to be checked very carefully. This holds true for right-sided subclavian artery lesions as well, whose treatment is believed to be a risky procedure due to the proximity of the common carotid artery [23].

Prognosis

To assess the success rate and the long-term follow-up of angioplasty or stenting, several studies were carried out. The primary technical success is achieved in about 98% of all observed cases [43], [79], [38]. Only in the case of occlusions was initial failure observed due to the inability of crossing the lesions. Common carotid artery stenosis should be primary stented due

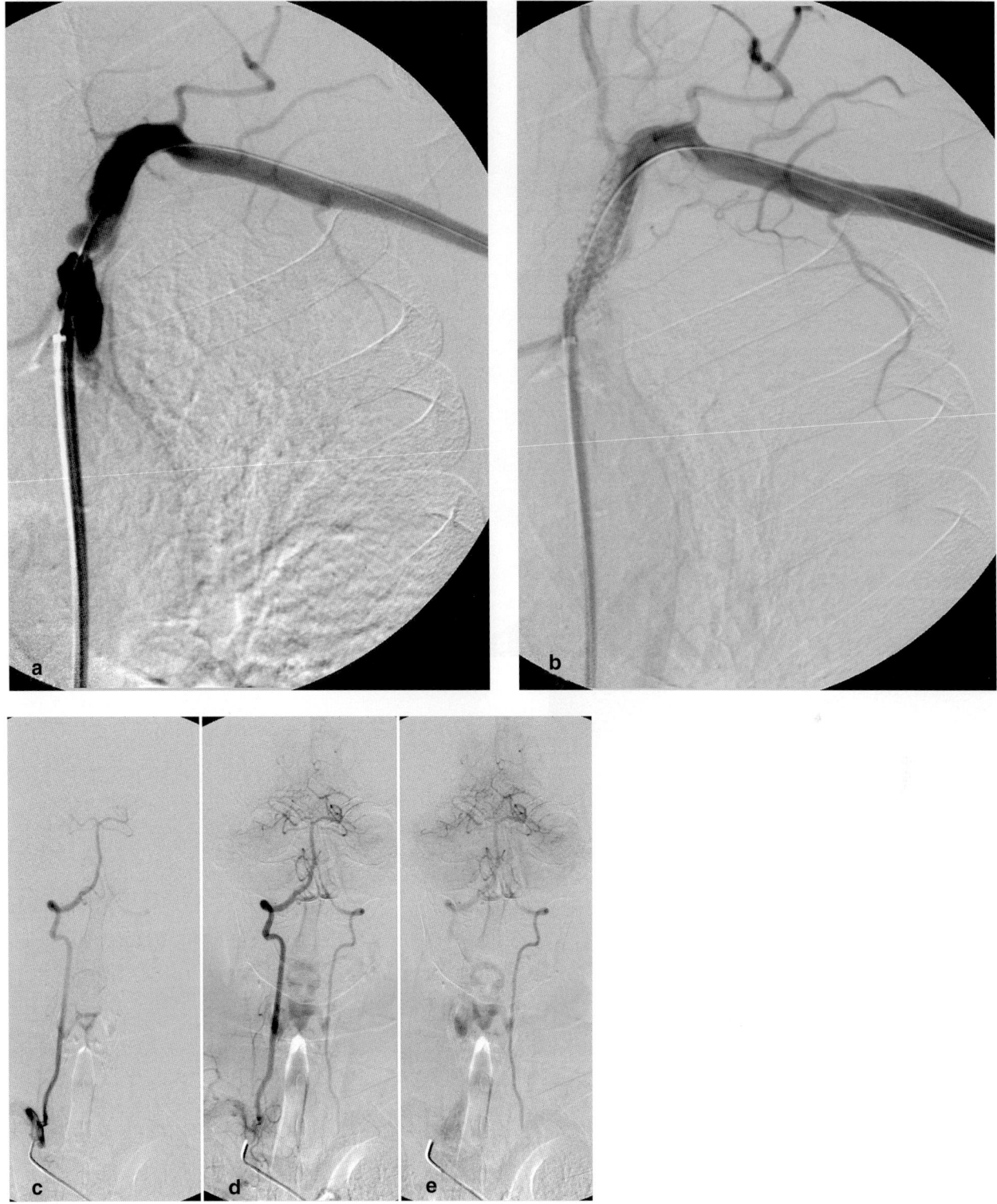

Fig. 5. Angiogram of a typical high-grade stenosis of the left subclavian artery (explanation see text).

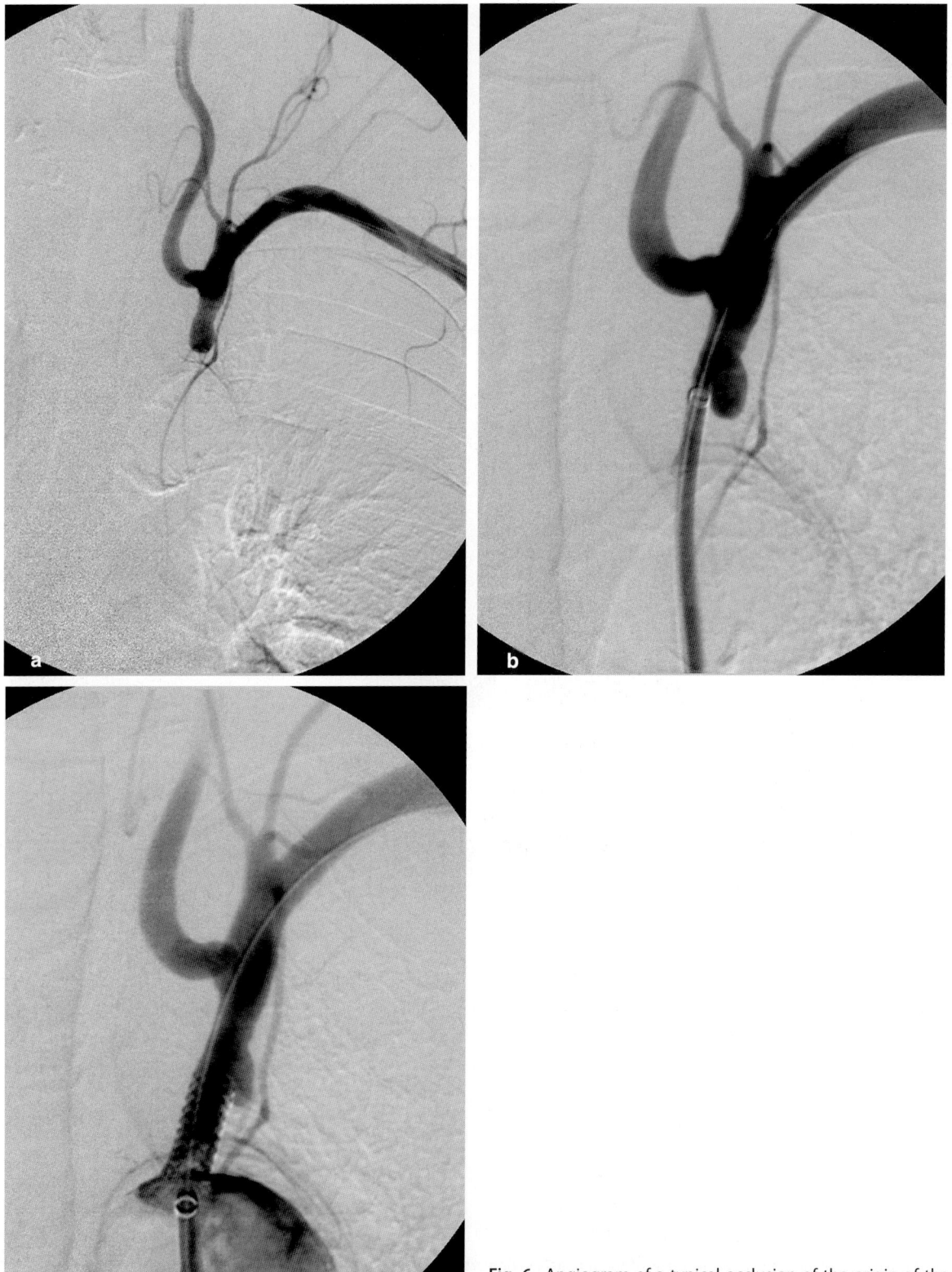

Fig. 6. Angiogram of a typical occlusion of the origin of the left subclavian artery (explanation see text).

to increased procedural safety, whereas lesions of the innominate artery or subclavian artery lesions can be dilated by angioplasty alone. However, stent placement must always be performed in case of a suboptimal angioplasty result. Primary stented lesions show a better 1-year patency rate (95% vs. 79%), but the long-term outcomes are slightly less favorable (59% vs. 68%) [79] than in angioplasty alone groups due to instent neointimal hyperplasia. The superior short-term outcome of stent treatment leads to the prevention of elastic vessel recoil [79]. Some authors did not see any difference in patency rate between stented and balloon-dilated alone lesions and report a general long-term patency rate of 89% [23]. Occluded lesions have as favorable a clinical outcome as stenotic lesions, despite the somewhat reduced initial technical success rate [23]. Patients with aortoarteritis should not undergo interventional therapy, due to the quite poor outcome. Considering all interventional methods, the local complication rate is known to be about 4.5%. Severe complications like periprocedural stroke or transient ischemic attacks are observed in up to 3.6%, whereas the incidence of neurological complications is lower in the treatment of the subclavian artery and higher in the treatment of the innominate artery or the common carotid artery [79], [11]. The reversed blood flow in the ipsilateral vertebral artery in patients with subclavian artery stenosis prevents vertebrobasilary ischemic events during the procedure. This reversed blood flow persists for several minutes after angioplasty [71]. The complication rate of the brachial approach is suggested to be higher than for the typical femoral approach. In some cases, a subclavian or innominate artery lesion can be more easily crossed from the brachial route.

It has been shown that the technical success rate for interventional methods is equivalent to that of surgical methods and a similar patency rate was also observed. However, the overall incidence of stroke is 3 ± 4% and of death 2 ± 2% in the published surgical studies. The risk of severe complications from surgery is at least 5%. A comparison of stenting over surgery demonstrates equal effectiveness, but fewer complications and suggests that stenting should be considered as the first-line therapy for subclavian or brachiocephalic obstruction [38].

Take home points

Atherosclerotic lesions of the extracranial brachiocephalic and common carotid artery stenosis should be preferably treated with percutaneous transluminal angioplasty or stenting. These techniques show high effectiveness and an excellent technical success rate as well as a good clinical outcome. Compared to surgery, angioplasty shows no greater risk of complications and even an overall lower complication rate. Except in cases of occlusions, technical success can be achieved in nearly every patient undergoing angioplasty. Common carotid artery lesions should be primary stented due to the safety of the technical procedure, whereas in subclavian or innominate artery lesions, the effectiveness of primary stenting versus angioplasty alone with respect to regarding the long-term patency rate is not yet proven. This suggests that primary stenting is not mandatory. However, if a suboptimal result occurs for dissection or residual stenosis under angioplasty alone, secondary stent treatment is mandatory. Attention also has to be paid to the origin of the vertebral artery to avoid dissection or covering it up. Usually, interventional therapy is performed via the femoral access, but an additional brachial route can be sometimes helpful when dealing with subclavian or innominate artery lesions. The risk of vertebrobasilary ischemic events is very low during the treatment of subclavian artery lesions due to the reversed blood flow in the ipsilateral vertebral artery. Antiplatelet therapy with clopidogrel or ticlopidine and acetylsalicylic acid is always mandatory after interventional treatment. Surgery is still indicated after unsuccessful interventional treatment or for the treatment of long segment occlusions, or if a history of embolization from incomplete occlusions or ulcerative plaques exists, or for lesions located very close to the vertebral origin.

Clinical examples

Fig. 5a shows a typical high-grade stenosis of the left subclavian artery. Using transfemoral access and after crossing the stenosis, a 7 French sheath was placed proximal to the stenosis. First, the stenosis was predilated with a 4 mm and a 5 mm diameter balloon-catheter. Then the sheath could be placed distal to the stenosis and a balloon-expandable stent 8 mm in diameter and 28 mm in length was correctly placed. The sheath was redrawn and then the stent was deployed. No restenosis remained (Fig. 5b). The patient suffered from the steal-syndrome with dizziness and precollapsing after arm exercises. Fig. 5c–e depict the steal phenomenon with a cross-flow from the left to the right vertebral artery and a resulting perfusion of the subclavian artery distal to the stenosis. After stent implantation no steal and no reversed blood flow was observed in the ipsilateral vertebral artery (Fig. 5f).

Fig. 6a is an angiogram of a typical occlusion of the origin of the left subclavian artery. The occlusion could be crossed via a transbrachial access, and than the guidewire could be drawn out of the additional transfemoral access. The sheath was introduced via the transfemoral access (Fig. 6b). The lesion could be treated successfully with a 8 mm in diameter balloon-expandable stent (Fig. 6c). The stent projects about 3 mm into the lumen of the aortic arch.

References

[1] Akins PT, Pilgram TK, Cross DT 3rd et al.: Natural history of stenosis from intracranial atherosclerosis by serial angiography. Stroke 29: 433–438 (1998).

[2] Alazzaz A, Thornton J, Aletich VA et al.: Intracranial percutaneous transluminal angioplasty for arteriosclerotic stenosis. Arch Neurol 57: 1625–1630 (2000).

[3] Arend WP, Michel BA, Bloch DA et al.: The American College of Rheumatology 1990 criteria for the classification of Takayasu arteritis. Arthritis Rheum 33: 1129–1134 (1990).

[4] Assadian A, Senekowitsch C, Rotter R et al.: Long-term results of covered stent repair of internal carotid artery dissections. J Vasc Surg 40: 484–487 (2004).

[5] Baumgartner RW, Mattle HP, Schroth G: Assessment of ./5 50% and < 50% intracranial stenoses by transcranial color-coded duplex sonography. Stroke 30: 87–92 (1999).

[6] Beletsky V, Nadarcishvili Z, Lynch J et al.: Canadian Stroke Consortium, Cervical arterial dissection: time for a therapeutic trial? Stroke 34: 2856–2860 (2003).

[7] Bogousslavsky J, Despland PA, Regli F: Spontaneous carotid dissection with acute stroke. Arch Neurol 44: 137–140 (1987).

[8] Bogousslavsky J, Barnett HJ, Fox AJ et al.: Atherosclerotic disease of the middle cerebral artery. Stroke 17: 1112–1120 (1986).

[9] Brewster DC, Moncure AC, Darling RC et al.: Innominate artery lesions: problems encountered and lessons learned. J Vasc Surg 2: 99–112 (1985).

[10] CAPRIE Steering Committee: A randomized, blinded, trial of clopidogrel versus aspirin in patients at risk of ischemic events (CAPRIE). Lancet 348: 1329–1339 (1996).

[11] Carotid artery stenting in clinical practice Results from the Carotid Artery Stenting (CAS)-registry of the Arbeitsgemeinschaft Leitende Kardiologische Krankenhausarzte (ALKK). Z Kardiol 94: 163–172 (2005).

[12] Cherry KJ Jr, McCullough JL, Hallett JW Jr et al.: Technical principles of direct innominate artery revascularization: a comparison of endarterectomy and bypass grafts. J Vasc Surg 9: 718–724 (1989).

[13] Chimowitz MI: Angioplasty or stenting is not appropriate as first-line treatment of intracranial stenosis. Arch Neurol 58: 1690–1692 (2001).

[14] Chimowitz MI, Kokkinos J, Strong J et al.: The Warfarin-Aspirin Symptomatic Intracranial Disease Study. Neurology 45: 1488–1493 (1995).

[15] Cohen J, Leker RR, Gotkine M et al.: Emergent stenting to treat patients with carotid artery dissection. Stroke 34: 254–257 (2003).

[16] Comerota AJ, Katz ML, Hosking JD et al.: Is transcranial Doppler a worthwhile addition to screening tests for cerebrovascular disease? J Vasc Surg 21: 90–97 (1995).

[17] Connors JJ 3rd, Wojak JC: Percutaneous transluminal angioplasty for intracranial atherosclerotic lesions: evolution of technique and short-term results. J Neurosurg 91: 415–423 (1999).

[18] Corston RN, Kendall BE, Marshall J: Prognosis in middle cerebral artery stenosis. Stroke 15: 237–241 (1984).

[19] Davis SM, Donnan GA.: Advances in Penumbra Imaging with MR. Cerebrovasc Dis [17 Suppl] 3: 23–27 (2004).

[20] De Bray JM, Lhoste P, Dubas F et al.: Ultrasonic features of extracranial carotid dissections: 47 cases studied by angiography. J Ultrasound Med 13: 659–664 (1994).

[21] de Rochemont Rdu M, Sitzer M, Zanella FE et al.: Stents in the treatment of intracranial atherosclerotic stenoses. Radiologe 44: 1004–1012 (2004).

[22] de Rochemont Rdu M, Turowski B, Buchkremer M et al.: Recurrent symptomatic high-grade intracranial stenoses: safety and efficacy of undersized stents-initial experience. Radiology 231: 45–49 (2004).

[23] De Vries JP, Jager LC, Van den Berg JC et al.: Durability of percutaneous transluminal angioplasty for ob-

structive lesions of proximal subclavian artery: long-term results. J Vasc Surg 41: 19–23 (2005).
[24] Diener HC, Cunha L, Forbes C et al.: European Stroke Prevention Study. 2. Dipyridamole and acetylsalicylic acid in the secondary prevention of stroke. J Neurol Sci 143: 1–13 (1996).
[25] Djouhri H, Guillon B, Brunnereau L: MR angiograhy for the long-term follow-up of dissecting aneurysms of the extracranial internal carotid artery. Am J Roentgenol 174: 1137–1140 (2000).
[26] Ducrocq X, Lacour JC, Debouverie M et al.: Cerebral ischemic accidents in young subjects. A prospective study of 296 patients aged 16 to 45 years. Rev Neurol 155: 575–582 (1999).
[27] Duong TQ, Fisher M: Applications of diffusion/ perfusion magnetic resonance imaging in experimental and clinical aspects of stroke. Curr Atheroscler Rep 6: 267–273 (2004).
[28] English JA, Carell ES, Guidera SA et al.: Angiographic prevalence and clinical predictors of left subclavian stenosis in patients undergoing diagnostic cardiac catheterization. Catheter Cardiovasc Interv 54: 8–11 (2001).
[29] Fanelli F, Salvatori FM, Ferrari R et al.: Stent repair of bilateral post-traumatic dissections of the internal carotid artery. J Endovasc Ther 11: 517–521 (2004).
[30] Feldmeier JJ, Merendaz C, Regli F: Symptomatic stenosis of the middle cerebral artery. Rev Neurol 139: 725–736 (1983).
[31] Ferrara F, Meli F, Raimondi F et al.: Subclavian stenosis/occlusion in patients with subclavian steal and previous bypass of internal mammary interventricular anterior artery: medical or surgical treatment? Ann Vasc Surg 18: 566–571 (2004).
[32] Gelal FM, Kitis O, Calli C et al.: Craniocervical artery dissection: diagnosis and follow-up with imaging and MR angiography. Med Sci Monit 10: 109–116 (2004).
[33] Gomez CR, Misra VK, Liu MW et al.: Elective stenting of symptomatic basilar artery stenosis. Stroke 31: 5–9 (2000).
[34] Gomez CR, Misra VK, Campbell MS et al.: Elective stenting of symptomatic middle cerebral artery stenosis. Am J Neuroradiol 21: 971–973 (2000).
[35] Gress DR, Smith WS, Dowd CF et al.: Angioplasty for intracranial symptomatic vertebrobasilar ischemia. Neurosurgery 51: 23–27; discussion 27–29 (2002).
[36] Gupta R, Schumacher HC, Mangla S et al.: Urgent endovascular revsacularization for symptomatic intracranial atherosclerosis stenosis. Neurology 61: 1729–1735 (2003).
[37] Gutierrez GR, Mahrer P, Aharonian V et al.: Prevalence of subclavian artery stenosis in patients with peripheral vascular disease. Angiology 52: 189–194 (2001).

[38] Hadjipetrou P, Cox S, Piemonte T et al.: Percutaneous revascularization of atherosclerotic obstruction of aortic arch vessels. J Am Coll Cardiol 33: 1238–1245 (1999).
[39] Hass WK, Easton JD, Adams HP Jr et al.: A randomized trial comparing ticlopidine hydrochloride with aspirin for the prevention of stroke in high-risk patients. Ticlopidine Aspirin Stroke Study Group. N Engl J Med 321: 501–507 (1989).
[40] Hennerici M, Klemm C, Rautenberg W: The subclavian steal phenomenon: a common vascular disorder with rare neurologic deficits. Neurology 38: 669–673 (1988).
[41] Henry M, Amor M, Henry I et al.: Percutaneous transluminal angioplasty of the subclavian arteries. J Endovasc Surg 6: 33–41 (1999).
[42] Houser OW, Mokri B, Sundt TM Jr et al.: Spontaneous cervical cephalic arterial dissection and its residuum: angiographic spectrum. Am J Neuroradiol 5: 27–34 (1984).
[43] Huttl K, Nemes B, Simonffy A et al.: Angioplasty of the innominate artery in 89 patients: experience over 19 years. Cardiovasc Intervent Radiol 25: 109–114 (2002).
[44] Johnson MB, Wilkinson ID, Wattam J et al.: Comparison of Doppler ultrasound, magnetic resonance angiographic techniques and catheter angiography in evaluation of carotid stenosis. Clin Radiol 55: 912–920 (2000).
[45] Kim SH, Qureshi AI, Levy EI et al.: Emergency stent placement for symptomatic acute carotid artery occlusion after endarterectomy. Case report. J Neurosurg 101: 151–153 (2004).
[46] Koch S, Rabinstein AA, Romano JG et al.: Diffusion-weighted magnetic resonance imaging in internal carotid artery dissection. Arch Neurol 61: 510–512 (2004).
[47] Kremer C, Mosso M, Georgiadis D et al.: Carotid dissection with permanent and transient occlusion or severe stenosis: long-term outcome. Neurology 60: 271–275 (2003).
[48] Lane D, Beevers M, Barnes N et al.: Inter-arm differences in blood pressure: when are they clinically significant? J Hypertens 20: 1089–1095 (2002).
[49] Lee JH, Kwon SU, Lee JH et al.: Percutaneous transluminal angioplasty for symptomatic middle cerebral artery stenosis: long-term follow-up. Cerebrovasc Dis 15: 90–97 (2003).
[50] Levy EI, Hanel RA, Boulos AS et al.: Comparison of periprocedure complications resulting from direct stent placement compared with those due to conventional and staged stent placement in the basilar artery. J Neurosurg 99: 653–660 (2003).
[51] Levy EL, Horowitz MB, Koebbe CJ et al.: Transluminal stent-assisted angioplasty of the intracranial vertebrobasilar system for medically refractory, posterior circulation ischemia: early results. Neurosurgery 48: 1215–1221 (2001).

[52] Leys D, Moulin TH, Stojkovic T et al.: DONALD Investigators. Follow-up of patients with history of cervical artery dissection. Cerebrovasc Dis 5: 43–49 (1995).
[53] Liu AY, Paulsen RD, Marcellus ML et al.: Long-term outcomes after carotid stent placement treatment of carotid artery dissection. Neurosurgery 45: 1368–1373; discussion 1373–1374 (1999).
[54] Lucas C, Moulin T, Deplanque D et al.: Stroke patterns of internal carotid artery dissection in 40 patients. Stroke 29: 2646–2648 (1998).
[55] Lutsep HL, Clark WM: Association of intracranial stenosis with cortical symptoms or signs. Neurology 12: 716–718 (2000).
[56] Lylyk P, Cohen JE, Ceratto R et al.: Angioplasty and stent placement in intracranial atherosclerotic stenoses and dissections. Am J Neuroradiol 23: 430–436 (2002).
[57] Lyrer P, Engelter S. Antithrombotic drugs for carotid artery dissection. Stroke 35: 613–614 (2004).
[58] Malek AM, Higashida RT, Phatouros CC et al.: Endovascular management of extracranial carotid artery dissection achieved using stent angioplasty. Am J Neuroradiol 21: 1280–1292 (2000).
[59] Melliere D, Becquemin JP, Benyahia NE et al.: Atherosclerotic disease of the innominate artery: current management and results. J Cardiovasc Surg 33: 319–323 (1992).
[60] Mori T, Kazita K, Chokyu K et al.: Short-term arteriographic and clinical outcome after cerebral angioplasty and stenting for intracranial vertebrobasilar and carotid atherosclerotic occlusive disease. Am J Neuroradiol 21: 249–254 (2000).
[61] Mori T, Fukuoka M, Kazita K et al.: Follow-up study after percutaneous transluminal cerebral angioplasty. Eur Radiol 8: 403–408 (1998).
[62] Mori T, Fukuoka M, Kazita K et al.: Follow-up study after intracranial percutaneous transluminal cerebral balloon angioplasty. Am J Neuroradiol 19: 1525–1533 (1998).
[63] Mori T, Mori K, Fukuoka M et al.: Percutaneous transluminal cerebral angioplasty: serial angiographic follow-up after successful dilatation. Neuroradiology 39: 111–116 (1997).
[64] Moritani T, Ekholm S, Westesson PL: Diffusion-Weighted MR Imaging of the Brain. Springer-Verlag Berlin Heidelberg New York (2004).
[65] Marks MP, Marcellus M, Norbash AM et al.: Outcome of angioplasty for atherosclerotic intracranial stenosis. Stroke 30: 1065–1069 (1999).
[66] Morris P: Intracranial Angioplasty and Stenting. In: Interventional and Endovascular Therapy of the Nervous System. Springer-Verlag NewYork, Inc. pp. 121–138 (2000).
[67] Mueller BT, Luther B, Waldemar H: et al. Surgical treatment of 50 carotid dissections: indications and results. J Vasc Surg 31: 980–988 (2000).
[68] North America Symptomatic Carotid Endarterectomy Trial Collaborators. Beneficial effect of carotid endarterectomy in symptomatic patients with high-grade carotid stenosis. N Engl J Med 325: 445–453 (1991).
[69] National Institute of Neurological Disorders and Stroke. Carotid endarterectomy for asymptomatic internal carotid artery stenosis. J Neurol Sci 129: 76–77 (1995).
[70] Parsons MW, Yang Q, Barber PA et al.: Perfusion magnetic resonance imaging maps in hyperacute stroke: relative cerebral blood flow most accurately identifies tissue destined to infarct. Stroke 32: 1581–1587 (2001).
[71] Rodriguez-Lopez JA, Werner A, Martinez R et al.: Stenting for atherosclerotic occlusive disease of the subclavian artery. Ann Vasc Surg 13: 254–260 (1999).
[72] Sacco RL, Kargman DE, Gu Q et al.: Race-ethnicity and determinants of intracranial atherosclerotic cerebral infarction. The Northern Manhattan Stroke Study. Stroke 26: 14–20 (1995).
[73] Schievink WI: Spontaneous dissection of the carotid and vertebral arteries. N Engl J Med 344: 898–906 (2001).
[74] Schievink WI: The treatment of spontaneous carotid and vertebral artery dissections. Curr Opin Cardiol 15: 316–321 (2000).
[75] Schievink WI, Björnsson J, Piepgras DG: Coexistence of fibromuscular dysplasia and cystic medial necrosis in a patient with Marfan's Syndrome and bilateral carotid artery dissections. Stroke 25: 2492–2496 (1994).
[76] Schievink WI, Mokri B, Piepgras DG: Spontaneous dissection of cervicocephalic arteries in childhood and adolescence. Neurology 44: 1607–1612 (1994).
[77] Schievink WI, Mokri B, O'Fallon WM: Recurrent spontaneous cervical-artery dissection. N Engl J Med 330: 393–397 (1994).
[78] Schievink WI, Mokri B, Whisnant JP: Internal carotid artery dissection in a community: Rochester, Minnesota, 1987–1992. Stroke 24: 1678–1680 (1993).
[79] Schillinger M, Haumer M, Schillinger S et al.: Risk stratification for subclavian artery angioplasty: is there an increased rate of restenosis after stent implantation? J Endovasc Ther 8: 550–557 (2001).
[80] Schumacher HC, Khaw AV, Meyers PM et al.: Intracranial angioplasty and stent placement for cerebral atherosclerosis. J Vasc Interv Radiol 15: 123–132 (2004).
[81] Schwarze JJ, Babikian V, DeWitt LD et al.: Longitudinal monitoring of intracranial arterial stenoses with transcranial Doppler ultrasonography. J Neuroimaging 4: 182–187 (1994).

[82] Segura T, Serena J, Castellanos M et al.: Embolism in acute middle cerebral artery stenosis. Neurology 56: 497–501 (2001).
[83] Shadman R, Criqui MH, Bundens WP et al.: Subclavian artery stenosis: prevalence, risk factors, and association with cardiovascular diseases. J Am Coll Cardiol 44: 618–623 (2004).
[84] Silbert PL, Mokri B, Schievink WI: Headache and neck pain in spontaneous internal carotid and vertebral artery dissections. Neurology 45: 1517–1522 (1995).
[85] SSYLVIA Study Investigators: Stenting of Symptomatic Atherosclerotic Lesions in the Vertebral or Intracranial Arteries (SSYLVIA): study results. Stroke 35: 1388–1392 (2004).
[86] Sztriha LK, Voros E, Sas K et al.: Favorable early outcome of carotid artery stenting without protection devices. Stroke 35: 2862–2866 (2004).
[87] The EC/IC-Bypass Study Group: Failure of extracranial-intracranial arterial bypass to reduce the risk of ischemic stroke. Results of an international randomized trial. N Engl J Med 313: 1191–1200 (1985).
[88] Thijs VN, Albers GW: Symptomatic intracranial atherosclerosis: outcome of patients who fail antithrombotic therpay. Neurology 55: 490–497 (2000).
[89] Warfarin-Aspirin Symptomatic Intracranial Disease (WASID) Trial Investigators: Design, progress and challenges of a double-blind trial of warfarin versus aspirin for symptomatic intracranial arterial stenosis. Neuroepidemiology 22: 106–117 (2003).
[90] Wityk RJ, Lehman D, Klag M et al.: Race and sex differences in the distribution of cerebral atherosclerosis Stroke 27: 1974–1980 (1996).
[91] Wong KS, Li H, Lam WW et al.: Progression of middle cerebral artery occlusive disease and its relationship with further vascular events after stroke. Stroke 33: 532–536 (2002).
[92] Wong KS, Gao S, Chan YL et al.: Mechanisms of acute cerebral infarctions in patients with middle cerebral artery stenosis: a diffusion-weighted imaging and microemboli monitoring study. Ann Neurol 52: 74–81 (2002).
[93] Wong KS, Huang YN, Gao S et al.: Intracranial stenosis in Chinese patients with acute stroke. Neurology 50: 812–813 (1998).
[94] Wylie EJ, Effeney DJ: Surgery of the aortic arch branches and vertebral arteries. Surg Clin North Am 59: 669–680 (1979).

Chapter 2.4

INTRACRANIAL MAGNETIC RESONANCE AND VASCULAR IMAGING IN PATIENTS WITH EXTRACRANIAL CAROTID STENOSIS

A. D. Mackinnon, A. D. Platts, and D. J. H. McCabe

Department of Radiology, St George's Hospital (ADM); Department of Neuroradiology (ADP), and University Department of Clinical Neurosciences (DJHMC), Royal Free and University College Medical School, Royal Free Hospital, London, UK; Department of Neurology (DJHMC), The Adelaide and Meath Hospital, incorporating the National Children's Hospital, Dublin, Ireland

Introduction to symptomatic and asymptomatic internal carotid artery stenosis and occlusion

The majority of transient ischemic attacks (TIAs) and ischaemic strokes are caused by thromboembolism from a stenosed large extracranial artery or occlusion of a large intracranial artery (atherothrombotic stroke), occlusion of a small intracranial artery (lacunar stroke), or embolism from the heart (cardioembolic stroke) [74]. In the remaining patients, the origin of the infarction is not established by investigation (TIA or ischaemic stroke of indeterminate aetiology), or less common causes for ischaemia or infarction are identified (e.g., sickle cell disease or vasculitis).

TIA or stroke in association with extracranial internal carotid artery (ICA) stenosis is a very important cause of morbidity and mortality in adults, and in one series, 25% of patients with carotid territory ischaemic stroke had ≥ 75% stenosis or occlusion of the ipsilateral ICA [6]. However, carotid artery territory TIA or stroke can occur in association with mild (0–49%), moderate (50–69%), or severe (70–99%) extracranial ICA stenosis, or ICA occlusion. Most patients with TIA or ischaemic stroke secondary to extracranial carotid artery stenosis present with clinical features of ipsilateral middle cerebral artery (MCA) rather than anterior cerebral artery (ACA) territory ischaemia or infarction, although exceptions do occur (see later). The majority of these patients are believed to have initial atherosclerotic plaque rupture with subsequent ipsilateral distal thromboembolism of platelet emboli and/or plaque fragments [24]. However, in some patients, acute thrombosis can occur on the plaque surface and cause extracranial ICA occlusion. Carotid occlusion may be asymptomatic if there is adequate intracerebral collateral circulation, but it may cause distal haemodynamic compromise especially in the presence of severe contralateral carotid stenosis or poor collateral circulation [91], [44]. In other patients with internal carotid artery occlusion, emboli may arise (i) from the occluded internal carotid stump, (ii) from the ipsilateral common or external carotid arteries via external carotid collaterals, or (iii) by transhemispheric passage from a contralateral internal carotid stenosis via the circle of Willis [44]. Embolic and haemodynamic mechanisms may cocontribute to the pathogenesis of cerebral ischaemia or infarction in some patients with ICA stenosis or occlusion [83]. All patients with symptomatic carotid stenosis or occlusion warrant aggressive secondary prevention to reduce the risk of subsequent TIA, stroke or other vascular events.

Asymptomatic stenosis (> 50%) of the extracranial carotid artery can be incidentally detected in approximately 4 to 8% of adults with non-invasive Doppler ultrasound screening [18]. These patients could potentially benefit from primary prevention strategies to prevent the morbidity or mortality associated with carotid territory TIA or stroke in the first instance.

In addition to the important group of patients with extracranial ICA stenosis, up to 10% of TIAs or ischaemic strokes may be attributed to atherosclerotic stenosis of a major intracranial artery [10]. Amongst Chinese patients, non-invasive imaging studies have suggested that intracranial stenosis may be found in 51% of patients presenting with TIAs, [35] and a third of patients presenting with acute stroke [93]. Atherosclerotic stenosis of a major intracranial artery is also an important cause of stroke in black and Hispanic patients [10]. Cerebral ischaemia or infarction in these patients may be secondary to thrombosis, thromboembolism, or distal haemodynamic compromise, and recurrent cerebrovascular events commonly occur despite the use of anti-thrombotic therapy [10].

Intracranial imaging can confirm or refute that the presenting symptoms and signs are secondary to carotid territory ischaemia or infarction, and may help to elucidate the aetiology and pathogenesis of the patient's TIA or stroke. This is important because the management of these patients is influenced by the presence or absence of prior symptoms [84], [21], [28], the severity and location of the stenosis in the symptomatic subgroup [44], [10], [71], [72], and the likely aetiopathogenesis of the symptoms. For example, despite the potential benefits of carotid endarterectomy in patients with severe carotid stenosis, better risk stratification of patients is required because certain subgroups derive less benefit from surgical treatment. One needs to operate on approximately 4 or 5 patients with symptomatic severe carotid stenosis within 2 weeks of symptom onset to prevent one stroke or death over the following 5 years [72]. In patients with asymptomatic > 60% carotid stenosis, one needs to perform a carotid endarterectomy on 17–19 patients to prevent one stroke or death over the following 5 years [21], [28]. These data illustrate the need to enhance our understanding of the pathogenic mechanisms responsible for carotid territory TIA or stroke, and the importance of identifying individual patients with carotid stenosis or occlusion who are at highest risk of recurrent symptoms during follow-up to facilitate improvements in stroke prevention. This might allow us to target 'lower risk' patients with asymptomatic or symptomatic severe carotid stenosis with more intense anti-thrombotic, anti-hypertensive or lipid-lowering therapy, while reserving surgical, endovascular or revascularisation therapy for those at 'higher risk'. Furthermore, this information could facilitate identification of, and intensification of antithrombotic treatment in, a subgroup of carotid stenosis patients who have ongoing embolism while awaiting carotid endarterectomy or stenting.

This chapter focuses on intracerebral imaging with T1- and T2-weighted, Diffusion-Weighted and Perfusion-Weighted Magnetic Resonance Imaging (MRI), and intracranial vascular imaging with intra-arterial catheter angiography, CT angiography (CTA), MR angiography (MRA), and transcranial Doppler ultrasonography (TCD) in the diagnostic work-up of patients with extracranial carotid stenosis. The role of TCD in detecting intracranial atherosclerotic ICA and MCA stenosis, and in monitoring patients with extracranial ICA stenosis will be discussed. Standard brain CT and Single-Photon Emission Computed Tomography (SPECT) imaging, T2* (gradient echo) and standard MRI of brain in patients with carotid territory haemorrhagic infarction, functional MR brain imaging, intracranial imaging of patients with carotid dissection, and Positron Emission Tomography (PET) have been dealt with in other chapters and will not be discussed further. The detailed investigation of patients with moyamoya disease is also beyond the scope of this chapter.

Magnetic Resonance Imaging (MRI) techniques to establish patterns and the likely aetiology of ischaemia or infarction in patients with carotid territory TIAs or stroke

It is our practice to perform intracranial structural brain imaging in all patients with carotid stenosis, especially in those patients who are being considered for carotid endarterectomy or endovascular treatment. Cranial MRI may localise the area of cerebral ischaemia or infarction, evaluate brain structure and function, and assess perfusion characteristics and large-vessel patency in a patient with a carotid territory TIA or ischaemic stroke. A standard MRI protocol for the investigation of a patient with a carotid territory TIA or stroke may include T1- and T2-

weighted and Fluid-Attenuated Inversion Recovery (FLAIR) sequences, Diffusion Weighted Imaging (DWI), Perfusion Weighted Imaging (PWI) and extra- and intracranial Magnetic Resonance Angiography (MRA).

T1- and T2-weighted MRI in patients with carotid territory TIA or stroke

T1- and T2-weighted MRI sequences form the core of almost every clinical MRI protocol, but are not the most sensitive techniques available to identify hyperacute cerebral ischaemia or infarction. One may detect 'absence of flow void' in an acutely occluded intracranial artery within 2 hours (and possibly within minutes) of onset of acute carotid territory ischaemic symptoms using T1- and T2-weighted MRI; T2-weighted sequences are more sensitive than T1-MRI at detecting this subtle abnormality [16] MR imaging following administration of gadolinium may identify abnormal enhancement (abnormally high signal) within the artery feeding the area of ischaemic cortex within the first 2 hours after symptom onset, presumably secondary to sluggish flow within the partially occluded vessel [94]. These changes are more easily seen on gadolinium- enhanced T1-weighted than T2-weighted MR images [94].

When cerebral blood flow falls to between 10 and 15 ml/100 g/minute, ischaemia-induced failure of the neuronal membrane sodium pump results in the intracellular accumulation of sodium and water with resultant neuronal swelling (cytotoxic oedema) [39]. Because T1-weighted MRI is useful for looking at normal brain anatomy, one may identify morphological swelling of the grey matter and subtle effacement of sulci on T1-weighted images in the acute phase after ischaemic stroke (within the first 2-4 hours), which is presumably secondary to cytotoxic oedema [94]. Although this can occur before high signal is seen on T2-weighted images, these changes may be very subtle and may not be reliably identified, and one cannot exclude acute cerebral infarction if T1-weighted MRI of brain is normal.

If severe cerebral ischaemia persists for more than 6 hours, the integrity of the capillary endothelial cells is compromised and intravascular fluid and protein leak into the extracellular space [39]. This leads to the development of vasogenic oedema which peaks at 24 to 48 hours [39]. T2-weighted imaging may identify high signal intensity change secondary to either cytotoxic or vasogenic oedema, but is much more commonly abnormal during the phase of development of vasogenic oedema (Fig. 1). Therefore, although T2 high signal change may be seen as early as

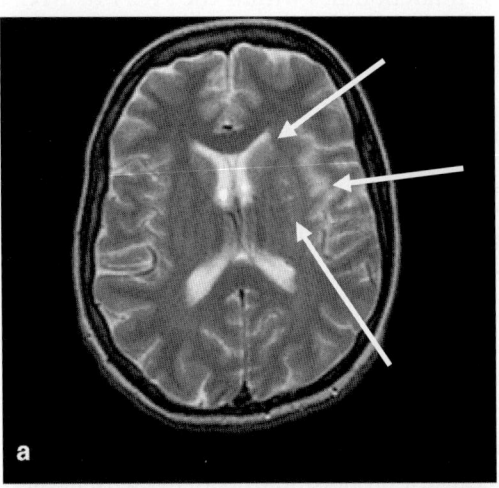

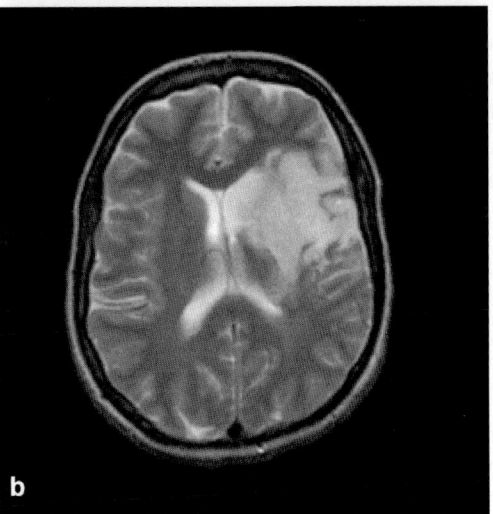

Fig. 1. a T2-weighted axial MRI: Subtle high signal intensity changes (arrows) involving the left frontal and insular cortex, left putamen and head of the left caudate nucleus 8 hours after onset of right hemiparesis and expressive dysphasia. **b** T2-weighted MRI brain 4 days later in same patient showing an established left MCA territory infarct.

6 to 8 hours after the onset of ischaemic symptoms, it is present in most, but not all, patients by 24 hours [94]. Corresponding low signal intensity change on T1-weighted MRI is rarely seen before 16 hours, and is only identified in some patients between 16 and 24 hours after onset of acute cerebral infarction, thus rendering low signal change on T1-weighted MRI a less sensitive marker of acute infarction than high signal change on T2-weighted images [94].

T1- and T2-weighted MRI can confirm that the area of infarction lies within the ACA or MCA territory in a symptomatic patient with ipsilateral carotid stenosis, thus implying that the stenosis caused the symptoms. However, T1- and T2-weighted MRI cannot identify acutely ischaemic tissue that is not destined to undergone irreversible infarction, and as stated above, may not actually identify all patients with acute cerebral infarction. Furthermore, because recent and long-standing cerebral infarcts both exhibit similar high signal intensity characteristics on T2-weighted images, one may not be able to differentiate between acute and established infarction with T2-weighted MRI unless the patient has developed acute oedema in association with a recent infarct. Because a proportion of patients with carotid stenosis have clinically asymptomatic established infarction on brain MRI, and others have co-existent small vessel disease or a potential cardiac source of embolism, additional MR imaging techniques may help to clarify whether the stenosis has caused the presenting symptoms or is likely to be incidental and asymptomatic.

Fluid-Attenuated Inversion Recovery (FLAIR) MRI

More recently, FLAIR MRI has been introduced to complement conventional T2-weighted sequences. FLAIR MRI provides a very heavily T2-weighted image of brain parenchyma and nullifies the signal from cerebrospinal fluid (CSF) [65]. FLAIR MRI is particularly useful in identifying periventricular and cortical infarcts which may be less obvious on conventional T2-weighted sequences because of partial volume effects and high CSF signal adjacent to the pathological region of interest (Fig. 2). Noguchi et al. identified high signal changes on FLAIR MRI, consistent with acute infarction, in 6 of 7 (86%) patients who were imaged within 3 hours of onset of ischaemic stroke [65]. Although FLAIR MRI may increase the likelihood of identifying acute carotid territory infarction compared with T1- or T2-weighted MRI, high signal abnormalities also persist on FLAIR MRI after the acute phase of cerebral infarction, and do not allow one to differentiate between recent or prior infarction. Ultimately, some infarcts may also appear as low signal intensity lesions on FLAIR if cavitation of the infarct occurs and the

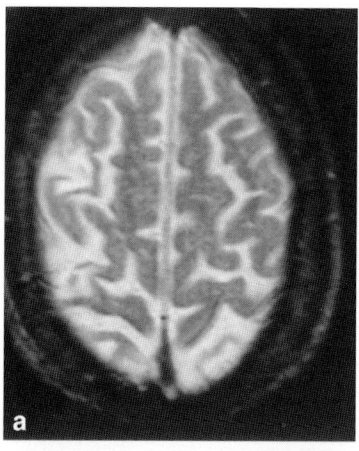

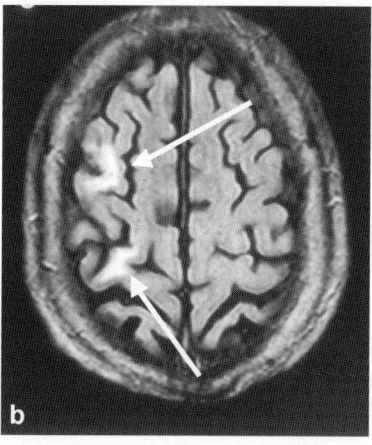

Fig. 2. a T2-weighted Turbo Spin Echo sequence at the high convexity level demonstrating equivocal high signal intensity changes in the right MCA territory; **b** FLAIR image at the same level demonstrating definite high signal intensity change involving the cortex in two separate gyral regions (white arrows) (Adapted from Brant-Zawadzki et al. [19]).

contents of the cavity approach the protein content of CSF.

Diffusion Weighted Imaging (DWI)

MRI can exploit the normal random motion of water molecules in the brain to produce image contrast [39]. In a Diffusion Weighted Imaging (DWI) protocol, the spatial location of each water molecule is effectively 'tagged' so that any net movement of water molecules during image acquisition results in a loss of signal and darkening of the images. This 'tagging' is achieved by a pair of very strong magnetic field gradients (diffusion gradients) which are typically added to a T2-weighted spin echo sequence [4]. These gradient pulses are designed to cancel each other out if there has been no movement of water molecules. Signal attenuation therefore occurs in normal tissues with random water motion, such as CSF; high signal change is seen on DWI in tissues that have restricted diffusion, e.g., with cytotoxic oedema associated with hyperacute cerebral ischaemia/infarction, and may also occur with subsequent vasogenic oedema in the later stages after cerebral infarction (see below).

Diffusion weighted scans are characterised by their b value (in s/mm^2) which is a function of the diffusion gradient strength, its duration, and the time interval between gradients. The conspicuity of the lesion on DWI relates to this b value. Although DW images are useful, the absolute intensities may not be a direct indicator of the diffusion coefficient. Factors that affect the diffusion coefficient on DWI include the T2 signal and the b value. DWI can be influenced by the 'T2 shine through effect' caused by high signal intensity changes on a corresponding T2-weighted MRI. However, each DW image has a corresponding Apparent Diffusion Coefficient (ADC) map which allows one to measure the degree of signal decay (slope of decay) rather than the absolute value, thus eliminating the influence of the T2 shine through effect on the ADC map. Areas which exhibit restricted diffusion and appear bright on a DW image have a low diffusion coefficient and appear hypointense or dark on an ADC map.

DWI has been shown to detect ischaemic lesions within minutes of the ictus in experimental animals, and within 30–90 minutes of acute stroke onset in humans [82]. Therefore, DWI is more sensitive than CT or conventional MRI at detecting acute cerebral ischaemia or infarction in the first few minutes and hours after symptom onset [64], [86], [22], [23], [5], [76], [42]. Acute ischaemic foci typically appear bright on DWI ('light bulb' sign) and dark on ADC maps (Fig. 3) [88]. High signal abnormalities on DWI may persist for up to 57 days (and very occasionally for up to 90 days) after ischaemic stroke, and then typically decrease in intensity [20]. Dark signal abnormality on an ADC map usually lasts for 10 days after ischaemic stroke onset, pseudonormalises, and may subsequently change to exhibit increased signal intensity [20]. However, dark signal abnormality on an ADC map may persist for up to a month in border-zone infarcts between the superficial and deep perforators of the middle cerebral artery, and should not be interpreted as indicating hyper-acute infarction in a patient with severe ipsilateral ICA stenosis [34].

It was initially felt that acute DWI signal changes on MRI represented irreversibly infarcted brain tissue. However, more recent longitudinal studies have shown that brain regions with initial abnormal signal intensity on DWI may regain normal signal intensity after recanalisation of the occluded artery [43] suggesting that cerebral ischaemia may also cause DWI signal change. This is supported by the observation that 45% of patients who had a hemispheric TIA in association with severe ipsilateral carotid stenosis had abnormal signal change on DWI in one series [42].

The additional information obtained from DWI in TIA and ischaemic stroke may influence clinical management. For example, an 85 year old man with severe right extracranial ICA stenosis who experiences a non-disabling stroke causing left arm and leg weakness, who is found to have an acute ischaemic lesion on DWI consistent with right pontine lacunar infarction, may not undergo carotid endarterectomy when the clinician concludes that the stenosis is asymptomatic. On the contrary, a patient with carotid stenosis who presents with a 'lacunar stroke syndrome' may be

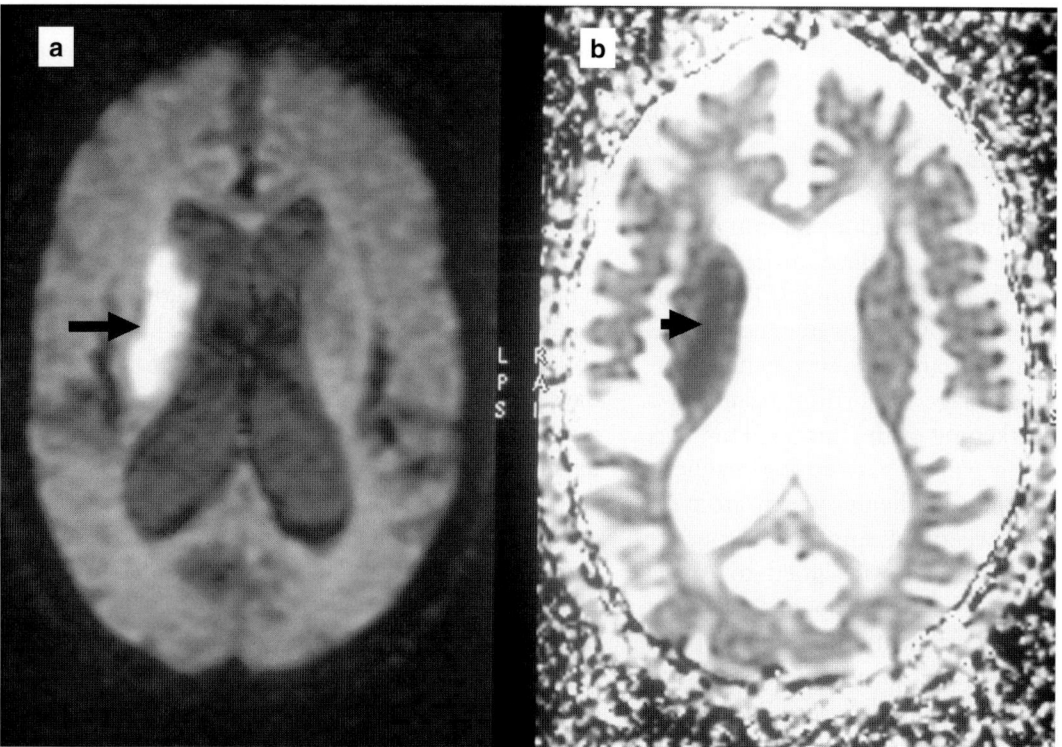

Fig. 3. **a** DWI in a patient with an acute right MCA territory infarct showing bright signal abnormality ('light bulb sign') in the right corona radiata (arrow); **b** Corresponding ADC map showing dark signal abnormality in the same region (arrowhead).

found to have a large subcortical infarct on DWI that could not be attributed to small vessel occlusion, thus allowing the clinician to conclude that the stenosis is "symptomatic" and warrants intervention [76]. Furthermore, some patients with severe carotid stenosis may have an alternative source of embolism; the finding of recent bilateral MCA and vertebrobasilar territory lesions on DWI would prompt a more intensive search for a cardio-embolic source of embolism that might require treatment with anticoagulation. Another important group of patients that might benefit from the information obtained from DWI are those with "clinically asymptomatic" severe extracranial ICA stenosis who have never had prior symptoms of TIA or stroke. The identification of recent ipsilateral MCA territory infarction on DWI in a "clinically asymptomatic" patient suggests that the stenosis has been "radiologically symptomatic" and may encourage the clinician to recommend carotid endarterectomy for stroke prevention if the potential benefits of treatment outweigh the risks in that individual. Although one must stress that there is no evidence from randomised controlled trials that clinically asymptomatic patients with cerebral infarction on MRI benefit more from carotid endarterectomy than patients without evidence of infarction on MRI, this is an issue that warrants further investigation.

DWI allows us to identify patterns of infarction in the acute stage after TIA or stroke, and can improve our understanding of the likely aetiopathogenesis of ischaemia or infarction in patients with extracranial carotid stenosis. Szabo et al. have utilised data from previous studies to describe 5 main patterns of infarction in patients with ischaemic stroke distal to an ipsilateral extracranial ICA stenosis or occlusion (Fig. 4) [83]:

(i) "**Territorial infarction**" involves the cerebral cortex and subcortical structures within the MCA, ACA or both vascular territories [83]. MCA infarcts may be considered to be "partial" if a distal MCA

Pattern	Description	Conventional Imaging Term	Example (DW MRI)
1	Large lesion involving the cortex	Territorial infarction	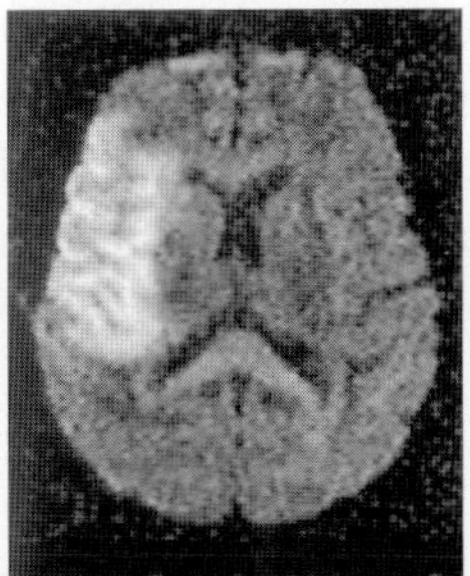
2	Subcortical lesion with or without additional smaller lesion(s)	Subcortical infarction	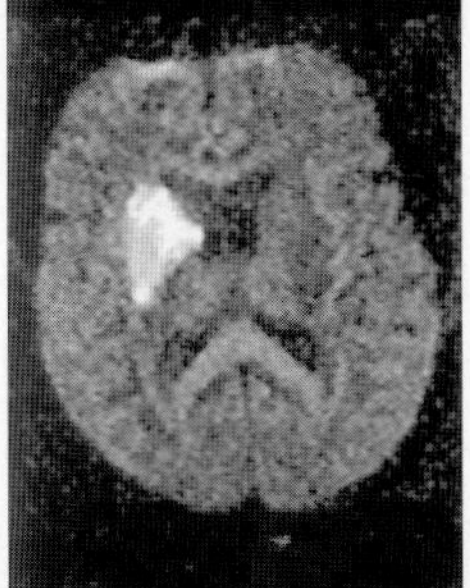
3	Large lesion involving the cortex with additional smaller lesion(s)	Territorial infarction with fragmentation	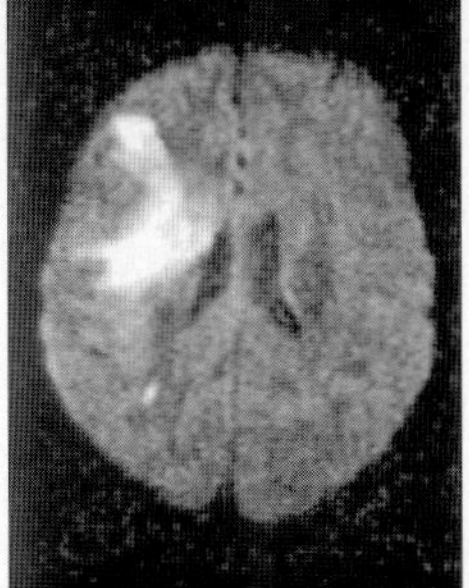
4	Several disseminated small lesions	...	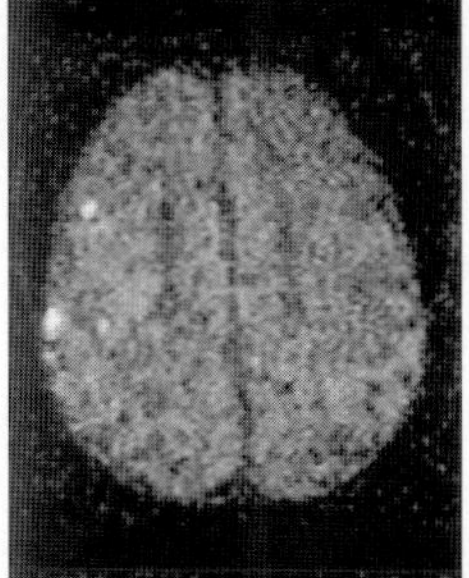
5	Small lesions in hemodynamic risk zones	Border zone infarction	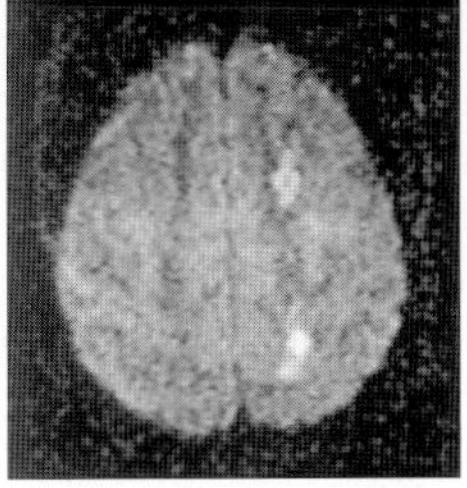

Fig. 4. Different patterns of infarction that one may see in patients with extracranial ICA stenosis (reproduced from [83]).

branch is occluded, and "large" if there is proximal occlusion at the level of the MCA bifurcation or trifurcation without an efficient collateral system (Fig. 5) [83]. "Complete" ACA and MCA territory infarction may occur in patients with embolisation and occlusion of the distal intracranial ICA [83].

(ii) "**Subcortical infarction**" involves the territory supplied by deep perforating branches originating from the distal intracranial ICA or the MCA trunk in the presence of adequate collateral supply to the cortex [83]. For example, embolic occlusion of the MCA trunk in the presence of patent superficial collaterals may cause a large striatocapsular infarct [83].

(iii) "**Territorial infarction with fragmentation**" represents a large territorial infarct with additional smaller lesions in either cortical or subcortical regions, presumably due to partial fragmentation of an embolus to the MCA [83].

(iv) Small "**disseminated lesions**" may be randomly distributed in the MCA territory and mainly involve the cortex [83]. This pattern of infarction may be secondary to fragmentation of a single MCA embolus, or may occur if multiple smaller emboli occlude smaller branches of the MCA [83].

(v) "**Border-zone infarction**" may also occur at the junction between two or more adjacent non-anastomosing arterial systems in patients with extracranial carotid stenosis [83], [61]. Two different patterns of border-zone infarction are recognised:

(a) "*Cortical (external) border-zone infarcts*" involve the cortical boundary zones that lie in the vascular territory supplied by the distal arterial branches of both the ACA and the MCA, the MCA and the posterior cerebral artery (PCA), or in the triple border-zone between the ACA, the MCA and the PCA; [61]. (b) "*Internal border-zone infarcts*" involve the white matter that lies in the vascular

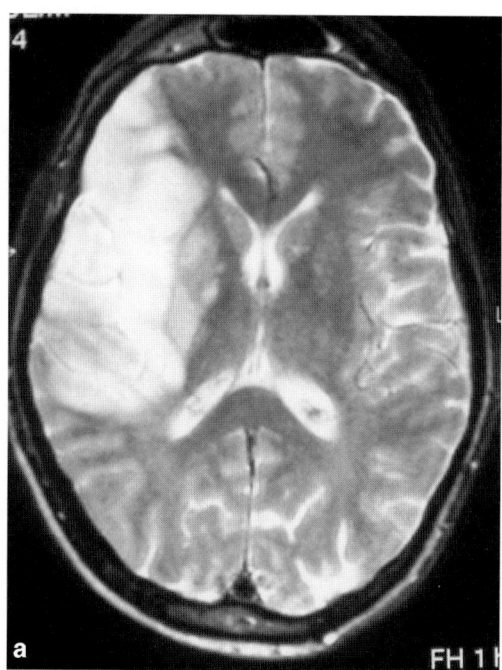

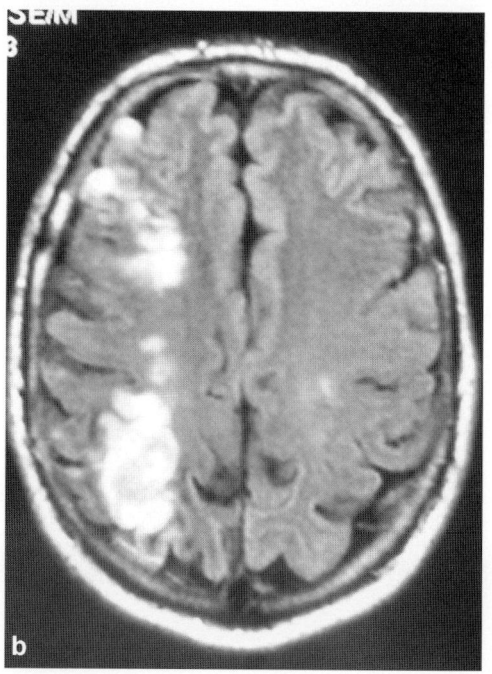

Fig. 5. Different patterns of infarction on MRI brain in two patients with extracranial internal carotid artery occlusion: **a** Axial T2-weighted MRI showing a right MCA territorial infarct with sparing of the right ACA territory. It is assumed that the right ACA territory has been spared because of collateral blood supply from the left carotid circulation via the anterior communicating artery; **b** Axial FLAIR MRI showing infarction in the border-zone between the MCA and the ACA territories, with relative preservation of parts of the fronto-parietal cortex; it is also possible that the patient had multiple emboli from the ICA stump to the MCA at the time of the occlusion. The relative sparing of the cortex suggests that the patient had a well developed superficial collateral supply e.g. from branches of the right external carotid artery.

territory between the arterial supply of the superficial arterial perforators (medullary perforating arteries) and the deep perforating arteries (lenticulostriate arteries) of the MCA [89], or in the centrum semiovale in the territory between the superficial arterial perforators of the MCA and ACA [61].

One might expect the first four patterns of ischaemia or infarction to occur predominantly in carotid stenosis patients with embolic occlusion of the intracranial ICA or MCA, and border-zone infarction to occur in patients with severe extracranial ICA stenosis with haemodynamic compromise secondary to poor collateral supply. However, because the size and location of the border-zones vary enormously between carotid stenosis patients, and even within individuals who develop increasingly severe carotid stenosis over time, it is difficult to be certain whether the cause of the ischaemic lesion on MR imaging is secondary to thromboembolic occlusion, 'low flow' with haemodynamic compromise, or a combination of both mechanisms [90]. A detailed history may provide some clues as to whether a carotid territory TIA is likely to secondary to thromboembolism or haemodynamic compromise. Haemodynamic TIAs are typically described as evolving over minutes (embolic TIAs are typically maximal within seconds of symptom onset), and may be associated with course jerking of the arm and/or leg contralateral to the stenosis in association with limb weakness or numbness. In patients with 'low flow retinopathy' distal to a unilateral severe extracranial ICA stenosis, monocular 'visual whiteout' may develop after exposure to bright sunlight and resolve over seconds to minutes when the patient leaves the bright surroundings. A haemodynamic mechanism is also more likely if TIA symptoms occur after standing or sitting up suddenly, after intake of antihypertensive medication, or if the symptoms only occur in very hot weather, after a hot bath or heavy meal [90]. One must accept that a patient with e.g. intracranial MCA branch stenosis who has an embolism to the MCA trunk from an extracranial ICA stenosis may present with a TIA that evolves in a manner that suggests 'haemodynamic' ischaemia.

It is also important to remember that because the lenticulostriate arteries arise from the MCA, occlusion of one of these 'end arteries' by an embolus from an extracranial ICA stenosis can also cause a clinical 'lacunar syndrome' with associated 'lacunar infarction' on brain imaging [37]. Therefore, screening for carotid stenosis in a patient with an anterior circulation lacunar TIA or stroke can be justified, although the pick-up rate is likely to be lower than in patients with classical large artery atherothrombotic TIA or stroke.

The following section reviews the imaging modalities that may improve our understanding of the potential mechanism(s) that may cause these different patterns of infarction in patients with extracranial ICA stenosis, and which may in turn inform clinical management decisions in this patient population.

Magnetic resonance Perfusion-Weighted Imaging (PWI)

Perfusion-Weighted Imaging (PWI) is an additional MRI technique that can provide some information about cerebral blood volume and blood flow [5] by exploiting magnetic susceptibility effects within the brain [39]. PWI involves rapidly injecting an intravenous bolus of gadolinium diethylenetriamine pentaacetic acid [70], which causes a transient reduction in signal within the cerebral blood vessels and brain parenchyma on T2*-weighted imaging [39]. Multi-slice images of the whole brain are typically acquired every 1 to 2 seconds, and sequential changes in signal intensity can be used to produce pixel-based colour maps, and to calculate a number of indices including the mean transit time of the bolus thorough the brain (MTT), the relative cerebral blood volume (rCBV) and the relative cerebral blood flow (rCBF) [39]. The relative cerebral blood flow is calculated by dividing the relative cerebral blood volume by the mean transit time (rCBF = rCBV/MTT). Prolongation of the mean transit time of the injected bolus is the earliest and most consistent sign of impaired cerebral perfusion [39]. When the MTT increases, autoregulatory mechanisms are activated which promote vasodilation and recruitment of collateral vessels, thus increasing cerebral blood volume and maintaining cerebral blood flow at a relatively constant level [39]. Thus, the response to impaired perfusion and prolongation of the

MTT provides some information about the brain's autoregulatory capacity and collateral reserve.

PWI has the potential to play a role in evaluating patients with extracranial ICA stenosis. However, it must be appreciated that PWI is semi-quantitative and cannot provide absolute values, but comparison of blood flow between the two hemispheres may provide information about the relative reduction in blood flow in the affected hemisphere [39]. In the presence of impaired perfusion distal to a severe unilateral ICA stenosis, relative cerebral blood volume in the affected hemisphere may be normal or increased if collateral supply is adequate, but may be decreased if collateral blood supply is insufficient and if maximum vasodilatory capacity has been exceeded [39]. This may allow one to speculate that recurrent stereotyped MCA territory TIAs in a patient with severe ipsilateral ICA stenosis are haemodynamic in origin if other non-invasive imaging modalities fail to provide evidence of embolism to the ipsilateral MCA (see section on TCD below). It follows that the data obtained from PWI may be less informative in patients with bilateral severe ICA stenosis who have impaired perfusion in the MCA or ACA territories on both sides. However, in some patients with bilateral ICA occlusion with collateral supply to the anterior circulation from extracranial collaterals, PWI may show impaired perfusion in the region of the cortical border-zones on both sides [39].

In acute carotid territory TIA or ischaemic stroke, perfusion of the affected brain region is impaired and can be detected with PWI. Initially, because DWI lesions were considered to represent areas of irreversible infarction, and because the perfusion defect was often larger than the lesion seen on DWI, it was assumed that the difference between the two defects, the "MR diffusion-perfusion mismatch zone", represented an area of ischaemic brain that had not yet undergone irreversible infarction (the ischaemic penumbra) [75]. Because more recent data have shown that DWI lesions may reverse following recanalisation of the feeding artery [43], the MR diffusion-perfusion mismatch model may overestimate the amount of irreversibly infarcted core tissue, thus underestimating the extent of the ischaemic penumbra.

How could these MR imaging studies provide useful information that could improve the care of patients with acute carotid territory TIA or stroke? Intravenous recombinant tissue plasminogen activator has been shown to improve the likelihood of a favourable outcome during follow-up if administered within 180 minutes of acute stroke onset, and may be of benefit in patients treated up to 270 minutes after symptom onset [27]. Ongoing studies, e.g. the Echoplanar Imaging Thrombolysis Evaluation Trial, are investigating the usefulness of combined DWI-PWI studies in selecting patients who may benefit from 'delayed thrombolytic therapy' if they seek medical attention outside of the usual three hour time period following stroke onset. Preliminary results from the Desmoteplase in Acute Ischemic Stroke trial suggest that DWI-PWI mismatch data may be used to select patients who may benefit from treatment with novel thrombolytic agents between 3 and 9 hours after acute ischaemic stroke onset, but larger trials are required to confirm these initial results [26]. Conversely, it may also be sensible to avoid thrombolytic therapy in patients with acute DWI lesions who have no residual perfusion deficit on PWI, because it is likely that these patients have already spontaneously recanalised the temporarily occluded feeding artery and may not derive any further benefit from thrombolysis. Furthermore, future PWI studies may facilitate identification of patients with acute MCA infarction who are likely to develop a malignant MCA syndrome secondary to more extensive MCA ischaemia than is predicted by DWI alone. If the results of ongoing trials, such as the Decompressive Surgery for the Treatment of Malignant Infarction of the Middle Cerebral Artery (DESTINY) trial are encouraging, the use of PWI in this setting deserves further study.

Intracranial vascular imaging with catheter angiography, CTA, and MRA in patients with extracranial carotid stenosis

Most clinicians request colour Doppler ultrasound imaging to initially establish the diagnosis of extracranial proximal ICA and carotid bifurcation stenosis. Colour Doppler ultrasound has a relatively high sensitivity and specificity in identifying severe extracranial ICA stenosis [62], [59], and the combination of Doppler ultrasound with other non-invasive imaging studies (e.g., extracranial MRA or CTA) improves the likelihood of 'accurately' identifying a severe ICA stenosis that might warrant intervention [66]. Because of the safety of non-invasive imaging techniques, many patients with proximal extracranial ICA stenosis do not have their stenosis severity measured with the "gold standard" technique of catheter angiography, and routine imaging of the intracranial circulation is not performed in many centres as part of the work-up of patients with carotid stenosis. Although standard cross-sectional CT and MRI images provide some information about the patency of the intracranial vessels, dedicated intracranial vascular imaging protocols are required to delineate the intracranial vessels in detail.

The potential benefits of intracranial imaging in patients with extracranial carotid stenosis include identification of:

- 'Tandem arterial stenosis' in the extracranial and intracranial ICA (Fig. 6)
- Intracranial atherosclerosis of the MCA, ACA, PCA, and their branches
- The response to intravenous or intra-arterial thrombolytic therapy
- The extent of the intracranial collateral arterial supply and
- Other pathological processes, including vasculitis or dissection, that may occasionally co-exist in patients with atherosclerosis.

Clinical examples of patients who could benefit from intracranial vascular imaging

Because colour Doppler ultrasound cannot visualise the distal extracranial ICA far above the angle of the mandible, one should suspect distal 'tandem' carotid stenosis in a patient with 'high-resistance flow' on Doppler waveform analysis of the proximal ICA, and distal extracranial and intracranial vascular imaging should be performed [73]. Intracranial vascular imag-

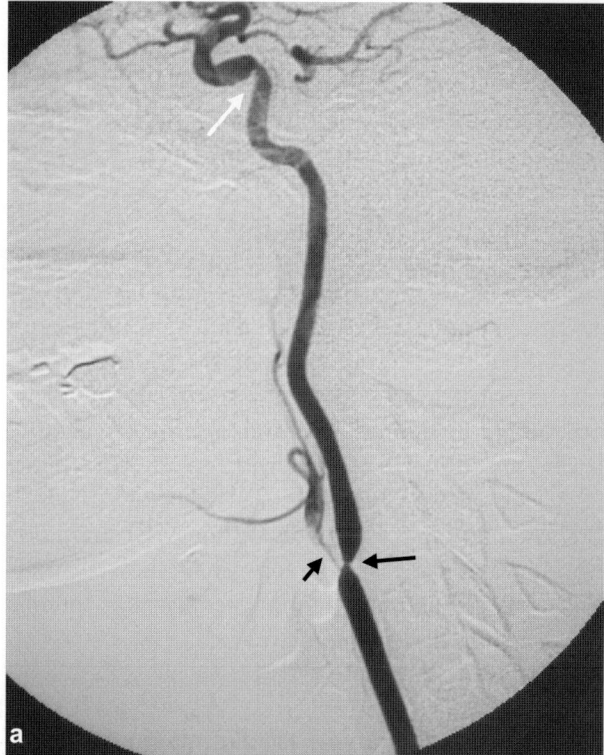

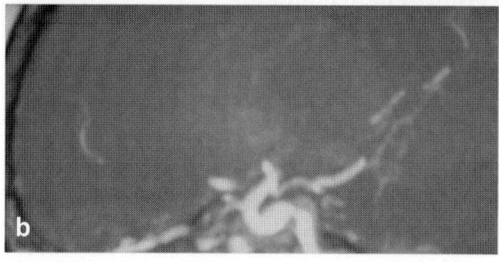

Fig. 6. a Intra-arterial digital subtraction angiogram with selective ICA injection showing > 80% stenosis of the origin of the extracranial internal carotid artery according to NASCET criteria (long black arrow). There is severe stenosis and trickle flow in the proximal external carotid artery (short black arrow), and there is a tandem stenosis of the proximal cavernous segment of the intracranial ICA (white arrow); b Intracranial time of flight MRA also showing the stenosis of the intracranial cavernous ICA.

ing should also be considered in patients at higher risk of having intracranial stenosis; e.g., the occurrence of 'haemodynamic' carotid territory TIAs in an Asian or black patient who only has moderate extracranial ICA stenosis warrants a search for co-existent intracranial stenosis that could be contributing to the symptoms. Intracranial vascular imaging may provide useful clinical information in a patient with mild carotid stenosis who is found to have proximal MCA occlusion on intracranial MRA 4 hours after stroke onset, because this patient may then be considered for intra-arterial thrombolysis. The degree of recanalisation of the occluded vessel can be re-assessed at a later date with non-invasive MRA. A patient with severe bilateral ICA stenosis who has recurrent posterior circulation ischaemic symptoms, but no evidence of proximal vertebral stenosis, would benefit from intracranial imaging to look for evidence of basilar artery stenosis and to assess intracranial collateral supply to the posterior and anterior circulation. If one encounters a patient with severe extracranial ICA stenosis who has multifocal bilateral ischaemic and haemorrhagic lesions on CT or MRI brain, intracranial catheter angiography may show features suggestive of vasculitis, and the stenosis may then be considered to be asymptomatic.

How might intracranial vascular imaging influence clinical management?

The information obtained from intracranial vascular imaging can influence clinical decision making in patients with carotid stenosis. In patients with carotid territory TIAs or stroke in association with tandem arterial stenosis affecting the extracranial and intracranial ICA, many clinicians would advise treatment of the extracranial stenosis first with either carotid endarterectomy or endovascular therapy. If TIAs or stroke recur in the absence of extracranial ICA restenosis, especially if one can detect emboli in the ipsilateral MCA on transcranial Doppler imaging and no other cause for the symptoms is identified, then one may conclude that the intracranial stenosis is causing the recurrent symptoms. This could lead to further intensification of best medical therapy or perhaps endovascular intervention, although it must be stressed that no randomised studies comparing these interventions have been published to date.

In the North American Symptomatic Carotid Endarterectomy Trial (NASCET), the presence of intracranial atherosclerotic disease on catheter angiography significantly influenced the risk of subsequent stroke only in patients with 85–99% extracranial ICA stenosis who were treated with best medical therapy alone; intracranial stenosis did not significantly impact on stroke risk in patients with < 50%, 50 to 69%, or 70 to 84% stenosis [41]. The three-year risk of ipsilateral stroke distal to an 85–99% extracranial ICA stenosis was significantly higher in those with *versus* those without intracranial atherosclerosis (45.7% *vs.* 25.3%, relative risk 1.8 [95% confidence interval 1.1–3.2]) [41]. In the same study, the three-year risk of ipsilateral stroke in surgically treated patients with 85–99% extracranial ICA stenosis was similar in those with and those without intracranial atherosclerosis (8.6% *vs.* 10%, relative risk 0.9, [95% confidence interval 0.2–3.0]). These data can be of use when counselling this subgroup of patients before carotid endarterectomy. Patients who have combined very severe extracranial and intracranial atherosclerosis have a very high risk of stroke if they are treated with best medical therapy alone, but the presence of intracranial stenosis does not appear to increase the hazard associated with surgery if they proceed to carotid endarterectomy.

A further study revealed that the presence of intracranial collateral supply to the symptomatic hemisphere in medically treated patients with symptomatic 70–99% extracranial ICA stenosis reduced the two-year absolute risk of ipsilateral hemispheric stroke by 16.5% (11.3 *vs.* 27.8%, p = 0.005) and the risk of ipsilateral hemispheric TIA by 17% (19.1 *vs.* 36.1%, p = 0.008) compared with patients who did not have collaterals [30]. Surgically treated patients with symptomatic 70–99% extracranial ICA stenosis who had collateral supply to the affected hemisphere had a lower peri-operative stroke risk in the 30 days after surgery compared with those patients without collaterals (1.1 *vs.* 4.9%) [30]. However, the presence of collaterals did not provide significant added protection against TIA or stroke in these surgically treated patients during prolonged follow-up at 2 years [30]. The beneficial effect of collateral supply was not evident in either the medically or surgically treated patient with near occlusion of the ICA. These data may also be useful in risk stratifying patients for carotid endarterectomy or endovascular therapy. For example, a patient with a recent non-disabling stroke in association with 70–99% ICA stenosis who has no collateral supply to the affected hemisphere should be considered for urgent carotid endarterectomy, but perhaps one should quote a higher peri-operative stroke risk than for a patient with good collateral supply.

If one suspects vasculitis in a patient with severe carotid stenosis, the appropriate management will be to investigate for an underlying cause, consider brain biopsy, and to treat the patient with immunosuppressive therapy rather than performing carotid endarterectomy.

Intracranial vascular imaging also provides information about the anatomy of, and the presence of any common anatomical variants of the circle of Willis. This may help clarify whether the patient has 'symptomatic' extracranial ICA stenosis or whether there is another likely source of embolism. If one identifies acute infarction on DWI in the ipsilateral frontal and occipital lobes in a carotid stenosis patient with a fetal origin of the PCA off the internal carotid artery, and no cardiac source of embolism is identified, one may conclude that the occipital embolus also arose from the ipsilateral stenosed ICA, thus indicating the need for carotid interventional therapy and obviating the need for anticoagulation. In contrast, if there is a normal configuration of the circle of Willis, and the PCA is supplied by the basilar artery, a thorough search for a cardiac source of embolism is essential.

Catheter angiography

As stated above, catheter angiography is considered to be the "gold standard" vascular imaging modality for visualising the intracranial circulation. Intravenous digital subtraction angiography has been largely abandoned because of poor resolution and increased complications, and will not be considered further in this chapter [1].
Intra-Arterial Digital Subtraction Angiography (I-ADSA) is an invasive test, usually performed via a transfemoral arterial route under local anaesthesia, although other puncture sites may be utilised. It is somewhat uncomfortable, usually requires hospital admission, and is associated with certain risks. Groin haematoma is the most frequent puncture site complication encountered, but is rarely associated with pseudo-aneurysm formation; local arterial dissection and distal arterial embolisation also occasionally occur, and patients should be informed that there is approximately a 1% overall risk of developing one of these "local" complications. Peri-procedural TIAs may occur in approximately 0.4% of patients (AD Platts, personal experience), and peri-procedural stroke in up to 2.5% of cases [47]. There is a degree of inter-operator variability, and it is not surprising that lower complication rates are achieved by more experienced operators [92]. Peri-procedural complication rates also depend on the angiographic technique used, with selective studies carrying lower complication rates than less selective arch aortic injection. Furthermore, the selection of patients for I-ADSA who have a high likelihood of severe intracranial atherosclerosis is likely to increase the risk of complications associated with the procedure, akin to the experience of catheter angiography in the investigation of patients with severe extracranial ICA stenosis [14]. Complication rates should be systemically recorded and monitored in each unit by continuous audit.

I-ADSA allows accurate measurement of the calibre of the residual arterial lumen and visualisation of plaque ulceration in the extracranial ICA and intracranial arterial circulation [41]. I-ADSA has a number of advantages over non-invasive intracranial imaging studies in that it:

– Provides images with high spatial and contrast resolution, with visualisation of peripheral arterial branches that are not easily seen on CTA or MRA (Fig. 7a and b)
– Provides information about dynamic arterial flow, although this is usually not quantifiable or reproducible
– Provides the radiologist with the unique ability to modify flow during the procedure in order to assess collateral blood supply via the circle of Willis and from extracranial collaterals (Fig. 7c).

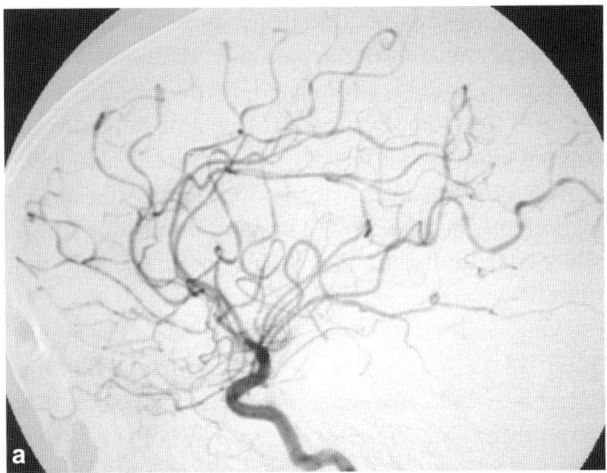
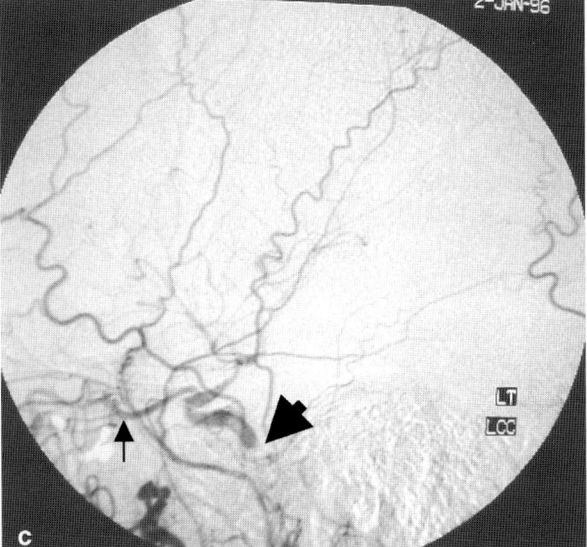
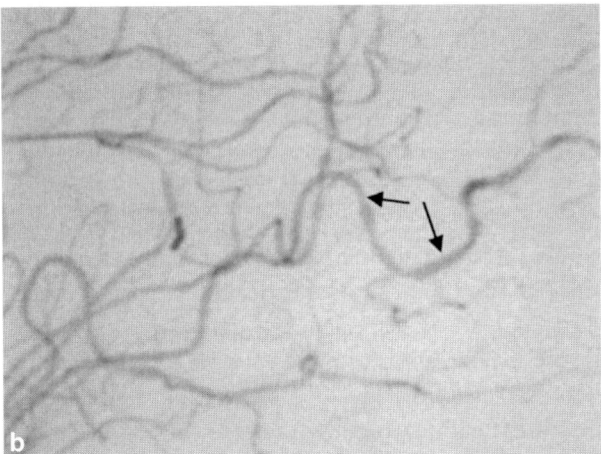

Fig. 7. a Selective intra-arterial carotid DSA (lateral projection) showing luminal irregularity with segmental narrowing and widening of branches of both the middle and anterior cerebral arteries. The patient presented with a haemorrhagic stroke after taking an unknown mixture of illicit substances, thought to include 'ecstasy' and cocaine. These peripheral arterial branches are rarely clearly visualised with current intracranial CTA or MRA imaging techniques; **b** High power view of the same patient showing stenotic and dilated segments of the angular branch of the middle cerebral artery (arrows); **c** I-ADSA following a left common carotid injection shows occlusion of the cervical internal carotid artery with refilling of the cavernous and supraclinoid internal carotid artery by reversed flow in the ophthalmic artery; the ophthalmic artery is supplied by branches of the external carotid artery. Large arrow, point of reconstitution of the intracranial cavernous ICA; Small arrow, reversed flow in the ophthalmic artery.

One of the limitations of I-ADSA is it does not directly image the vessel wall itself or allow one to identify the exact site of disease within the affected vessel wall. Furthermore, if peri-procedural complication rates are not kept to a minimum, the potential benefit from intervention in a patient with extracranial ICA stenosis, especially in those with asymptomatic severe carotid stenosis, may be outweighed by the combined short-term risks of angiography and revascularisation.

'Non-invasive' intracranial angiography

Intracranial CTA and MRA currently offer lower spatial resolution and less clear visualisation of the intracranial vessels than I-ADSA, but the peri-procedural morbidity associated with CTA or MRA is substantially lower. However, the adverse impact of the lower accuracy of these relatively 'non-invasive' imaging studies of the intracranial circulation in patients with extracranial ICA stenosis is uncertain.

CT Angiography (CTA)

CTA involves the intravenous administration of a non-ionic iodinated contrast agent, that is typically injected at a rate of 3ml per second [39]. The patient is transported through the gantry of a spiral multi-detector CT scanner by a motorised table, and the rotating detector ring of the scanner acquires 3D data at a time that coincides with the phase of high intra-arterial contrast enhancement (first pass imaging). Post-processing of the acquired data sets allows one to construct 3D CT angiographic images, on which one can visualise the intracranial vessels and quantify the degree of stenosis of an intracranial artery. More rapid table movement obviously allows a larger field of imaging to be covered, but leads to more movement blurring artefact in the acquired images (Z-axis blur). Industry developments are focusing on producing wider blocks of detectors that will sample a larger area than that covered by the currently available spiral CT scanners, thus minimising the need for table movement with the goal of improving imaging quality.

The advantages of CTA include the fact that it can be performed in conjunction with standard CT brain imaging, it is a relatively non-invasive test which can be performed on an out-patient basis, and current 'leading-edge' machines can cover a region of interest from the aortic arch to the intracranial middle cerebral arteries.

However, there are some limitations and disadvantages of CTA as an intracranial vascular imaging technique. Patients undergoing CTA probably have approximately a 0.04% risk of experiencing a severe adverse reaction, and a 0.004% risk of experiencing a very severe adverse reaction to the iodinated contrast agent [63]. Patients who are treated with metformin should discontinue therapy for 48 hours peri-procedurally, and an iso-osmolar contrast agent needs to be used in elderly diabetic patients with elevated serum creatinine levels to minimise the risk of contrast-induced renal failure. Therefore, clinicians must follow the guidelines for patient' preparation laid down by the local Radiology department.

CTA does not allow one to visualise sequential vessel opacification over time, thus rendering investigation of collateral intracranial blood supply more difficult than with catheter angiographic studies. This is because filling of collateral vessels may be delayed, and although patent, these collateral channels may not be opacified with CTA. Therefore, one cannot exclude the possibility that collateral channels exist, even if they are not identified with intracranial CTA. Because CT is very sensitive at detecting calcium, heavy calcification of a stenosed intracranial artery may also impede visualisation of the residual lumen of the vessel and hinder grading of the severity of an intracranial stenosis [32]. CTA may not always clearly visualise the lumen of the intra-cavernous portion of the ICA because the degree of enhancement of the cavernous sinus may be similar to the enhancement of the adjacent intra-cavernous carotid artery; this may obscure visualisation of the artery [32]. It may also be difficult to isolate the petrosal intra-osseous segment of the intracranial ICA from the surrounding bone using automated reconstruction techniques, and time-consuming post-processing of the images from this region is required on an angiographic workstation [80].

One small prospective series reported that intracranial CTA was reliable at identifying intracranial ICA or MCA trunk occlusion that was subsequently confirmed on intra-arterial DSA [45]. However, a subsequent small retrospective study that compared the sensitivity of intracranial CTA with I-ADSA suggested that CTA may be a sensitive test for identifying severe (70 to 99%) stenosis or occlusion of the intracranial MCA or ACA, but not for identifying severe stenosis of the intracranial ICA [80]. Therefore, larger prospective studies are required to adequately assess the sensitivity and specificity of intracranial CTA in identifying intracranial anterior circulation stenosis or occlusion in patients with extracranial carotid artery stenosis.

Despite these technical limitations, CTA is likely to play an increasingly important role in imaging the intracranial circulation in patients with extracranial ICA stenosis in future, especially in view of the ready availability of this test.

Magnetic Resonance Angiography (MRA)

In carotid stenosis patients without a contraindication to MRI, the combination of MRI and

MRA allows the comprehensive evaluation of the brain structure, perfusion, and vasculature. There are three main MR techniques used to image the intracranial vessels, and all of these techniques can also visualise the extracranial vessels during the same imaging session:

- Phase contrast MRA (PC-MRA)
- Time-of-flight MRA (ToF-MRA)
- Contrast enhanced MRA (CE-MRA)

Each technique has its own limitations and produces artefacts which the interpreting Radiologist must be familiar with. Some are common to all techniques, such as movement artefact, whereas others are technique-specific. These are summarised below:

(i) PC-MRA

PC-MRA applies a magnetic field to create a phase shift in protons within a predetermined range of flow velocities [11]. The magnitude of the phase shift is used to create an image, with high signal representing flowing protons within the predetermined velocity range. Background structures are then suppressed to allow construction of a PC-MR angiogram [11]. PC-MRA may allow depiction of slow flow within a large intracranial artery and flow within smaller intracranial vessels.

One of the limitations of PC-MRA is that the technique provides images with poor spatial resolution. Furthermore, PC-MRA only detects phase shift caused by flow within a predetermined velocity range. If an extracranial or intracranial ICA stenosis causes an alteration in flow velocity above or below the predetermined velocity range, the distal intracranial vessel segment will not be detected and visualised. Therefore, incorrect velocity encoding at the beginning of the imaging protocol may lead to the false impression that an intracranial artery is occluded, when in fact, flow may only be reduced within the patent vessel. The technique is also limited by being insensitive to the direction of flow, and although this may be useful when one is imaging flow in a tortuous intracranial artery, venous blood flow may potentially obscure images of the arterial anatomy. For these reasons, we do not routinely use PC-MRA in the investigation of intracranial arterial stenosis, and mainly reserve this technique for the investigation of cerebral venous sinus thrombosis.

(ii) ToF-MRA

Time of flight ("in-flow") MRA is a gradient-echo short T1 sequence in which protons in flowing blood that enter the magnetic imaging field generate a strong signal, whereas protons in stationary background tissue are suppressed, thus generating a high intensity signal within blood vessels [11]. With 2D ToF MRA, the image is built up from thin slices which have been sequentially acquired, whereas 3D ToF MRA acquires the data for the whole imaging slab at the same time. In comparison with 2D ToF MRA, the 3D technique is less susceptible to degradation by movement artefact, there is an improved signal-to-noise ratio, and shorter radio-frequency pulses can be used leading to better suppression of signal from background structures, such as fat within the orbit and dorsum sella. For these reasons, the 3D ToF MRA technique is usually preferred to 2D ToF MRA for visualisation of the intracranial arterial circulation.

Current ToF-MRA techniques provide familiar angiogram type images that can easily be reconstructed and manipulated by the reporting Radiologist. One can visualise the intracranial ICA, the MCA, the ACA and their first branches only. This is useful in identifying stenosis or occlusion of the ICA, proximal MCA or ACA, but peripheral branch occlusion will not be reliably identified with this technique (Fig. 8a). Although 3D ToF-MRA still has relatively poor spatial resolution in comparison with I-ADSA, the new generation of 3 Tesla MRI scanners should significantly improve the spatial resolution of the acquired images compared with those obtained on a 1.5 Tesla MRI scanner. Current demonstrations suggest that at least one higher order of peripheral vessels will be visualised with 3 Tesla MR imaging.

ToF-MRA has a number of methodological limitations that one must be aware of:

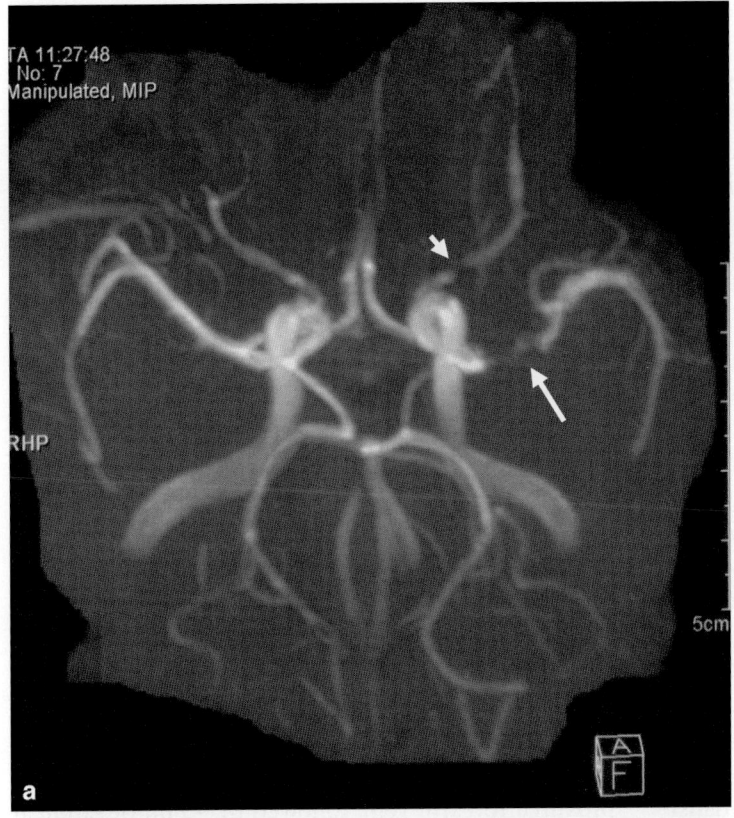

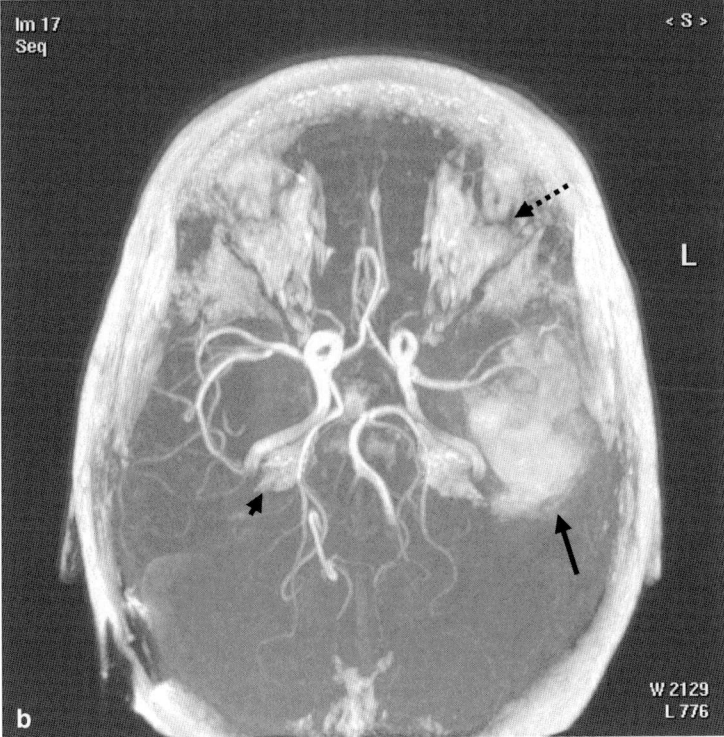

Fig. 8. a Intracranial ToF-MRA showing a proximal left MCA stenosis (large white arrow) in a patient with a left hemispheric MCA infarct of undetermined aetiology. The minor irregularity of the left ophthalmic artery (arrowhead) suggests that an ICA embolus fragmented and partially occluded both vessels; **b** Intracranial ToF MRA in a patient with a recent left MCA territory intracranial haemorrhage. The haematoma appears hyperintense on this T1-weighted imaging sequence (T1 shortening), thus obscuring adequate visualisation of this distal branches of the left MCA (long black arrow) compared with the normal distal branches of the right MCA. One cannot exclude either an aneurysm or a focal stenosis of the distal left MCA with this technique at this stage after symptom onset. This image also shows hyperintesnity from fat within the petrous apex (arrowhead) and the orbits (dashed arrow) which can easily be removed by post-processing of the images.

- **'In plane flow saturation'**: ToF MRA is most sensitive at detecting flow perpendicular to the plane of data acquisition, and the signal obtained from blood flowing in vessels aligned at lesser angles to the acquisition plane is less intense and must not be erroneously interpreted as indicating stenosis of that vessel. In addition, vessels which run parallel to the plane of data acquisition may not have detectable flow within them at all, thus resulting in absent arterial segments which must not be interpreted as being occluded. This most commonly occurs in the MCA and its branches.
- **'In slab saturation'**: ToF-MRA data are acquired in 'slabs' or 'chunks'. When the flowing blood traverses one of these slabs, the signal intensity from the flowing blood at the periphery of the slab temporarily decreases, resulting in an abrupt change in signal intensity and an inhomogeneous signal return from the artery being studied. This may also give the false impression of a focal stenosis in the vessel, and hence the importance of studying the source images that are used to generate the ToF-MRA.
- **'Susceptibility artefact'**: ToF-MRA is intrinsically vulnerable to inhomogeneity in the local magnetic environment. The interfaces between air and soft tissue at the skull base are a frequent source of this artefact, and one should not over-interpret loss of signal in the ICA in this region as indicating stenosis or occlusion.
- **'T1 shortening'**: Tissue with intrinsically short T1 signal will be seen on the acquired ToF MRA images. Subcutaneous and orbital fat can easily be removed by post processing techniques, but blood products, e.g., within an intracerebral haematoma or a haemorrhagic infarct, will remain on the reconstructed image and may obscure precise visualisation of local vascular anatomy (Fig. 8b).
- **Overestimation of stenosis severity:** This has been reported to occur especially in the intra-cavernous portion of the intracranial ICA [32].

(iii) CE-MRA

Gadolinium chelates produce signal change on T1-weighted MRI sequences (T1 shortening) in proportion to their concentration in blood. Unlike PC-MRA or ToF-MRA, contrast enhanced intracranial MRA simply depends on local intravascular T1 shortening caused by the presence of gadolinium within a vessel, and does not rely on velocity-dependent or inflow phase shifts. Therefore, movement and flow artefacts are minimised, and even vessels which run in the plane of imaging are well visualised. For these reasons, CE-MRA is usually the intracranial MR angiographic imaging modality of choice to visualise the intracranial vessels when intracranial arterial stenosis is suspected.

The timing from the injection of contrast to the onset of image acquisition is critical to the success of CE-MRA [11]. During the study, an initial small 'timing bolus' of 3 ml of gadolinium may be administered manually or via an automated pump, and the time taken for the bolus to reach the intracranial circulation is calculated. Alternatively, one can use an automated 'bolus detection' and 'scan triggering' scheme to precisely begin image acquisition once the bolus arrives in the arteries being studied [11]. Typically, a 40 ml bolus of gadolinium is injected into a proximal forearm vein, followed by 40 ml of saline at a rate of 3 ml/s. Image acquisition begins as the contrast arrives in the intracranial arterial circulation, so that visualisation of intracerebral veins is avoided. A 3D volume ultrashort T1-weighted acquisition sequence is used, and the imaging parameters are set to minimise the signal return from background tissues, and to focus on the profoundly short T1 signal change from the gadolinium bolus within the artery. If one is imaging the intracranial circulation in a patient with extracranial ICA stenosis, it is important to appreciate that CE-MRA has poorer spatial resolution than I-ADSA, although the image quality is often better that that seen with non-enhanced MRA. However, if the image acquisition is not precisely timed to coincide with the arrival of the injected gadolinium bolus, then the arteries may be under-filled or the images obscured by 'venous phase contamination'. Furthermore, CE-MRA is also susceptible to TI shortening effects, as outlined above.

Therefore, if the clinical history, or the results of extracranial imaging studies suggest that intracranial vascular imaging could facilitate clinical decision making in a patient with asymptomatic or symptomatic extracranial ICA stenosis, the options are to screen the patient with I-ADSA, CTA or MRA. Although I-ADSA is the gold standard vascular imaging technique, MRA (especially CE-MRA or ToF-MRA) or CTA are safer and allow one to obtain information about brain structure and vascular anatomy in one sitting. If further information is required that is likely to influence clinical management, e.g. delineation of collateral arterial blood supply in a patient with critical ICA stenosis, or the exclusion of intracranial vasculopathy involving smaller arterioles that one cannot visualise with current non-invasive arterial imaging techniques, one should proceed to I-ADSA. The imaging technique of choice is clearly determined by local availability and local expertise, and it is important to realise that certain CT and MRI systems provide better quality vascular imaging than others. When the Neuroradiologist is informed about the precise information that the clinician requires from the test, he/she can decide which non-invasive imaging test should be performed or whether one should proceed directly to catheter angiography. Advances in intracranial CTA and MRA techniques in future are likely to reduce the need for I-ADSA in many carotid stenosis patients in whom intracranial vascular imaging is needed.

Transcranial doppler ultrasound (TCD)

Development and applications of TCD

Transcranial Doppler Ultrasound (TCD) allows non-invasive measurement of blood flow velocity in the basal intracerebral vessels [57]. Although Doppler ultrasound was first applied to patients in the 1960s, Aaslid et al. first described successful insonation of the middle cerebral artery in 1982 [2]. Since then, TCD has been used for a number of different purposes, including measurement of dynamic cerebrovascular responses, intra- and peri-procedural monitoring in patients with carotid stenosis, detection of intra-cranial stenosis, and detection of vasospasm after subarachnoid haemorrhage [57]. More recently, it has been appreciated that TCD can also be used for cerebral emboli detection [81] and hence the potential usefulness of TCD in investigating and monitoring patients with carotid stenosis or occlusion.

TCD technique

To enable sufficient transmission of ultrasound waves and successful insonation of the basal intracerebral vessels through the skull bones, a low frequency transducer (usually 2 MHz) is used [57]. An aqueous gel is applied to the transducer to improve ultrasound transmission by maintaining an air-free contact between the transducer and the patient. TCD takes advantage of specific areas of the bony cranium that tend to be relatively thin (acoustic windows) to investigate the intracranial vasculature (Fig. 9a–c). Arterial localisation is achieved by the use of pulsed Doppler that allows one to determine the depth of the insonated vessel and the direction of blood flow within the vessel. A typical TCD spectra obtained from insonating the MCA is shown in Fig. 9d. One may insonate the terminal ICA, MCA, ACA and proximal PCA via a transtemporal window above the zygomatic arch. (Fig 9b) [57]. However, TCD may also be performed through a transorbital acoustic window which allows insonation of the distal internal carotid artery and the ophthalmic artery, or via a transforaminal approach to insonate the distal vertebral arteries and the basilar artery (Fig. 9c) [57]. For obvious reasons, the transtemporal approach is most commonly preferred for investigating patients with extracranial carotid stenosis or suspected anterior circulation intracranial stenosis.

Advantages and limitations of conventional TCD

Conventional TCD has a number of advantages as a method of evaluating patients with carotid stenosis and occlusion. It is relatively cheap; it is non-invasive and thus allows relatively prolonged monitoring and

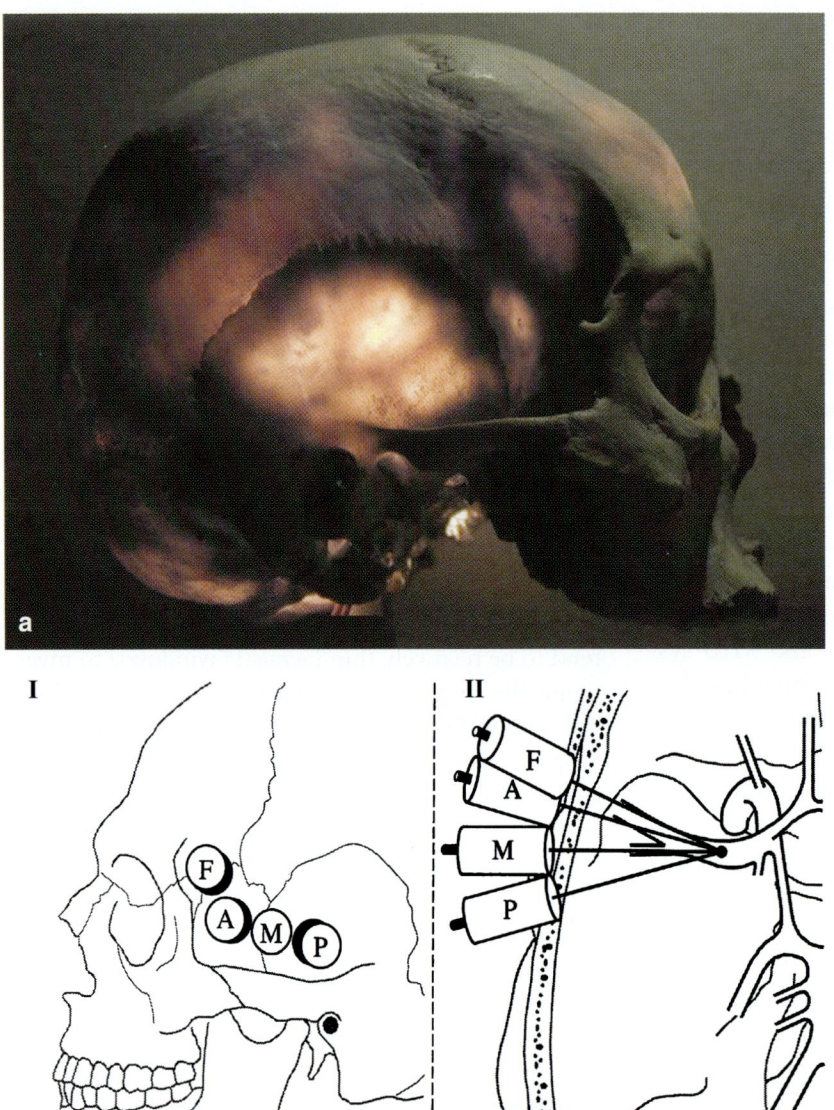

Fig. 9. a Photograph of skull illuminated from the inside. The relatively translucent area represents the transtemporal acoustic window, an area of thin bone above the zygomatic arch (Reproduced with permission from Rune Aaslid, 2005:). **b I** Insonation of the MCA via the transtemporal window. The transtemporal window can be divided into four distinct areas: Posterior (*P*), Middle (*M*), Anterior (*A*), and Frontal (*F*) windows. In practice, the operator often commences insonation via the posterior window because this is the region which usually affords best access to the MCA. **II** Transducer angulations vary according to which transtemporal window is being utilized (adapted from *Fujioka KA, Douville CM: Anatomy and freehand examination. In Transcranial Doppler* (Newell DW, Aaslid R, eds.), *pp. 9–32. New York; Raven Press, 1992;* **c** The transtemporal (transducer probe), transorbital (thick white arrow) and transforaminal (via the foramen magnum, dashed white arrow) windows are the three natural acoustic windows that allow penetration of the ultrasound beam into the cranium and insonation of the major intracranial arteries. Most investigators use the transtemporal window for insonation of the anterior, middle, and posterior cerebral arteries. Original drawing by Rune Aaslid (reproduced with permission). **d** Typical Doppler spectral waveform obtained from insonation of the MCA using an ambulatory TCD device. Velocity (cm/s) is plotted on the y-axis, and time (s) on the x-axis. The insonation depth is 50 mm and the direction of flow is towards the transducer.

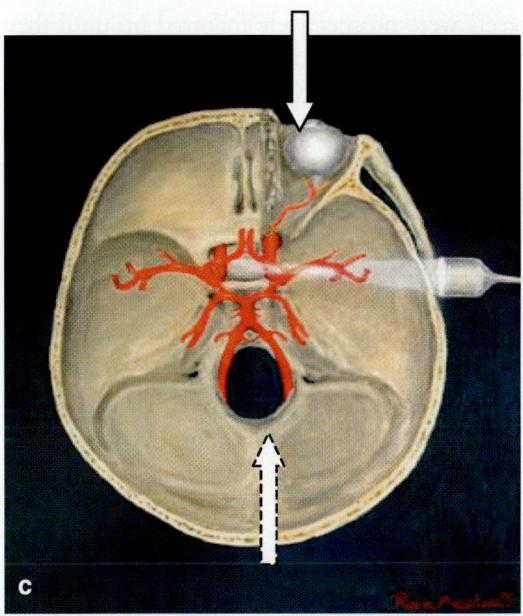

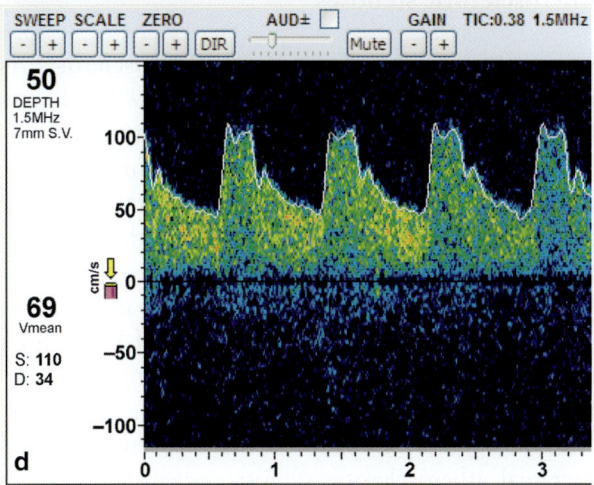

Fig. 9. (Continued)

repeated measurements. It also has high temporal resolution making it an ideal tool to study rapid changes in cerebral haemodynamics and to detect cerebral emboli from a proximal source [57].

Its limitations include the reliance on a trained technician to position the device and interpret the data; and the poor spatial resolution of the technique does not allow one to obtain clinically useful information about the calibre of an intracranial vessel [57]. The non-portability of conventional TCD limits its recording time to approximately one hour, which is sufficient for performing cerebral haemodynamic studies but a short time window to allow one to assess cerebral embolisation. Recently, ambulatory TCD has become available which allows prolonged recordings of up to 8 hours [49], [48]. Another limitation of TCD is the inability of the ultrasound waves to pass across the temporal bone in 3–5% of patients [31]. With advancing age, especially in females, hyperostosis of the temporal bone occurs [8], [50], and this increases the percentage of patients who have an inadequate acoustic window [38]. The inability to obtain an adequate acoustic window is also more common in black and Asian subjects.

Principles of cerebral haemodynamic measurements using TCD

As stated earlier, some patients with severe carotid stenosis or occlusion may have cerebral haemodynamic compromise which may predispose to, or contribute to, the pathogenesis of TIA or ischaemic stroke. When collateral circulation is insufficient to maintain cerebral blood flow, the low resistance intracranial arterioles respond by vasodilating (cerebral autoregulation), and their ability to vasodilate further in response to an administered vasodilator is reduced. Haemodynamically compromised brain regions can be identified by the finding of increased oxygen extraction on PET studies [16]. However, one can also investigate for haemodynamic compromise by measuring vasodilatory reserve or reactivity [68]. Increased inspired carbon dioxide (CO_2) in air, or acetazolamide (a carbonic anhydrase inhibitor) are the most commonly used vasodilating stimuli [68]. SPECT studies can be performed to measure cerebral blood flow (CBF) before and after administration of a vasodilator [9]. However, PET and SPECT studies are expensive, not necessarily widely available, and the patient is exposed to ionising radiation.

TCD is a simpler method of assessing cerebrovascular vasodilatory reserve or reactivity [67]. However, TCD measures blood flow velocity and not absolute blood flow, and the technique is only valid in estimating changes in cerebral blood flow if the vessel diameter does not change during the intervention. It has been demonstrated by cerebral angiography that there is very little or no change in the MCA diameter after the administration of concentrations of CO_2 that are used in TCD studies [36], and therefore, measurement of cerebrovascular reactivity with TCD in response to CO_2 appears to be a valid technique. However, high doses of CO_2 occasionally cause hypertension which may lead to an increase in cerebral perfusion and a 'passive' increase in the recorded velocity in the MCA [19]. This may give the erroneous impression that cerebral autoregulation is preserved, when it fact it may be impaired [19] thus emphasising the importance of monitoring blood pressure during the procedure to control for this potential confounder [57].

TCD technique of carbon dioxide reactivity

Blood flow velocity in the middle cerebral artery (MCA) is monitored with TCD while the patient breathes air, and then during the inhalation of a mixture of 5–8% carbon dioxide and air [57]. Similar studies can be performed before and after the administration of acetazolamide. In normal subjects, there is a marked increase in blood flow velocity of < 50%, that is dependent on the concentration of CO_2 administered [58]. An increase in MCA velocity of < 20% in response to inhalation of 8% CO_2 has been considered to represent exhausted cerebrovascular reactivity [51].

CO_2 reactivity in patients with severe carotid stenosis and occlusion

In keeping with PET and SPECT studies, a minority of patients with severe carotid stenosis or carotid occlusion, essentially those with poor collateral supply, have markedly impaired CO_2 reactivity [67], which may improve in some patients following carotid endarterectomy [29]. Markus and Cullinane performed baseline CO_2 reactivity studies in 48 patients with carotid occlusion who had been asymptomatic for at least 3 months, and 59 patients with 70–99% carotid stenosis who had been clinically asymptomatic for at least 2 years [51].

The subjects were prospectively followed-up until they experienced a TIA, stroke, died, or the study terminated. Exhausted ipsilateral MCA reactivity was a significant predictor of an increased risk of ipsilateral TIA and stroke during follow-up in the whole group, and also in the carotid occlusion and asymptomatic carotid stenosis subgroups independently. Similar to PET [25] and SPECT [46] studies, the evaluation of cerebral haemodynamic reserve using TCD may facilitate identification of a sub-group of high risk patients with carotid stenosis or occlusion who may benefit from revascularization procedures, especially in centres without access to PET or SPECT. However, randomized controlled intervention trials are required to formally test this hypothesis.

TCD for the detection of intracranial atherosclerotic stenoses

As stated earlier, intracranial atherosclerosis is an important cause of TIA and stroke, and may co-exist with extracranial carotid stenosis. However, the true prevalence of intracranial atherosclerotic stenosis of the ICA and its branches may have been underestimated because of the traditional dependence on invasive vascular imaging techniques to diagnose intracranial stenosis in the past, and the fact that many patients with TIA or stroke do not have intracranial vascular imaging performed at all.

Although TCD may be used to screen for intracranial atherosclerotic stenosis, especially affecting the middle cerebral artery, the test is neither 100% sensitive [15] nor specific [69] at identifying intracranial MCA stenosis when compared with cerebral angiography. In an acute atherothrombotic stroke in a patient with known extracranial ICA stenosis, one cannot determine whether an alteration in flow velocity in the ipsilateral intracranial ICA or MCA is secondary to the presence of an embolus in the vessel or a fixed atherosclerotic stenosis. If the TCD recording returns to normal on repeat testing after a suitable time interval, one can conclude that the vessel was temporarily occluded or narrowed by embolic material that was subsequently either lysed or washed distally.

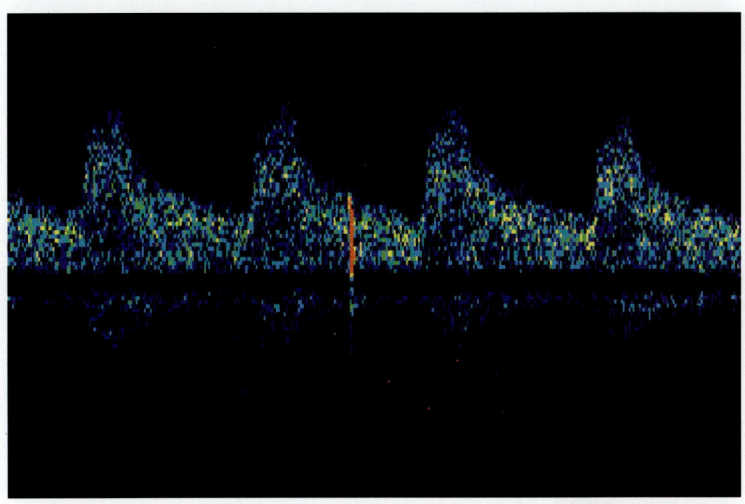

Fig. 10. The typical appearance of an Embolic Signal (vertical red line) within the Middle Cerebral Artery Doppler spectral waveform.

With the availability of intracranial CTA, MRA and DSA, we do not use TCD as an initial screening test for intracranial atherosclerotic stenosis of the ICA or its branches in adults. However, TCD is a very useful non-invasive initial screening test for distal intracranial non-atherosclerotic ICA or MCA stenosis in children with sickle cell disease, because the results of this test may predict stroke risk in this patient population [79]. TCD may also be used for ongoing monitoring of sickle cell disease patients with intracranial stenosis who have been shown to benefit from chronic transfusion therapy [3].

Intra-operative and peri-operative TCD monitoring in patients with carotid stenosis

The high temporal resolution and non-invasive nature of TCD make it ideally suited to intraoperative and perioperative monitoring of patients undergoing carotid endarterectomy (CEA) or carotid endovascular therapy (angioplasty and stenting) [57]. During carotid endarterectomy, if collateral blood supply is inadequate, the ipsilateral MCA velocity may dramatically fall during cross clamping of the extracranial ICA [57] with the resultant risk of TIA or stroke secondary to haemodynamic compromise. These patients may then have a shunt inserted by the surgeon before proceeding further with the operation. Similarly, during carotid endovascular therapy, the MCA velocity may fall during inflation of the angioplasty balloon, or secondary to vasospasm induced by stimulation of the vessel wall by a catheter tip, a carotid stent, or a distal neuroprotective filter device. In these patients, TCD may influence the clinical management of the patient. The Interventional Neuroradiologist may temporarily postpone further deployment of the stent until the MCA velocity returns towards the baseline value, and any neuroprotective filter would be removed as soon as possible. TCD can also detect cerebral emboli during and after CEA and carotid stenting (see below).

TCD for embolic signal detection

Because thromboembolism is believed to be the underlying mechanism responsible for TIA or stroke in most patients with extracranial ICA carotid stenosis, the ability to detect emboli in patients with asymptomatic and symptomatic ICA stenosis may allow one to risk stratify patients who are being considered for CEA, and may improve our understanding of the pathogenesis of TIA or stroke in individual patients.

Ultrasound offers the unique ability to detect emboli as they pass through the circulation [58]. Embolic signals secondary to 'solid' embolic material, presumed to be composed of platelet-platelet aggregates, thrombus or plaque fragments, were de-

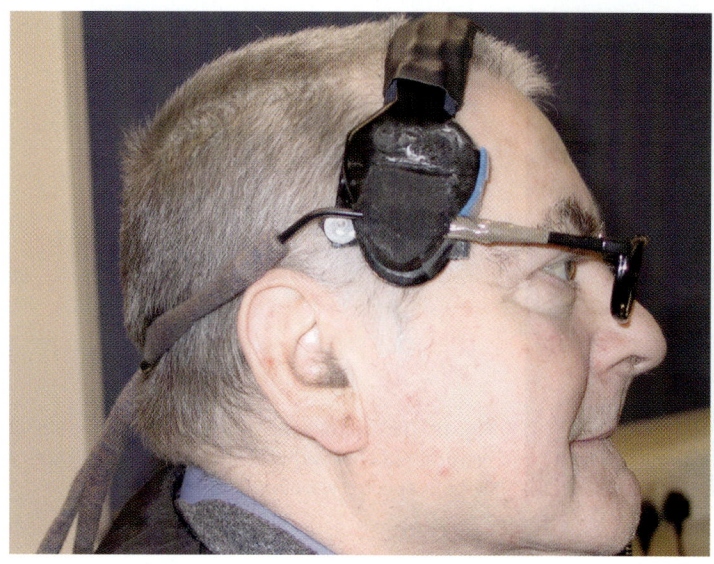

Fig. 11. A patient undergoing ambulatory TCD recording; the transducer is held in place by the frame of a pair of spectacles and the Doppler unit is carried in a jacket pocket that the patient wears for the duration of the recording.

tected by TCD monitoring during carotid endarterectomy in 1990 [81]. Over the last decade, TCD has been used to detect and monitor asymptomatic embolisation in patients with a variety of vascular diseases including carotid stenosis [78]. intracranial stenosis [17], valvular heart disease and atrial fibrillation [85], [13] recent myocardial infarction, and during and immediately after both carotid endarterectomy [81], [40], and angioplasty [53].

Embolic signals have a characteristic appearance on the Doppler spectrum (Fig. 10), and standardised identification criteria were drawn up by the Consensus Committee of the Ninth International Cerebral Hemodynamic Symposium in 1995 [12]. Embolic signals appear as short duration (usually < 300 ms), high intensity signals due to the fact that more ultrasound is scattered and reflected by the embolus than by the surrounding red blood cells [57]. They are also predominantly unidirectional, and accompanied by a characteristic "chirping sound" on audio recording. In contrast, artefacts produced by transducer movement, eating, or talking, result in predominantly bidirectional signals which have an intensity increase that is maximal at low velocities.

These asymptomatic embolic signals are considerably more frequent than clinical embolic events [52]. A one hour TCD recording of the ipsilateral middle cerebral artery can detect embolic signals in up to 28% of asymptomatic [60] and 50% of symptomatic > 50% carotid stenosis patients [60], [56]. Embolic signals may be detected more frequently in symptomatic than asymptomatic subjects [55], and are more common in symptomatic patients in the early compared with the late phase after symptom onset [60], [56], [77]. They are also more common in patients with plaque ulceration compared with those without plaque ulceration on angiographic [87] or histological examination [79].

There is increasing evidence that the presence of embolic signals is an independent risk factor for subsequent ipsilateral TIA and stroke in patients with asymptomatic and symptomatic > 60% ICA stenosis [60]. A recent prospective study of 200 consecutively recruited, recently symptomatic patients with > 50% ICA stenosis has demonstrated that the presence of embolic signals independently predicts short-term ipsilateral stroke risk [56].

Recently, advances in technology have reduced the size of the TCD recording equipment and have enabled prolonged ambulatory recordings for 5–8 hours to be performed (Fig. 11) [48]. Ambulatory TCD recordings may allow better estimation of the 'true embolic load' to be determined, with the identification of embolic signals in up to 75% of patients with symptomatic ≥ 50% ICA stenosis [48]. In a small study of 15 patients with asymptomatic ≥ 50%

ICA stenosis, embolic signals were detected in 27% of patients during a single 8-hour recording, and 47% of patients after a second 8-hour recording [48]. Ambulatory TCD may also provide novel insights into the pattern of embolisation from an extracranial ICA stenosis, for example, the considerable temporal variability in embolisation and the presence of clustering of embolic signals [48].

The additional information obtained from TCD regarding ongoing embolisation has the potential to facilitate better risk stratification and advances in treatment of patients with extracranial ICA stenosis. Although patients with TIA or non-disabling stroke in the vascular territory supplied by a severe (70–99%) symptomatic carotid stenosis should ideally be operated on within 2 weeks, this is not always possible in some countries because of limited resources. Additional information on active embolisation might allow one to identify patients with symptomatic severe ICA stenosis who are likely to derive most benefit from hyperacute surgical or endovascular treatment, or who may benefit from more intensive antithrombotic therapy whilst awaiting intervention. In addition, because the potential benefit from carotid endarterectomy is lower in patients with moderate (50–69%) symptomatic ICA stenosis [72], the presence of embolic signals may identify a high risk subgroup who may benefit from carotid endarterectomy within the first 2 weeks after symptom onset. However, larger studies are required to determine whether TCD is a reliable method of predicting which patients are likely to benefit from interventional or best medical treatment of carotid stenosis.

The ongoing prospective multicentre, international Asymptomatic Carotid Emboli Study (ACES) is assessing the frequency of embolic signals in patients with asymptomatic carotid stenosis, and this study will provide further information about whether the presence of embolic signals predicts stroke risk in these patients. These data may also facilitate selection of asymptomatic severe carotid stenosis patients who may benefit from carotid endartectomy for primary stroke prevention.

Because embolic signals detected on TCD are considerably more frequent than clinical events, and have been shown to be an independent predictor of subsequent TIA and stroke, they have the potential to be used as a surrogate marker to assess the effectiveness of novel antithrombotic therapies. The Clopidogrel and Aspirin for Reduction of Emboli in Symptomatic Carotid Stenosis (CARESS) trial has shown that short-term clopidogrel and aspirin combination antiplatelet therapy was significantly more effective than aspirin monotherapy at preventing asymptomatic embolisation in patients with symptomatic > 50% carotid stenosis [54]. Larger prospective studies are also required to determine whether a reduction in the frequency of embolic signals following alteration of antiplatelet therapy truly correlates with a reduction in the subsequent risk of TIA or stroke during follow-up.

Summary

Over the past 30 years, there have been marked advances in intracerebral imaging techniques which have improved our understanding of the pathogenesis of TIA and stroke, and facilitated rapid confirmation of cerebral ischaemia or infarction in patients with atherosclerotic carotid stenosis. MRI can help to confirm or refute the clinical impression that an extracranial ICA stenosis caused the TIA or stroke syndrome, and may influence clinical management decisions in the acute and subacute stages after symptom onset. Intra-arterial catheter angiography is still the "gold standard" test for imaging the intracranial vessels, but it must be performed by experienced radiologists who regularly audit their practice because of the risks associated with this investigation in carotid stenosis patients who often have widespread atherosclerosis. Non-invasive intracranial vascular imaging techniques, including MRA, CTA and TCD, allow visualisation of the large intracranial arteries, and further technical advances in this field are likely to further reduce the need for catheter angiography in future. Future noninvasive imaging studies are likely to improve our ability to risk stratify carotid stenosis patients to facilitate optimisation of medical, surgical, endovascular, or revascularisation therapy.

References

[1] Aaron JO, Hesselink JR, Oot R, Jones RL, Davis KR, Taveras JM: Complications of intravenous DSA performed for carotid artery disease: a prospective study. Radiology 153: 675–678 (1984).

[2] Aaslid R, Markwalder TM, Nornes H: Noninvasive transcranial Doppler ultrasound recording of flow velocity in basal cerebral arteries. Journal of Neurosurgery. 57: 769–774 (1982).

[3] Adams RJ, McKie VC, Hsu L, Files B, Vichinsky E, Pegelow C et al.: Prevention of a first stroke by transfusions in children with sickle cell anemia and abnormal results on transcranial Doppler ultrasonography. N Engl J Med 339: 5–11 (1998).

[4] Baird AE, Warach S: Magnetic resonance imaging of acute stroke. J Cereb Blood Flow Metab 18: 583–609 (1998).

[5] Beauchamp NJ Jr, Barker PB, Wang PY, vanZijl PC: Imaging of acute cerebral ischemia. Radiology 212: 307–324 (1999).

[6] Bogousslavsky J, Van Melle G, Regli F.: The Lausanne Stroke Registry: analysis of 1,000 consecutive patients with first stroke. Stroke 19: 1083–1092 (1988).

[7] Brant-Zawadzki M, Atkinson D, Detrick M, Bradley WG, Scidmore G: Fluid-attenuated inversion recovery (FLAIR) for assessment of cerebral infarction. Initial clinical experience in 50 patients. Stroke 27: 1187–1191 (1996).

[8] Bruno A, Biller J, Silvidi JA: A reason for failure to obtain transcranial Doppler flow signals. Hyperostosis of the skull. Stroke 19: 274 (1988).

[9] Burt RW, Witt RM, Cikrit DF, Reddy RV: Carotid artery disease: evaluation with acetazolamide-enhanced Tc-99m HMPAO SPECT. Radiology 182: 461–466 (1992).

[10] Chimowitz MI, Lynn MJ, Howlett-Smith H, Stern BJ, Hertzberg VS, Frankel MR et al.: Comparison of warfarin and aspirin for symptomatic intracranial arterial stenosis. N Engl J Med 352: 1305–1316 (2005).

[11] Clifton AG: MR angiography. Br Med Bull 56: 367–377 (2000).

[12] Consensus Committee of the Ninth International Cerebral Hemodynamic Symposium. Basic identification criteria of Doppler microembolic signals. Stroke 26: 1123 (1995).

[13] Cullinane M, Wainwright R, Brown A, Monaghan M, Markus HS: Asymptomatic embolization in subjects with atrial fibrillation not taking anticoagulants: a prospective study. Stroke 29: 1810–1815 (1998).

[14] Davies KN, Humphrey PR: Complications of cerebral angiography in patients with symptomatic carotid territory ischaemia screened by carotid ultrasound. J Neurol Neurosurg Psychiatry 56: 967–972 (1993).

[15] de Bray JM, Daugy J, Legrand MS, Pulci S: Acute middle cerebral artery stroke and transcranial Doppler sonography. Eur J Ultrasound 7: 31–36 (1998).

[16] Derdeyn CP, Yundt KD, Videen TO, Carpenter DA, Grubb RL Jr, Powers WJ: Increased oxygen extraction fraction is associated with prior ischemic events in patients with carotid occlusion. Stroke 29: 754–758 (1998).

[17] Diehl RR, Samii C, Diehl A: Dynamics and embolic activity of symptomatic intra-cranial cerebral artery stenoses. Acta Neurologica Scandinavica 106: 173–181 (2002).

[18] Dodick DW, Meissner I, Meyer FB, Cloft HJ: Evaluation and management of asymptomatic carotid artery stenosis. Mayo Clin Proc 79: 937–944 (2004).

[19] Dumville J, Panerai RB, Lennard NS, Naylor AR, Evans DH: Can cerebrovascular reactivity be assessed without measuring blood pressure in patients with carotid artery disease? Stroke 29: 968–974 (1998).

[20] Eastwood JD, Engelter ST, MacFall JF, Delong DM, Provenzale JM: Quantitative assessment of the time course of infarct signal intensity on diffusion-weighted images. Am J Neuroradiol 24: 680–687 (2003).

[21] Executive Committee for the Asymptomatic Carotid Atherosclerosis Study. Endarterectomy for asymptomatic carotid artery stenosis. JAMA 273: 1421–1428 (1995).

[22] Fiebach J, Jansen O, Schellinger P, Knauth M, Hartmann M, Heiland S et al.: Comparison of CT with diffusion-weighted MRI in patients with hyperacute stroke. Neuroradiology 43: 628–632 (2001).

[23] Fiebach JB, Schellinger PD, Jansen O, Meyer M, Wilde P, Bender J et al.: CT and diffusion-weighted MR imaging in randomized order: diffusion-weighted imaging results in higher accuracy and lower interrater variability in the diagnosis of hyperacute ischemic stroke. Stroke 33: 2206–2210 (2002).

[24] Golledge J, Greenhalgh RM, Davies AH: The symptomatic carotid plaque. Stroke 31: 774–81 (2000).

[25] Grubb RL Jr, Derdeyn CP, Fritsch SM, Carpenter DA, Yundt KD, Videen TO et al.: Importance of hemodynamic factors in the prognosis of symptomatic carotid occlusion. JAMA 280: 1055–1060 (1998).

[26] Hacke W, Albers G, Al Rawi Y, Bogousslavsky J, Davalos A, Eliasziw M et al.: The Desmoteplase in Acute Ischemic Stroke Trial (DIAS): a phase II MRI-based 9-hour window acute stroke thrombolysis trial with intravenous desmoteplase. Stroke 36: 66–73 (2005).

[27] Hacke W, Donnan G, Fieschi C, Kaste M, von Kummer R, Broderick JP et al.: Association of outcome with early stroke treatment: pooled analysis of ATLANTIS, ECASS, and NINDS rt-PA stroke trials. Lancet 363: 768–774 (2004).

[28] Halliday A, Mansfield A, Marro J, Peto C, Peto R, Potter J et al.: Prevention of disabling and fatal strokes

by successful carotid endarterectomy in patients without recent neurological symptoms: randomised controlled trial. Lancet 363: 1491–1502 (2004).
[29] Hartl WH, Janssen I, Furst H: Effect of carotid endarterectomy on patterns of cerebrovascular reactivity in patients with unilateral carotid artery stenosis. Stroke 25: 1952–1957 (1994).
[30] Henderson RD, Eliasziw M, Fox AJ, Rothwell PM, Barnett HJ: Angiographically defined collateral circulation and risk of stroke in patients with severe carotid artery stenosis. North American Symptomatic Carotid Endarterectomy Trial (NASCET) Group. Stroke 31: 128–132 (2000).
[31] Hennerici M, Rautenberg W, Sitzer G, Schwartz A: Transcranial Doppler ultrasound for the assessment of intracranial arterial flow velocity – Part 1. Examination technique and normal values. Surg Neurol 27: 439–448 (1987).
[32] Hirai T, Korogi Y, Ono K, Nagano M, Maruoka K, Uemura S et al.: Prospective evaluation of suspected stenoocclusive disease of the intracranial artery: combined MR angiography and CT angiography compared with digital subtraction angiography. Am J Neuroradiol 23: 93–101 (2002).
[33] Hoppe C: Defining stroke risk in children with sickle cell anaemia. Br J Haematol 128: 751–766 (2005).
[34] Huang IJ, Chen CY, Chung HW, Chang DC, Lee CC, Chin SC et al.: Time course of cerebral infarction in the middle cerebral arterial territory: deep watershed versus territorial subtypes on diffusion-weighted MR images. Radiology 221: 35–42 (2001).
[35] Huang YN, Gao S, Li SW, Huang Y, Li JF, Wong KS et al.: Vascular lesions in Chinese patients with transient ischemic attacks. Neurology 48: 524–525 (1997).
[36] Huber P, Handa J: Effect of contrast material, hypercapnia, hyperventilation, hypertonic glucose and papaverine on the diameter of the cerebral arteries. Angiographic determination in man. Invest Radiol 2: 17–32 (1967).
[37] Inzitari D Eliasziw M, Sharpe BL, Fox AJ, Barnett HJ: Risk factors and outcome of patients with carotid artery stenosis presenting with lacunar stroke. North American Symptomatic Carotid Endarterectomy Trial Group. Neurology 54: 660–666 (2000).
[38] Itoh T, Matsumoto M, Handa N, Maeda H, Hougaku H, Hashimoto H et al.: Rate of successful recording of blood flow signals in the middle cerebral artery using transcranial Doppler sonography. Stroke 24: 1192–1195 (1993).
[39] Jager HR: Diagnosis of stroke with advanced CT and MR imaging. Br Med Bull 56: 318–333 (2000).
[40] Jansen C, Ramos LM, van Heesewijk JP, Moll FL, van Gijn J, Ackerstaff RG: Impact of microembolism and hemodynamic changes in the brain during carotid endarterectomy. Stroke 25: 992–997 (1994).
[41] Kappelle LJ, Eliasziw M, Fox AJ, Sharpe BL, Barnett HJ: Importance of intracranial atherosclerotic disease in patients with symptomatic stenosis of the internal carotid artery. The North American Symptomatic Carotid Endarterectomy Trail. Stroke 30: 282–286 (1999).
[42] Kastrup A, Schulz JB, Mader I, Dichgans J, Kuker W: Diffusion-weighted MRI in patients with symptomatic internal carotid artery disease. J Neurol 249: 1168–1174 (2002).
[43] Kidwell CS, Saver JL, Mattiello J, Starkman S, Vinuela F, Duckwiler G et al.: Thrombolytic reversal of acute human cerebral ischemic injury shown by diffusion/perfusion magnetic resonance imaging. Ann Neurol 47: 462–469 (2000).
[44] Klijn CJ, Kappelle LJ, Tulleken CA, van Gijn J: Symptomatic carotid artery occlusion. A reappraisal of hemodynamic factors. Stroke 28: 2084–2093 (1997).
[45] Knauth M, von Kummer R, Jansen O, Hahnel S, Dorfler A, Sartor K: Potential of CT angiography in acute ischemic stroke. Am J Neuroradiol 18: 1001–1010 (1997).
[46] Kuroda S, Houkin K, Kamiyama H, Mitsumori K, Iwasaki Y, Abe H: Long-term prognosis of medically treated patients with internal carotid or middle cerebral artery occlusion: can acetazolamide test predict it? Stroke 32: 2110–2116 (2001).
[47] Leow K,.Murie JA: Cerebral angiography for cerebrovascular disease: the risks. Br J Surg 75: 428–430 (1988).
[48] Mackinnon AD, Aaslid R, Markus HS: Ambulatory transcranial Doppler cerebral embolic signal detection in symptomatic and asymptomatic carotid stenosis. Stroke 36: 1726–1730 (2005).
[49] Mackinnon AD, Aaslid R, Markus HS: Long-term ambulatory monitoring for cerebral emboli using transcranial Doppler ultrasound. Stroke 35: 73–78 (2004).
[50] Marinoni M, Ginanneschi A, Forleo P, Amaducci L: Technical limits in transcranial Doppler recording: inadequate acoustic windows. Ultrasound Med Biol 23: 1275–1277 (1997).
[51] Markus H, Cullinane M: Severely impaired cerebrovascular reactivity predicts stroke and TIA risk in patients with carotid artery stenosis and occlusion. Brain 124: 457–467 (2001).
[52] Markus H: Monitoring embolism in real time. Circulation 102: 826–828 (2000).
[53] Markus HS, Clifton A, Buckenham T, Brown MM: Carotid angioplasty. Detection of embolic signals during and after the procedure. Stroke 25: 2403–2406 (1994).
[54] Markus HS, Droste DW, Kaps M, Larrue V, Lees KR, Siebler M et al.: Dual Antiplatelet Therapy With Clopidogrel and Aspirin in Symptomatic Carotid Stenosis Evaluated Using Doppler Embolic Signal Detection. The Clopidogrel and Aspirin for Reduction of Emboli in Symptomatic Carotid Ste-

nosis (CARESS) Trial. Circulation 111: 2233–2240 (2005).
[55] Markus HS, Thomson ND, Brown MM: Asymptomatic cerebral embolic signals in symptomatic and asymptomatic carotid artery disease. Brain 118: 1005–1011 (1995).
[56] Markus HS, MacKinnon A: Asymptomatic embolization detected by Doppler ultrasound predicts stroke risk in symptomatic carotid artery stenosis. Stroke 36: 971–975 (2005).
[57] Markus HS: Transcranial Doppler ultrasound. Br Med Bull 56: 378–388 (2000).
[58] Markus HS: Transcranial Doppler ultrasound. J Neurol Neurosurg Psychiatry 67: 135–137 (1999).
[59] McCabe DJ, Pereira AC, Clifton A, Bland JM, Brown MM: Restenosis after carotid angioplasty, stenting, or endarterectomy in the Carotid and Vertebral Artery Transluminal Angioplasty Study (CAVATAS). Stroke 36: 281–286 (2005).
[60] Molloy J, Markus HS: Asymptomatic embolization predicts stroke and TIA risk in patients with carotid artery stenosis. Stroke 30: 1440–1443 (1999).
[61] Momjian-Mayor I, Baron JC: The pathophysiology of watershed infarction in internal carotid artery disease: review of cerebral perfusion studies. Stroke 36: 567–577 (2005).
[62] Moneta GL, Edwards JM, Chitwood RW, Taylor LM Jr, Lee RW, Cummings CA et al.: Correlation of North American Symptomatic Carotid Endarterectomy Trial (NASCET) angiographic definition of 70% to 99% internal carotid artery stenosis with duplex scanning. J Vasc Surg 17: 152–157 (1993).
[63] Morcos SK: Acute serious and fatal reactions to contrast media: our current understanding. Br J Radiol 78: 686–693 (2005).
[64] Mullins ME, Schaefer PW, Sorensen AG, Halpern EF, Ay H, He J et al.: CT and conventional and diffusion-weighted MR imaging in acute stroke: study in 691 patients at presentation to the emergency department. Radiology 224: 353–360 (2002).
[65] Noguchi K, Ogawa T, Inugami A, Fujita H, Hatazawa J, Shimosegawa E et al.: MRI of acute cerebral infarction: a comparison of FLAIR and T2-weighted fast spin-echo imaging. Neuroradiology 39: 406–410 (1997).
[66] Patel SG, Collie DA, Wardlaw JM, Lewis SC, Wright AR, Gibson RJ et al.: Outcome, observer reliability, and patient preferences if CTA, MRA, or Doppler ultrasound were used, individually or together, instead of digital subtraction angiography before carotid endarterectomy. J Neurol Neurosurg Psychiatry 73: 21–28 (2002).
[67] Ringelstein EB, Sievers C, Ecker S, Schneider PA, Otis SM: Noninvasive assessment of CO_2-induced cerebral vasomotor response in normal individuals and patients with internal carotid artery occlusions. Stroke 19: 963–969 (1988).
[68] Ringelstein EB, Van Eyck S, Mertens I: Evaluation of cerebral vasomotor reactivity by various vasodilating stimuli: comparison of CO_2 to acetazolamide. J Cereb Blood Flow Metab 12: 162–168 (1992).
[69] Rorick MB, Nichols FT, Adams RJ: Transcranial Doppler correlation with angiography in detection of intracranial stenosis. Stroke 25: 1931–1934 (1994).
[70] Rosen BR, Belliveau JW, Vevea JM, Brady TJ: Perfusion imaging with NMR contrast agents. Magn Reson Med 14: 249–265 (1990).
[71] Rothwell PM, Eliasziw M, Gutnikov SA, Fox AJ, Taylor DW, Mayberg MR et al.: Analysis of pooled data from the randomised controlled trials of endarterectomy for symptomatic carotid stenosis. Lancet 361: 107–116 (2003).
[72] Rothwell PM, Eliasziw M, Gutnikov SA, Warlow CP, Barnett HJ: Endarterectomy for symptomatic carotid stenosis in relation to clinical subgroups and timing of surgery. Lancet 363: 915–924 (2004).
[73] Rouleau PA, Huston J III, Gilbertson J, Brown RD Jr, Meyer FB, Bower TC: Carotid artery tandem lesions: frequency of angiographic detection and consequences for endarterectomy. Am J Neuroradiol 20: 621–625 (1999).
[74] Sacco RL, Ellenberg JH, Mohr JP, Tatemichi TK, Hier DB, Price TR et al.: Infarcts of undetermined cause: the NINCDS Stroke Data Bank. Ann Neurol 25: 382–390 (1989).
[75] Schlaug G, Benfield A, Baird AE, Siewert B, Lovblad KO, Parker RA et al.: The ischemic penumbra: operationally defined by diffusion and perfusion MRI. Neurology 53: 1528–1537 (1999).
[76] Schulz UG, Briley D, Meagher T, Molyneux A, Rothwell PM: Diffusion-weighted MRI in 300 patients presenting late with subacute transient ischemic attack or minor stroke. Stroke 35: 2459–2465 (2004).
[77] Siebler M, Sitzer M, Rose G, Bendfeldt D, Steinmetz H: Silent cerebral embolism caused by neurologically symptomatic high-grade carotid stenosis. Event rates before and after carotid endarterectomy. Brain 116: 1005–1015 (1993).
[78] Siebler M, Sitzer M, Steinmetz H: Detection of intracranial emboli in patients with symptomatic extracranial carotid artery disease. Stroke 23: 1652–1654 (1992).
[79] Sitzer M, Muller W, Siebler M, Hort W, Kniemeyer HW, Jancke L et al.: Plaque ulceration and lumen thrombus are the main sources of cerebral microemboli in high-grade internal carotid artery stenosis. Stroke 26: 1231–1233 (1995).
[80] Skutta B, Furst G, Eilers J, Ferbert A, Kuhn FP: Intracranial stenoocclusive disease: double-detector heli-

cal CT angiography versus digital subtraction angiography. Am J Neuroradiol 20: 791–799 (1999).
[81] Spencer MP, Thomas GI, Nicholls SC, Sauvage LR: Detection of middle cerebral artery emboli during carotid endarterectomy using transcranial Doppler ultrasonography. Stroke 21: 415–423 (1990).
[82] Symms M, Jager HR, Schmierer K, Yousry TA: A review of structural magnetic resonance neuroimaging. J Neurol Neurosurg Psychiatry 75: 1235–1244 (2004).
[83] Szabo K, Kern R, Gass A, Hirsch J, Hennerici M: Acute stroke patterns in patients with internal carotid artery disease: a diffusion-weighted magnetic resonance imaging study. Stroke 32: 1323–1329 (2001).
[84] The European Carotid Surgery Trialists Collaborative Group. Risk of stroke in the distribution of an asymptomatic carotid artery. Lancet 345: 209–212 (1995).
[85] Tong DC, Bolger A, Albers GW: Incidence of transcranial Doppler-detected cerebral microemboli in patients referred for echocardiography. Stroke 25: 2138–2141 (1994).
[86] Urbach H, Flacke S, Keller E, Textor J, Berlis A, Hartmann A et al.: Detectability and detection rate of acute cerebral hemisphere infarcts on CT and diffusion-weighted MRI. Neuroradiology 42: 722–727 (2000).
[87] Valton L, Larrue V, Arrue P, Geraud G, Bes A: Asymptomatic cerebral embolic signals in patients with carotid stenosis. Correlation with appearance of plaque ulceration on angiography. Stroke 26: 813–815 (1995).
[88] van Everdingen KJ, van der Grond J, Kappelle LJ, Ramos LM, Mali WP: Diffusion-weighted magnetic resonance imaging in acute stroke. Stroke 29: 1783–1790 (1998).
[89] Warlow CP, Dennis MS, van Gijn J, Hankey GJ, Sandercock PAG, Bamford JM et al.: Where is the lesion? In: Warlow CP, Dennis MS, van Gijn J, Hankey GJ, Sandercock PAG, Bamford JM et al., eds. Stroke. A practical guide to management, pp 80–145. Oxford: Blackwell Science Ltd. (1996).
[90] Warlow CP, Dennis MS, van Gijn J, Hankey GJ, Sandercock PAG, Bamford JM et al.: What caused this transient or persisting ischaemic event? In: Warlow CP, Dennis MS, van Gijn J, Hankey GJ, Sandercock PAG, Bamford JM et al. eds. Stroke. A practical guide to management, pp 190–257. Oxford: Blackwell Science Ltd. (1996).
[91] Whisnant JP, Basford JR, Bernstein EF, Cooper ES, Dyken ML, Easton JD et al.: Special report from the National Institute of Neurological Disorders and Stroke. Classification of cerebrovascular diseases III. Stroke 21: 637–676 (1990).
[92] Willinsky RA, Taylor SM, TerBrugge K, Farb RI, Tomlinson G, Montanera W: Neurologic complications of cerebral angiography: prospective analysis of 2,899 procedures and review of the literature. Radiology 227: 522–528 (2003).
[93] Wong KS, Huang YN, Gao S, Lam WW, Chan YL, Kay R: Intracranial stenosis in Chinese patients with acute stroke. Neurology 50: 812–813 (1998).
[94] Yuh WT, Crain MR, Loes DJ, Greene GM, Ryals TJ, Sato Y: MR imaging of cerebral ischemia: findings in the first 24 hours. Am J Neuroradiol 12: 621–629 (1991).

FROM IMAGING TO THERAPY IN CAROTID ARTERY STENOSIS

Chapter 3

FROM IMAGING TO THERAPY IN CAROTID ARTERY STENOSIS: FROM THE SURGICAL POINT OF VIEW

K. Bettermann and J. F. Toole

Wake Forest University School of Medicine, Winston-Salem, USA

Ischemic stroke results from a multitude of causes but more than 30% are due to atherosclerosis of arteries providing blood to the brain. More than 67% of all atherosclerotic carotid lesions are located in the extracranial cerebral circulation with 38% percent of those being found in the region of the carotid bifurcation [9], [38]. Atheromatous plaques in the bifurcation occur frequently as flow characteristics of blood are altered at arterial branching points causing turbulence and shear stress [74]. Less common locations are in the carotid siphon, at the origin of the ophthalmic artery or in both locations (tandem lesions).

Historical perspective

As early as in 1658 Wepfer described "corpra fibrosa" in the wall of arteries as well as intra- and extracranial carotid thrombosis as cause of ischemic stroke [71]. After him Baillie in 1677 and Thomas Willis mentioned calcified plaques in the arteries of the neck causing cerebral infarction being also one of the first to describe transient ischemic attack (TIA), stroke in evolution, and completed infarction [6], [73]. Despite these early observations that extracranial atherosclerosis is a major source for cerebral ischemic events, physicians surprisingly focused more on intracranial disease as reason for stroke until the 1950s. It was believed that stroke was not so much due to artery to artery embolism from a neck lesion, but due to intracranial artery disorders such as vasospasm. Therefore early unsuccessful surgical approaches for stroke prevention were limited to stellate ganglion block, cervical sympathetectomy, ligation of the carotid artery bifurcation and intracranial internal carotid artery ligations using metallic clips. In 1905 Chiari revived the concept that occlusive disease of the extracranial arteries can result in stroke describing ulcerating plaque in the bifurcation found during his pathological studies [18] and then Hunt [41] noted that the extracranial portions of the carotid arteries should be carefully examined in patients with TIA and ischemic stroke. With the development of cerebral angiography in 1927 by Moniz [51], it became apparent that extracranial occlusive disease was a major cause for ischemic stroke. Thereafter correction had to await the development of vascular surgery during World War II.

The modern concept of carotid endarterectomy for stroke prevention started in the 1950s. C. Miller Fisher in 1951 and then in 1954 published his landmark articles showing a clear relation of extracranial carotid disease and stroke and predicting that one day vascular surgery would be essential for prevention of ischemic stroke [30], [29]. Based on his publication in 1951, Carrea et al. [17] performed the first partial resection of an internal carotid stenosis followed by a bypass from the external to the distal internal carotid artery in 1951. The first successful carotid endarterectomy was performed by DeBakey in 1953 [21] and Strulley et al., performed the first reconstruction of an occluded internal carotid artery in 1953 [68]. This was followed by one of the most important interventions in carotid surgery performed by Eastcott et al. in 1954 [24] who resected a stenosed bifurcation and restored flow by end-to-end anastomosis between the common carotid and internal artery in a patient with a left hemispheric transient ischemic attacks. This procedure was done under general anesthesia using hypothermia. These accomplishments laid the groundwork for carotid endarterectomy (CEA) as we know it today and which is currently challenged by carotid artery stenting.

Non-invasive visualization of the vascular anatomy of the brain became possible with the development of head computed tomography (CT) by Hounsfield and Cormack [40], [19] during the 1970s and magnetic resonance imaging (MRI) during the 1980s by Manfield in Britain [46] and Lauterbur in the U.S. [44] who were both awarded the Nobel Prize in 2003.

The development of Neurosonology by Reid and Spencer in 1972 [57] and Blue, McKinney and Barnes in 1972 demonstrated its diagnostic validity correlating carotid ultrasound B-mode images with conventional arteriography [10]. Olinger in 1969, [56] based on previous work by Herz and Bliss [39] published one of the first reports on the visualization of carotid arteries by B-mode ultrasound imaging and Miyazaki and Kato [50] furthered transcranial Doppler as a diagnostic tool for stroke patients by recording changes in blood flow velocities through the intact human skull. Advancement of CT- and MR-angiography since the 1980s and their wide availability add an accumulating body of essential information important for the modern management of patients with carotid stenosis.

Atherosclerosis

Despite intense research over the last 50 years the initial injury that results in the activation of the complex cascade of atherosclerosis remains unknown. Probably the initial step of atherothrombotic plaque formation is a combination of genetic predisposition and environmental factors which result in endothelial dysfunction [66]. Chronic subtle endothelial injury may be caused by increased intravascular pressure, shear stress or turbulent blood flow leading to increased endothelial permeability, leukocyte adhesion, and accumulation of LDL cholesterol into the vessel wall. Lipid accumulation stimulates the release of cytokines, inhibits nitrous oxide production and stimulates vascular smooth muscle cells that migrate from the media to the intimal layer. There the vascular muscle cells proliferate and induce extracellular matrix proteins including collagen and proteoglycans which in turn stimulate platelet adhesion, activation of platelets and macrophages mediating a chronic inflammatory response. Chronic smooth cell proliferation remodels the vascular wall with subsequent further intra- and extra-cellular accumulation of lipids in the vessel wall. Remodeling of the artery can lead to compensatory expansion of the arterial wall with increase in the wall volume by plaque formation. Typical plaques are characterized by an increased lipid content consisting of a large necrotic core surrounded by a thin protective fibrous cap which makes them rupture releasing showers of arterial emboli.

Plaque accumulation can also cause negative remodeling, with little or no expansion of the arterial wall, but steady progression of luminal stenosis. Plaques are stable over relatively long periods of time, but as they progress can lead to hemodynamic compromise secondary to diminished flow and perfusion pressure resulting in cerebral infarction if, for example, there is an uncompensated fall in systemic blood pressure with subsequent reduction in cerebral perfusion pressure. Advanced imaging techniques have been developed to assess not only the degree of the carotid stenosis and the cerebral vasomotor perfusion reserve but also allowing analysis of plaque morphology and composition [20], [4], [16], [22].

Recurrence of cerebral ischemic events

Medical, endovascular and surgical interventions aimed at atherothrombotic plaque stabilization or plaque removal play a significant role for stroke prevention. The rationale for carotid endarterectomy is based on the natural course of the disease and the recurrence rate of ischemic events in patients with previous TIA or cerebral infarction observed in large epidemiological studies [65], [48], [72]. For patients with an ischemic infarction, the risk of recurrence is 4–8% within the first month, 12–13% at one year and 20–29% after 5 years. The cumulative five year risk is about 9% annually. The risk of ischemic stroke following an initial TIA is 3–10% in the first month, 10–14% after one year and 25–40% in the next five years which means that about one-third of all patients presenting with TIA or stroke will develop a major cerebral infarction over the course of five years following their initial event [64], [65], [13]. This risk might even be higher in certain populations with traditional atherosclerotic risk factors such as hypertension, diabetes mellitus or coronary artery disease and among patients with TIAs due to extracranial carotid stenosis [61], [5]. Patients with large ulcerated plaques in the internal carotid artery also have a higher risk of stroke [53], [28].

The stroke risk of patients having had a TIA is probably higher than reported as many of those patients do not seek medical attention after the first TIA. In general the awareness of TIA as a medical emergency in the general population is poor and even in patients hospitalized for another cause, stroke and TIA are frequently missed and treatment is delayed due to seemingly benign and evanescent phenomena such as pure sensory symptoms, dizziness, transitory ataxia or visual changes.

Therefore it is imperative that candidates appropriate for endarterectomy are identified early so that screening for stroke risk and appropriate management is initiated. Auscultation of the carotid arteries for bruits is important as the presence of bruits warrants further diagnostic workup. Overall the degree of stenosis does not correlate well with the loudness of the murmur. The most ominous murmur is soft, high pitched, and present throughout the entire cardiac cycle. Murmurs originating from the internal versus the external carotid artery are characterized by their presence in both systole and diastole and their increase in intensity or duration with compression of the superficial temporal, facial or occipital arteries, during which blood is diverted from the external to the internal carotid artery. Screening approaches use different imaging modalities alone or in combination including conventional carotid duplex ultrasound, measurement of ankle-brachial indices, or CT based measurement of coronary artery calcium as measures for generalized atherosclerosis [49], [55].

Decision regarding endarterectomy, stenting or medical treatment including combinations thereof requires judgment and experience to reach a correct prognosis and degree of stenosis whether it is symptomatic or asymptomatic and needs to address the patient's age, gender, co-morbidities, especially concomitant coronary artery disease or contralateral carotid artery disease, degree of stenosis identified by reliable imaging and presence or absence of minor stroke, TIA or leukoariosis and clinical silent stroke present on brain MRI.

Neuroimaging studies for the diagnosis of carotid stenosis

Atherosclerotic occlusive disease of the carotids can be evaluated by the use of carotid duplex sonography, MRA, CTA or angiography. Non-invasive studies play an essential role in the diagnosis. However, all techniques require validation and quality control within individual centers to guarantee high specificity and sensitivity.

Carotid duplex examination for evaluation of the major extracranial arteries is performed by real-time B-mode studies and duplex and color flow imaging and has the ability to detect and characterize atherothrombotic plaque, measure intimal media thickness (IMT) and to determine the degree of vascular stenosis and collateral supply. IMT measurements, electron-beam computed tomography (EBCT,) magnetic resonance coronary angiography and flow-mediated arterial dilation by ultrasound are used to evaluate patients with subclinical atherosclerosis at risk for ischemic events early and to monitor the effectiveness of medical interventions [8], [59].

Carotid duplex studies in combination with TCD provide information on flow dynamics, the presence or absence of collateral circulation and its effectiveness as well as an estimation of the cerebral vascular reserve. Furthermore they help detect emboli which may originate from the heart, the aortic arch, or the carotid itself. In the near future advancement of this technology will allow the analysis of plaque constituents and markers of inflammation in order to assess the risk of an embolic stroke [7]. Current carotid and TCD studies are supplementary to MRA or CTA and are excellent tools when validated against cerebral angiography at the institution where the studies are performed and when used under strict guidelines provided by credentialing bodies and technical quality control. However, ultrasound is operator dependent and can overestimate the degree of carotid stenosis if a contralateral high grade stenosis or occlusion is present [15].

Cerebral angiography is now performed less frequently because it does not give exact assessment of plaque size and morphology which newer MRA and CTA based techniques are capable of producing. Cerebral angiography is associated with a combined mortality and morbidity of 0.5–4% in patients with atherosclerosis so that many medical centers today perform CEA based on MRA, CTA or carotid duplex studies alone. MRA has some limitations due to possible over-estimation of the degree of stenosis and the production of flow artifacts which might result in misclassification of patients. CTA is advantageous because it is not dependent on blood flow velocity providing more precise assessment of high grade stenosis but it requires intravenous contrast which can have serious side effects.

In the near future the development of higher resolution MRI, new contrast materials and biomarkers for detecting chronic inflammatory changes in patients with substantial atherosclerotic disease will improve the assessment of patients at risk for ischemic events [62], [69], [12], [70]. However, at this time the indication for CEA depends on the patient's co-morbidity, life expectancy, gender, symptoms and the degree of carotid stenosis measured by appropriate imaging studies. Precise measurement of the degree of carotid stenosis is essential to decide which patient benefits the most from CEA.

Measurement of stenosis

Several different methods have been used to assess the degree of carotid stenosis using cerebral angiography. The major clinical trials for CEA in symptomatic carotid stenosis, the European Carotid Surgery Trial [26] and the North American Symptomatic Carotid Endarterectomy Trial [5] used different reference points. ECST chose the area of the smallest vessel lumen for measurement, whereas NASCET measured the smallest lumen at the level of stenosis comparing it with the carotid artery lumen distal to the bulb, as previously described by Blaisdell and colleagues [9]. A severe 70–99 % stenosis based on NASCET criteria corresponds to a 85–99% stenosis in ECST and a moderate stenosis of 50–69% in NASCET corresponds to a 75–84% stenosis in ECST. It is surprising that the two differed given that the benefit of surgery correlates directly with the degree of stenosis.

The American Asymptomatic Carotid Artery Study [2] followed the NASCET method, measuring the minimal residual lumen at the side of stenosis (MRL) and the distal lumen (DL) at which the arterial walls became parallel on arteriogram, calculating the degree of stenosis as $100 \times (1-(MRL/DL))$ whereas the European Asymptomatic Carotid Surgery Trial [3] used only B mode carotid ultrasound to estimate the degree of stenosis.

CEA for stroke prevention

Most patients with carotid artery disease are identified after they had a TIA or stroke. Less frequently patients at risk for ischemic stroke from carotid artery disease are identified by screening examinations during which a carotid bruit was noticed and had prompted further investigation. In the United States, more than 130,000 carotid endarterectomies were performed in 1996 with an increase in number in 2000. The proportion of patients operated who have never had symptoms, but who have extracranial carotid disease increased from 16% between 1990 and 1994 to 45% in the years between 1995 and 2000 [11]. Although the proportion of patients who undergo CEA for asymptomatic lesions continues to rise, the controversy continues regarding decision whether these patients should undergo surgery, stenting or should only be medically managed.

At this point this decision of is mainly based on the presence or absence of neurological symptoms. However, in clinical practice this criterion seems somewhat arbitrary as many patients who appear to be asymptomatic clinically have had clinical silent strokes on their imaging study within the watershed regions or the vascular territory of the affected carotid artery [54], [14]. Inapparent ischemic events may be due to the fact that some strokes are localized in areas not causing any clinical symptoms, that TIAs occur while the patient is asleep or that patients do not report their transient symptoms. Symptoms of a TIA are often vague and the diagnosis depends merely on the patient's subjective history. Patients with amaurosis fugax usually seek medical attention immediately, whereas those with more diffuse transient episodes such as sensory symptoms, ataxia, dizziness, or mild difficulties finding words may not seek medical attention. Additionally in patients with a previous history of migraine the differential diagnosis from complicated migraines, simple partial seizures or pre-syncopal events is often impossible.

The amount of clinically silent infarctions is apparently much higher than had been previously anticipated when head CT or brain MRI are used to assess patients with carotid stenosis. Even in clinically asymptomatic patients with high grade carotid stenosis cranial CT has shown that up to 15% of these patients had ischemic strokes and MRI studies have demonstrated that up to 20% had cerebral infarctions in the affected internal carotid territory. A relatively high proportion of patients with silent brain MRI lesions and asymptomatic carotid stenosis have cognitive impairment [47] indicating that asymptomatic carotid disease is not as benign as often presumed. Furthermore, TCD studies have demonstrated that asymptomatic patients frequently have microemboli originating from the carotid arteries when the ipsilateral middle cerebral artery is monitored [45], [67] and that plaque composition is an important predictor for distal embolization [63]. Further imaging studies using high resolution MRI, advanced imaging software for data analysis and improved contrast agents help to determine which patients are at highest risk for cerebral ischemic events.

In the future analysis of plaque morphology and composition will be equally as important as the degree of stenosis.

Symptomatic carotid stenosis

Guidelines are provided by the major medical associations such as American Heart Association, how to manage patients with symptomatic carotid stenosis based on two clinical trials [26], [5]. According to the results of ESCT and NASCET patients should undergo carotid endarterectomy if they have symptomatic stenosis $\geq$ 70 % as measured by the ECST method or $\geq$ 85% measured by the NASCET method, if they have no significant co-morbidities, a high risk for stroke and access to an experienced surgical team with a low complication rate. Higher peri-operative complication rates were observed in both studies in patients with the cerebral ischemic versus retinal ischemic events, in patients presenting with crescendo TIA or stroke in evolution, in patients with symptomatic coronary artery disease and in women. Goal is to reduce the risk of postoperative ipsilateral ischemic stroke by CEA to 1% or less per year.

NASCET demonstrated an absolute risk reduction of 12.5% from CEA for patients with 70–99% stenosis and only a 5% absolute risk reduction for patients with a 50–69% stenosis. Similarly, ECST showed an absolute risk reduction of 11.6% for 70–99% stenosis and only a 4.6% absolute risk reduction for patients with 50–69% stenosis. CEA in patients with occlusion did not result in any significant benefit, but higher surgical risk for major complication or death. Subsequent meta-analysis pooling data from ECST and NASCET [25] and using the degree of stenosis as measured by the Blaisdell method showed an absolute risk reduction of 15.9% over two years, with number needed to treat of six patients to see benefit of CEA, in those with 70–99% stenosis. The absolute risk reduction was 4.6% over five years with number needed to treat of 22 for those patients with 50–69% stenosis. Interestingly, a high degree of absolute risk reduction by CEA was additionally found for contralateral ischemic stroke over five years in patients with a 70–99 % stenosis.

In a sub-analysis of symptomatic men older than 75 years with diabetes mellitus, those with degree of stenosis ≥ 90% without occlusion, those with large ulcerated plaques causing stenosis and those with contralateral carotid occlusion showed a benefit from CEA. Meta-analysis of ECST and NASCET data also indicated that patients with near occlusion showed an absolute risk reduction of 5.6% over two years, but conversely worse outcome with negative risk reduction of −1.7% over five years. However, the number of cases for long-term follow-up was too few to allow a reliable long-term assessment.

Asymptomatic carotid stenosis

Despite several multi-center trials and meta-analyses of data collected in patients with asymptomatic carotid disease, how to best manage these patients continues to be controversial. Data are now available from two large prospective multi-center trials, the Asymptomatic Carotid Atherosclerosis Study (ACAS) and the European Asymptomatic Carotid Surgery Trial (ACST). As previously observed in symptomatic carotid artery disease, the risk for stroke increased in both studies with increasing degree of stenosis from about 1–2% annually in patients with a 50–75% asymptomatic stenosis to 6% per year with a 75–90% stenosis to more than 8% yearly in patients with ≥ 90% stenosis. ACAS enrolled 1,662 patients with 60–99% stenosis with clinical follow-up of 2.7 years as the study was terminated early by the safety monitoring board after significant differences between the surgical and the medical treatment arms had been observed. Therefore data to the planned 5 year duration of the study had to be extrapolated which was later often criticized as weakness of the study. The absolute risk reduction for ipsilateral stroke and perioperative death and stroke in all patients undergoing surgery was 5.9% with number needed to treat of 17 over 2.7 years. The absolute risk reduction for men over five years was 8% with number needed to treat of 12.5, whereas women only had an absolute risk reduction of 1.4% over five years with number needed to treat of 71. A comparable gender difference regarding the potential benefit of CEA was also observed in ACST. The reason for these differences remain obscure and may be related to the smaller vessel caliber in women.

The ACST study enrolled 3,120 patients with carotid artery stenosis of ≥ 60% diagnosed by carotid duplex imaging. 1,284 patients had a carotid stenosis of < 80%. The absolute risk reduction for all types of stroke was 5.4% for patients undergoing CEA with number needed to treat of 19 over a follow-up period of nearly 3.4 years. The stroke risk for those patients was reduced for ipsilateral as well as for contralateral stroke following CEA. The absolute risk reduction for men was 8.2% and 4.1% for women. Patients between 65 to 74 years had a similar rate of absolute risk reduction whereas patients older than 75 years seemed to have a less significant absolute risk reduction of 3.3%. ACST like ACAS, demonstrated that patients with ≥ 60% stenosis measured by the Blaisdell method may benefit from carotid endarterectomy if the perioperative surgical risk is minimal in order to achieve an optimal risk/benefit ratio.

A major critique point of both studies was that ACAS and ACST had much lower than average mortality and morbidity rates for CEA and perioperative complications because only selected surgeons and patients were involved in these studies and that this does not necessarily reflect the perioperative risks observed in a community hospital. In ACAS the operative mortality was low at 0.14% and the risk of stroke and death was only 1.5%. In contrast it has been reported that the risk of stroke and death can be up to three times higher than in ACAS and the operative mortality can be as much as 8% higher than in ACAS in the community setting [5]. Many therefore suggest a watch and wait approach in patients with asymptomatic carotid stenosis of less than 80% and to monitor the effects of optimal medical management by regular assessment of plaque progression by carotid duplex studies every six to twelve months. If atherosclerosis progresses despite best medical therapy and risk factor modification, these patients probably should undergo CEA if the perioperative risk is low.

Coronary artery disease and CEA

Atherosclerosis is a generalized disease affecting not only the carotid arteries but often concomitantly the coronary arteries, the abdominal aorta and the peripheral arteries. This is especially true for the elderly, a population segment which is rapidly growing. Many patients who initially presented for carotid artery stenosis actually have significant morbidity or mortality due to diseases of other vascular beds mandating a more comprehensive evaluation by additional imaging studies. In three months of admission for TIA or cerebral infarction the risk for myocardial infarction and cerebrovascular death is 2 to 5% and about 30% within two years. Asymptomatic coronary artery disease in this population is high with about 20–40% and up to 25–60% of patients with symptomatic and asymptomatic carotid artery stenosis having inducible myocardial ischemia [4].

Asymptomatic patients selected for CEA must undergo a thorough preoperative cardiac evaluation and if significant disease is found, patients should be considered for percutaneous angioplasty and possibly stenting prior to CEA. Whether these patients should undergo carotid stenting, simultaneous CABG and CEA or staged surgeries and which if either procedure should be performed first is controversial [34], [58].

Carotid artery stenting

Indication for carotid stenting remains controversial, until the completion of multi-center trials which compare indications, efficacy and safety with conventional carotid endarterectomy [27], [23] Moreover follow-up studies will be necessary to assess stent durability. In order to accomplish this it is important for interventionalists to monitor efficacy, quality and complication rates locally, nationally and internationally.

Imaging study for choice of the interventional approach

Carotid Duplex, angiography, CTA and MRA help to measure the degree of stenosis and characterize the atheromatous lesion allowing choice of the most appropriate interventional technique. Depending on the composition and morphology of the plaque, the shape of the interior wall, the extent and distribution of atheromatous plaques and the remaining vascular lumen different techniques for CEA including conventional open endarterectomy with or without patching (vein or Dacron patch), selective endarterectomy, inversion endarterectomy or angioplasty followed by stenting are feasible. Atheromatous plaque in the carotid artery bifurcation are often associated with significant ipsilateral stenosis in the siphon. Frequently, the intracranial lesion is surgically inaccessible and might require endovascular intervention. If the intracranial stenosis exceeds the degree of the stenosis in the proximal arterial segment, CEA should be avoided because it does not improve flow through the distal segment.

Timing of surgery

There is still some controversy regarding the timing of carotid surgery following cerebral infarction. Data from NASCET and ECST indicate that within one month hemispheric TIA or ischemic infarction have a high risk of recurrent ischemic events and may therefore benefit from early surgery. Therefore, many authors now suggest that CEA be performed within two weeks following the cerebral ischemic event [60]. In the presence of a large cerebral infarction, however, there is increased risk for hyperperfusion injury and subsequent intracranial hemorrhage due to disturbance of the blood brain barrier and impairment of vascular cerebral autoregulation. In these surgery should be delayed for 4 to 6 weeks [36]. Timing of surgery for patients with stroke in evolution or in those with crescendo TIAs is controversial. A meta-analysis of CEA studies published between 1980 and 2000 shows that the mortality rate and stroke risk is about 20% when stroke in evolution or crescendo TIA undergo immediate endarterectomy [42]. On the other hand postponing CEA may place patients at risk for recurrent cerebrovascular events. Neuroimaging studies such as diffusion and perfusion weighted MRI, acetazolamide SPECT or TCD studies assessing cerebral vascular reactivity may help to identify those patients who would actually benefit from immediate CEA.

Complications of CEA and the role of neuroimaging

Most peri-operative complications are due to carotid embolism or ischemia induced by cross clamping of the artery. Other complications are due to a residual flap at the CEA site, the development of post-operative thrombus and hyperperfusion syndrome, especially in the presence of a large infarction with a dysfunctional blood-brain barrier and impaired cerebral autoregulation. Reperfusion injury causes cerebral edema and/or intracranial hemorrhage and occurs in about 1%. Transcranial color coded ultrasound using echo contrast agents, acetazolamide SPECT, PET or PW/DW weighted MRI or spin labeling perfusion MR can be used to identify early signs of hyperperfusion syndrome following CEA [43], [1], [33] possibly allowing early intervention such as strict blood pressure control, seizure prophylaxis and temporary discontinuation of antithrombotic therapy which is now routinely initiated immediately following the intervention.

Restenosis

Despite complete plaque removal, restenosis occurs in up to 8% of patients of which about 3% of patients become symptomatic requiring a second intervention. Based on biopsy studies, recurrent arterial lesions were shown to be often due to intimal smooth muscle cell proliferation and not progression of atherothrombic plaque. Restenosis usually occurs within the first three to six months and is usually due to intimal hyperplasia which can sometimes regress spontaneously. Histologically, smooth muscle cells and fibroblasts proliferate and start to deposit collagen rich matrix tissue into the arterial wall. This results in stenosis covered with a smooth surface which typically does not lead to disturbed laminar flow as occurs with irregular atherosclerotic plaque,

and the potential for embolic events is therefore relatively low. Late restenosis occurs after two years and these lesions have a higher thromboembolic potential. Reported rates for restenosis were 10% after two years and 17% after 10 years following CEA. [31]. Women were shown to have a greater risk which is possibly due to smaller vessel caliber size and/or the different hormonal environment. It has been therefore recommended that all women should undergo patch angioplasty which can significantly reduce the risk for restenosis in follow-up studies [31], [52].

Classic risk factors for atherosclerosis should be closely monitored and modified to diminish the risk of recurrent stenosis. Imaging plays an essential role for detecting restenosis and especially relatively inexpensive and non-invasive imaging tools such as ultrasound should be routinely used for monitoring of CEA patients.

Perioperative ultrasound imaging

Over 2,000,000 CEAs have been performed worldwide since 1954. Intraoperative monitoring using carotid duplex and TCD studies are now more frequently performed at many medical centers to minimize the risk of poor surgical outcome. Real time B-mode imaging performed intraoperatively to evaluate the CEA site can detect residual flaps, suture line stricture, plaque residuals or plaque dislodgement as potential source for thrombotic vessel occlusion or distal embolization. Doppler spectrum analysis allows early detection of turbulent flow and restenosis. In a pilot study performed by Gaunt et al. [35] the perioperative stroke risk could be lowered from 4% to 1% using intraoperative TCD monitoring and angioscopy. TCD can detect embolization occurring during the dissection phase of an unstable plaque allowing the surgeon to modify the procedural technique and can help in the decision if and when to use a shunt. TCD monitoring also allows constant volume flow measurements to maintain perfusion rates at 15 cm per second which is thought to be the approximate threshold to prevent loss of neuronal electrical function. TCD monitoring allows assessment of intraoperative shunt function and identification of thrombus formation. Following endarterectomy TCD can be used to assess the intracranial collateral flow and velocities.

Further post-surgical carotid duplex studies, in our opinion, should be performed after two to six weeks following endarterectomy to evaluate the CEA site and to differentiate between recurrent and residual stenosis. Long-term neuro-ultrasound studies should then be performed every six months for one year and then annually for follow-up for the development of restenosis. The role of the IMT measurement to detect restenosis early is being currently investigated. If restenosis develops, endovascular angioplasty and stenting are the usually preferred interventions to avoid complications from secondary CEA such as permanent cranial nerve palsies, vascular damage or complications associated with wound healing.

Carotid occlusion

Patients with occlusion are managed differently than patients with high-grade stenosis as they do not benefit from CEA. Neuroimaging plays a central role to identify these patients. Carotid duplex is an excellent method to identify patients with carotid stenosis; however it is limited in the presence of a string sign as it cannot differentiate between severe stenosis and carotid occlusion. MRA is limited in this situation as time of flight imaging is flow velocity dependent, thus leading to overestimation of the degree of stenosis. MRA can show a flow void suggesting total carotid occlusion when in fact vascular flow is diminished. CTA might overcome these difficulties, but the gold standard remains cerebral angiography which also allows assessment of collateral flow.

The procedural risk from CEA for occlusion is especially high in patients with occlusion on one side and high grade stenosis in the other side. In unilateral occlusion occurring within one week, flow can be reestablished in less than 20% of cases. The risk is especially great in patients with large cerebral infarction where mortality rates up to 50% have been reported [32]. Patients with internal carotid artery occlusion might be candidates for EC/IC bypass which is currently under investigation [37]. To identify patients who might benefit tests for cerebral vascular perfusion reserve are performed using PET, TCD with hyperventilation, acetazolamide administration or CO_2 inhalation or acetazolamide-SPECT studies can also help identify patients with impaired cerebral vascular perfusion reserve due to insufficient collateral flow and impaired autoregulation who may benefit from a bypass.

Neuroimaging also plays an essential role for identifying patients with multiple vascular lesions. Patients frequently have multiple vascular lesions within vascular territories leading to more difficult decision making. Patients with bilateral carotid stenosis have a higher risk of mortality and morbidity because it increases with the number of surgeries necessary. In patient with bilateral carotid stenosis it is generally recommended to perform a carotid endarterectomy only on the symptomatic side and to closely monitor the patient for disease progression of the other with serial carotid duplex studies and long-term follow-up. If both carotid arteries have a high grade stenosis, usually the side with the greater stenosis is reconstructed first, followed by the other in four to six weeks. Simultaneous surgery of both carotid arteries should be avoided due to the increased risk of mortality and morbidity and higher complication rates due to tissue swelling or potential bilateral recurrent laryngeal nerve palsy causing airway obstruction.

Conclusion

Neuroimaging plays an essential role in identifying patients with significant carotid stenosis early and to select those who will benefit most from surgery. Patients with symptomatic carotid stenosis ≥ 70% by ESCT or ≥ 80% by NASCET criteria should undergo CEA in the absence of significant comorbidities, if they are at high risk for stroke and have access to an experienced surgical team with low complication rates. Patients with asymptomatic stenosis with a hemodynamic significant stenosis of

≥ 60% who are otherwise at a high risk for stroke should be considered for carotid endarterectomy, if the surgical and perioperative mortality and morbidity can be kept low at less than 3%. In the future endovascular stents may replace carotid endarterectomy or may be an important "add-on modality" to carotid endarterectomy. However, currently trial data and long-term follow-up data are missing to assess if carotid stenting results in comparable long-term outcomes for stroke prevention. Currently endovascular approaches are favored for recurrent stenosis, carotid stenosis associated with radiation injury or in patients with high operative risk from multiple co-morbidities especially in the elderly population.

Intraoperative and postsurgical monitoring with ultrasound in patients undergoing stenting or CEA is crucial to prevent complications and to identify those who develop restenosis. In the future, new neuroimaging approaches combined with the development of new biomarkers of active inflammatory atherosclerotic disease will become available. IMT measurements with carotid duplex ultrasound as well as CT measurement of coronary artery calcium among other approaches will help to identify those patients at high risk for stroke. Evaluation of patients presenting with carotid bruit by ultrasound studies remains important. Advances of nuclear imaging, the development of new contrast materials and new MRI and CT based imaging sequences and software applications will be used to identify patients with unstable plaques. These methods will allow us to detect rapidly advancing atherosclerosis and will be essential to select who should undergo CEA or stenting based on plaque characterization and molecular imaging of vessel wall metabolism. These new advances may hopefully allow a paradigm shift from surgical and endovascular interventions following a oftentimes devastating ischemic cerebral event to early screening and medical treatment for primary stroke prevention.

References

[1] Ances BM, McGarvey JL, Abrahams JM et al.: Continuous arterial spin labeled perfusion magnetic resonance imaging in patients before and after carotid endarterectomy. J Neuroimaging 14: 133–138 (2004).

[2] Asymptomatic Carotid Atheroslcerosis Study Group (ACAS): Study design for randomized prospective trial of carotid endarterectomy for asymptomatic atherosclerosis. Stroke 20: 844–849 (1989).

[3] Asymptomatic Carotid Surgery Trial (ACST) Collaborative Group: Prevention of disabling and fatal strokes by successful carotid endarterectomy in patients without recent neurological symptoms: randomized controlled trial. Lancet 163: 1491–1502 (2004).

[4] Adams GJ, Greene J, Vick III GW et al.: Tracking regression and progression of atherosclerosis in human carotid arteries using high-resolution magnetic resonance imaging. Magn Reson Imag 22: 1249–1258 (2004).

[5] Alamowitch S, Eliasziw M, Algra A, Meldrum H, Barnett HJM: for the North American Symptomatic Carotid Endarterectomy Trial (NASCET) group (2001) Risk, causes and prevention of ischaemic stroke in elderly patients with symptomatic internal-carotid-artery stenosis. Lancet 357: 1154–1160 (2001).

[6] Baillie M: The Morbid Anatomy of Some of the Most Important Parts of the Human Body. London: J. Johnson and G. Nicol (1793).

[7] Bhatia V, Bhatia R, Dhindsa S, Virk A: Vulnerable plawues, inflammation and newer imaging modalities. J Postgrad Med 49: 361–368 (2003).

[8] Bisoendial RJ, Hovingh GK, de Groot E, Kastelein JJP, Lansberg PJ, Stroes ESG: Measurement of subclinical atherosclerosis: beyond risk factor assessment. Curr Opin Lipidol 13: 595–603 (2002).

[9] Blaisdell FW, Hall AD, Thomas AN et al.: Cerebrovascular occlusive disease: Experience with panarteriography in 300 consecutive cases. Calif Med 103: 321–329 (1965).

[10] Blue SK, McKinney WM, Barnes R et al.: Ultrasonic B-mode scanning for study of extracranial vascular disease. Neurology 22: 1079–1085 (1972).

[11] Bond R, Rerkasem K, Rothwell PM: Systematic review of the risks of carotid endarterectomy in relation to the clinical indication for and timing of surgery. Stroke 34: 2290–2301 (2003).

[12] Boyle JJ: Macrophage activation in atherosclerosis: pathogenesis and pharmacology of plaque rupture. Curr Vasc Pharmacol 3: 63–68 (2005).

[13] Broderick J, Brott T, Kothari R et al.: The Greater Cincinnati/Northern Kentucky Stroke Study: preliminary first-ever and total incidence rates of stroke among blacks. Stroke 29: 415–421 (1998).

[14] Brott T, Tomsick T, Feinberg W et al.: Baseline silent cerebral infarction in the Asymptomatic Carotid Atherosclerosis Study. Stroke 25: 1122–1129 (1994).

[15] Busuttsil SJ, Franklin DP, Youkey JR et al.: Carotid duplex overestimation of stenosis due to severe contralateral disease. Am J Surg 172: 144–147 (1996).

[16] Cappendijk VC, Cleutjens KBJM, Kessels AGH et al.: Assessment of human atherosclerotic carotid plaque components with multisequence MR imaging: Initial experience. Radiology 234: 487–492 (2005).

[17] Carrea R, Molins M, Murphy G: Surgery of spontaneous thrombosis of the internal carotid in the neck: carotido-carotid anastomosis. Case report and analysis of the literature on surgical cases. Medicina (B Aires) 1: 20–29 (1955).

[18] Chiari H: Über das Verhälten des Teilungswinkels der Carotis communis bei der Endasteritis chronic deformans. Verh Deutsch Path Ges 9: 326 (1905).

[19] Cormack AM: Representation of a function by its line integrals, with some radiological applications. J Appl Phys 34: 2722 (1963).

[20] Corot C, Petry KG, Trivedi R et al.: Macophage imaging in central nervous system and in carotid atherosclerotic plaque using ultrasmall superparamagnetic iron oxide in magnetic resonance imaging. Invest Radiol 39: 619–625 (2004).

[21] DeBakey ME: Successful carotid endarterectomy for cerebrovascular insufficiency. Nineteen-year follow-up. JAMA 233: 1083–1085 (1975).

[22] Denzel C, Balzer K, Muller KM, Lell M, Lang W: Imaging techniques for showing the morphology and surface structure of extracranial internal carotid artery plaques. Dtsch Med Wochenschr 130: 1267–1272 (2005).

[23] Douglas JS, Weintraub WS, Holms D: Rationale and design of the randomized, multicenter, cilostazol for RESTenosis (CREST) trial. Clin Cardiol 26: 451–454 (2003).

[24] Eastcott HHG, Pickering GW, Robb CG: Reconstruction of internal carotid artery in a patient with intermittent attacks of hemiplegia. Lancet 2: 994–996 (1954).

[25] Eckstein HH, Schumacher H, Dorfler A et al.: Carotid endarterectomy and intracranial thrombolysis: simultaneous and staged procedures in ischemic Stroke J Vasc Surg 29: 459–471 (1999).

[26] European Carotid Surgery Trialist's Collaborative Group (ESCT): MRC European Carotid Surgery Trial: interim results for symptomatic patients with severe (70–99%) or with mild (0–29%) carotid stenosis. Lancet 337: 1235–1243 (1991).

[27] EVA-3S Investigators: Carotid angioplasty and stenting with and without cerebral protection. Clinical alert from the endarterectomy versus angioplasty in patients with symptomatic severe carotid stenosis (EVA-3S) trial. Stroke 35: e18–e21 (2004).

[28] Fisher M, Paganini-Hill A, Martin A et al.: Carotid plaque pathology. Thrombosis, Ulceration, and Stroke Pathogenesis. Stroke 36: 253–257 (2005).

[29] Fisher CM: Occlusion of the carotid arteries. Further experiences. Arch Neuro Psych 72: 187–204 (1954).

[30] Fisher CM, Adams RD: Observations on brain embolism. J Neuropath Exper Neurol 10: 92–94 (1951).

[31] Frericks H, Kievit J, Vaalen JM: Carotid recurrent stenosis and risk of ipsilateralstroke: A systematic review of the literature. Stroke 29: 244–250 (1998).

[32] Friedman SG, Riles TS, Lamparello PJ, Imparato AM, Sakwa MP: Surgical therapy for the patient with internal carotid artery occlusion and contralateral stenosis. J Vasc Surg. 6: 856–861 (1987).

[33] Fujimoto S, Toyoda K, Inoue T et al.: Diagnostic impact of transcranial color-coded real-time sonography with echo contrast agents for hyperperfusion syndrome and carotid endarterectomy. Stroke 35: 1852–1856 (2004).

[34] Gasparis AP, Ricotta L, Cuadra SA et al.: High risk carotid endarterectomy: fact or fiction. J Vasc Surg 37: 40–46 (2003).

[35] Gaunt ME, Smith JL, Ratliff DA, Bell RP, Naylor AR: A comparison of quality control methods applied to carotid endarterectomy. Eur J Vasc Endovasc Surg 11: 34–11 (1996).

[36] Giordano JM, Trout HH 3rd, Kozloff L, DePalma RG: Timing of carotid artery endarterectomy after Stroke J Vasc Surg 2: 250–255 (1985).

[37] Grubb RL Jr, Powers WJ, Derdeyn CP, Adams HP Jr, Clarke WR: The carotid occlusion surgery study. Neurosurg Focus 15: e9 (2003).

[38] Hass WK, Fields WS, North RR et al.: Joint study of extracranial arterial occlusion: II. Arteriography, techniques, sites, and complications. JAMA 203: 961–968 (1968).

[39] Herz CH: Ultrasonic engineering in heart diagnosis. Am J Cardiol 19: 6–17 (1967).

[40] Hounsfield GN: A method of and apparatus for examination of a body by radiation such as X-ray or gamma radiation. Patent Specification 1283915 (1972).

[41] Hunt JR: The role of the carotid arteries in the causation of vascular lesions of the brain, with remarks on certain special features of the symptomatology. Amer J Med Sci 147: 704 (1914).

[42] Inzitari D, Eliasziw M, Gates P et al.: The causes and risk of stroke in patients with asymptomatic internal-carotid-artery stenosis. North American Symptomatic Carotid Endarterectomy Trial Collaborators. N Engl J Med 342: 1693–1700 (2000).

[43] Karapanayiotides T, Meuli R, Devuyst G et al.: Postcarotid endartectomy hyperfusion or reperfusion syndrome. Stroke 36: 21.26 (2005).

[44] Lauterbur PC: Image formation by induced local interactions–examples employing nuclear magnetic-resonance. Nature 242(5234): 190–191.

[45] Mackinnon AD, Aaslid R, Markus HS: Ambulatory transcranial Doppler cerebral embolic signal detection

in symptomatic and asymptomatic carotid stenosis. Stroke 36: 1726–1730 (2005).
[46] Mansfield P: Multi-planar image-formation using NMR spin echoes. J Phys C Solid State Phys 10: L55–L58 (1977).
[47] Mathiesen EB, Waterloo K, Joakimsen O et al.: Reduced neuropsychological test performance in asymptomatic carotid stenosis: The Tromso Study. Neurology 62: 695–701 (2004).
[48] Matsumoto N, Whisnant JP, Kurland LT et al.: Natural history of stroke in Rochester, Minnesota, 1955 through 1969: An extension of a previous study, 1945 through 1954. Stroke 4: 20–29 (1973).
[49] McDermott MM, Liu K, Criqui MH et al.: Ankle-brachial index and subclinical cardiac and carotid disease: the multi-ethnic study of atherosclerosis. Am J Epidemiol 162: 33–41 (1005).
[50] Miyazaki M, Kato K: Measurement of cerebral blood flow by ultrasonic Doppler technique. Hemodynamic comparisons of right and left arotid arteries in patients with hemiplegia. Jap Circ J 29: 383 (1965).
[51] Moniz E: Diagnostic des tumeurs cérébrales et épreuve de encephalographie artérielle. Paris: Masson et Cie, (1931).
[52] Moore WS, Mohr JP, Najafi H, Robertson JT, Stoney RJ, Toole JF: Carotid endarterectomy: practice guidelines. Report of the Ad Hoc Committee to the Joint council of the Society for Vascular surgery and the North American Chapter of the International Society for Cardiovascular Surgery. J Vasc Surg 15: 469–479 (1992).
[53] Moore WS, Boren C, Malone JM et al.: Natural history of nonstenotic, asymptomatic ulcerative lesions of the carotid artery.
[54] Norris JW, Zhu CZ: Silent stroke and carotid stenosis. Stroke 23: 483–485 (1992).
[55] Ohnesorge BM, Hofmann LK, Flohr TG, Schoepf UJ: CT for imaging coronary artery disease: defining the paradigm for its application. Int J Cardiovasc Imaging 21: 85–104 (2005).
[56] Olinger C: Ultrasonic carotid echoarteriography AJR 106: 282–295 (1969).
[57] Reid JM, Spencer MP: Ultrasonic Doppler techniques for imaging blood vessels. Science 176: 1235–1236 (1972).
[58] Ricotta JJ, DeWeese JA: Is routine carotid ultrasound surveillance after carotid endarterectomy worthwhile? Am J Surg 172: 140–143 (1996).
[59] Riley WA, Evans GW, Sharrett AR, Burke GL, Barnes RW: Variation of common carotid artery elasticity with intimal-medial thickness: the ARIC Study. Atherosclerosis Risk in Communities. Ultrasound Med Biol 23: 157–164 (1997).
[60] Rothwell PM, Eliasziw M, Gutnikov SA et al.: for the Carotid Endarterectomy Trialists Collaboration. Endarterectomy for symptomatic carotid stenosis in relation to clinical subgroups and timing of surgery. Lancet 363: 915–924 (2004).
[61] Russo LS Jr: Carotid system transient ischemic attacks: clinical, racial, and angiographic correlations. Stroke 12: 470–473 (1981).
[62] Rutt BK, Clarke SE, Fayad ZA: Atherosclerotic plaque characterization by MR imaging. Curr Drug Targets Cardiovasc Haematol Disord 4: 147–159 (2004).
[63] Sabetai MM, Tegos TJ, Clifford C et al.: Carotid plaque echogenicity and types of silent CT-brain infarcts. Is there an association in patients with asymptomatic carotid stenosis? Int Angiol 20: 51–57 (2001).
[64] Sacco RL, Shi T, Zamanillo MC et al.: Predictors of mortality and recurrence after hospitalized cerebral infarction in an urban community: The Northern Manhattan Stroke Study. Neurology 44: 626–34 (1994)
[65] Sacco RL, Wolf PA, Kannel WB et al.: Survival and recurrence following Stroke The Framingham study. Stroke 13: 290–295 (1982)
[66] Schoen FJ: Blood Vessels. In: Kumar, Robbins, Cotran (eds). Pathologic Basis of Disease. 7th ed. Amsterdam: Elsevier 2005. p 512
[67] Siebler M, Kleinschmidt A, Sitzer M et al.: Cerebral microembolism in symptomatic and asymptomatic high-grade internal carotid artery stenosis. Neurology 44: 615–618 (1994)
[68] Strully KJ, Hurwitt ES, Blankenberg HW: Thrombo-endarterectomy for thrombosis of the internal carotid artery in the neck. J Neurosurg 10: 474–482 (1953)
[69] Trivedi RA, U-King-Im J-M, Graves MJ et al.: MRI-derived measurements of fibrous-cap and lipid-core thickness: the potential for identifying vulnerable carotid plaques in vivo. Neuroradiology 46: 738–743 (2004)
[70] Vemuganti R, Dempsey RJ: Carotid atherosclerotic plaques from symptomatic stroke patients share the molecular fingerprints to develop in a neoplastic fashion: a microarray analysis study. Neuroscience 131: 359–374 (2005)
[71] Wepfer, JJ: Observationes anatomicae, ex cadaveribus eorum, quos sustulit apoplexia, cum exercitatione de ejus loco affecto. Schaffhausen, Joh. Caspari Suteri. (1658)
[72] Whisnant JP, Fitzgibbons JP, Kurland LT et al.: Natural history of stroke in Rochester, Minnesota, 1945 through 1954. Stroke 2: 11–22 (1971)
[73] Willis T: Pathologiae cerebri et nervosa generic specimen. Cited by Schoenberg BS, Mellinger JF, Schoenberg DG. Cerebrovascular disease in infants and children: a study of incidence, clinical features, and survival. Neurology 28: 763–768 (1978)
[74] Zarins CK, Giddens DP, Bharadvaj BK et al.: Carotid bifurcation atherosclerosis. Quantitative correlation of plaque localization with flow velocity profiles and wall shear stress. Circ Res 53: 502–514 (1983).

Additional articles reviewed but not cited in text

Allen BT, Anderson CB, Rubin BG et al.: The influence of anesthetic technique on preoperative complications after carotid endarterectomy. J Vasc Surg 19: 834–843 (1994).

Baker WH, Howard VJ, Howard G et al.: Effect of contralateral occlusion on long-term efficacy of endarterectomy in the Asymptomatic Carotid Atherosclerosis Study (ACAS). Stroke 31: 2330–2334 (2000).

Barnett HJM, Taylor DW, Eliasziw M et al.: for the North American Symptomatic Carotid Endarterectomy Trial Collaborators. Benefit of carotid endarterectomy in patients with symptomatic moderate or severe stenosis. N Engl J Med 339: 1415–1425 (1998).

Blakeley DD, Oddone EZ, Hasselblad V et al.: Noninvasive carotid artery testing. A meta-analytic review. Ann Intern Med 122: 360–367 (1995).

Blaser T, Hofmann K, Buerger T et al.: Risk of stroke, transient ischemic attack, and vessel occlusion before endarterectomy in patients with symptomatic severe carotid stenosis. Stroke 33: 1057–1062 (2002).

Bond R et al.: High morbidity and mortality due to endarterectomy. Cerebrovasc Dis 16: 1–125 (2003).

Brown MM, Hacke W: Carotid artery stenting: the need for randomised trials. Cerebrovasc Dis 18: 57–61 (2004).

Caplan LR, Skillman J, Ojemann R et al.: Intracerebral hemorrhage following carotid endarterectomy: a hypertensive complication? Stroke 9: 457–460 (1978).

CASANOVA Study Group: Carotid surgery versus medical therapy in asymptomatic carotid stenosis. Stroke 22: 1229–1235 (1991).

CASANOVA Study Group: Carotid surgery versus medical therapy in asymptomatic carotid stenosis. J Neurol 237: 129–161 (1990).

Dosick SM, Whalen RC, Gale SS, Brown OW: Carotid endarterectomy in the stroke patient: computerized axial tomography to determine timing J Vasc Surg 2: 214–219 (1985).

Elgersma OE, Wust AF, Buijs PC et al.: Multidirectional depiction of internal carotid arterial stenosis: three-dimensional time-of-flight MR angiography versus rotational and conventional digital subtraction angiography. Radiology 216: 511–516 (2000).

European Carotid Surgery Trialist's Collaborative Group. Endarterectomy for moderate symptomatic carotid stenosis: interim results from the MRC European Carotid Surgery Trial. Lancet 347: 1591–1593 (1996)

Endarterectomy for asymptomatic carotid artery stenosis. Executive Committee for the Asymptomatic Carotid Atherosclerosis Study JAMA 273: 1421–1428 (1995).

European Carotid Surgery Trialist's Collaborative Group (ESCT): Randomized trial of endarterectomy7 for recently symptomatic carotid stenosis: Final results of the MRC European Carotid Surgery Trial (ECST). Lancet 351: 1379–1387 (1998).

Eckstein H-H, Heider P, Wolf O et al.: Kontroversen in der Behandlung von Karotisstenosen. Studienstand und evidence-based medicine. Der Chirug 7: 672–680 (2004).

Finlay JM, Tucker WS, Ferguson GG et al.: Guidelines for the use of carotid ndarterectomy: Current recommendations from the Canadian Neurosurgical Society. Can Med Assoc J 157: 653–659 (1997).

Fiorani P, Sbarigia E, Speziale F et al.: General anesthesia versus cervical block and perioperative complications in carotid artery surgery. Eur J Vasc Endovasc Surg. 13: 37–42 (1997).

Fisher CM, Adams RD: Observations on brain embolism. J Neuropath & Exper Neurol 10: 92–94 (1951).

Fleck JD, Biller J: Carotid endarterectomy for symptomatic and asymptomatic carotid stenosis: In Gorelick PB, Alter M. (eds) The Prevention of Stroke. New York: Panthenon pp 223–232 (2002).

Fisher CM Clinical picture of cerebral arteriosclerosis. Minn Med. 38: 839–851 (1955).

Garcia JH, Khang-Loon H: Carotid atherosclerosis. Definition, pathogenesis, and clinical significance. Neuroimaging Clin N Am. 6: 801–810 (1996).

Gassecki AP, Ferguson GG, Eliasziw M et al.: Early endarterectomy for severe carotid artery stenosis after a non-disabling stroke: Results from the North American Symptomatic Carotid Endarterectomy Trial. J Vasc Surg 20: 288–295 (1994).

Halm EA, Chassin MR, Tuhrim S et al.: Revisiting the appropriateness of carotid endarterectomy. Stroke 34: 1464–1471 (2003).

Hankey GJ, Warlow CP, Molyneux AJ: Complications of cerebral angiography for patients with mild carotid territory ischaemia being considered for carotid endarterectomy. J Neurol Neurosurg Psychiatry 53: 542–548 (1990).

EBG: Zusatze zu Benj Bell's Abhandlung von den Geschwuren und deren Behandlung. Germany. 1793

RW 2nd. Carotid artery stenting. Surg Clin North Am. 84: 1281–1294 (2004)

Howard G, Howard VJ: Stroke incidence, mortality, and prevalence. In: Gorelick PB, Alter M (eds) The Prevention of Stroke. New York: Panthenon Publishing. pp 1–11 (2002).

Johnston DC, Goldstein LB: Clinical carotid endarterectomy decision making: Noninvasive vascular imaging versus angiography. Neurology 56: 1009–1015 (2001).

Johnson SC, Fayad PB, Gorelick PB et al.: Prevalence and knowledge of transient ischemic attacks among US adults. Neurology 60: 1429–1434 (2003).

Kallmes DF, Omary RA, Dix JE, Evans AJ, Hillman BJ: Specificity of MR angiography as a confirmatory test of carotid artery stenosis. AJNR Am J Neuroradiol 17: 1501–1506 (1996).

Khanna HL, Garg AG: Seven hundred seventy-four carotid [774] endarterectomies for strokes and transient ischaemic attacks: comparison of results of early vs. late surgery. Acta Neurochir Suppl (Wien) 42: 103–106 (1988).

Krishnamurthy S, Tong D, McNamara KP, Steinberg GK, Cockroft KM. Early carotid endarterectomy after ischemic stroke improves diffusion/perfusion mismatch on magnetic resonance imaging: report of two cases. Neurosurgery 52: 238–242 (2003).

Levi CR, O'Malley HM, Fell G et al.: Transcranial Doppler detected cerebral microembolism following carotid endarterectomy: High microembolic signal loads predict postoperative cerebral ischaemia. Brain 120: 621–629 (1997).

Marcus HS, Thomson ND, Brown MM: Asymptomatic cerebral embolic signals in symptomatic and asymptomatic carotid artery disease. Brain 118: 1005–1011 (1995).

Maroulis J, Karkanevatos A, Papakostas K et al.: Cranial nerve dysfunction following carotid endarterectomy. Int Angiol 19: 237–241 (2000).

Mattos MA Summer DS, Bohannon WT et al.: Carotid endarterectomy in women: challenging the results from ACAS and NASET. Ann Surg 234: 438–446 (2001).

Mayberg MR, Winn HR: Endarterectomy for asymptomatic carotid artery stenosis. Resolving the controversy. JAMA 273: 1459–1461 (1995).

McPherson CM, Woo D. Cohen PL et al.: Early carotid endarterectomy for critical carotid artery stenosis after thrombolysis therapy in acute ischemic stroke in the middle cerebral artery. Stroke 32: 2075–2080 (2001).

Mohr JP, Caplan LR, Melski JW et al.: The Harvard Cooperative Stroke Registry: a prospective registry. Neurology 28: 754–762 (1978).

Nederkoorn PJ, vab der Graaf Y, Hunink MG: Duplex ultrasound and magnetic resonance angiography compared with digital subtraction angiography in carotid artery stenosis: A systemic review. Stroke 34: 1324–1332 (2003).

Pan XM, Saloner D, Reilly LM et al.: Assessment of carotid artery stenosis by ultrasonography, conventional angiography, and magnetic resonance angiography: correlation with in vivo measurement of plaque stenosis. J Vasc Surg 21: 82–89 (1995).

Rautenberg W, Mess W, Hennerici M: Prognosis of asymptomatic carotid occlusion. J Neurol Sci 98: 213–220 (1990).

Ringleb PA, Kunze A, Allenberg JR. et al.: The Stent-Supported Percuatneous Angioplasty of the Carotid Artery vs. Endarterectomy Trial. Cerebrovasc Dis 18: 66–68 (2004).

Rothwell PM, Gutnikov SA, Warlow CP: European Carotid Surgery Trialist's Collaboration. Reanalysis of the final results of the European Carotid Surgery Trial. Stroke 34: 514–523 (2003).

Rothwell PM: Analysis of agreement between measurements of continuous variables: general principles and lessons from studies of imaging of carotid stenosis. J Neurol 247: 825–834 (2000).

Russo LS Jr: Carotid system transient ischemic attacks: clinical, racial, and angiographic correlations. Stroke 12: 470–473 (1981).

Sacco RL Shi T, Zamanillo MC, Kargman DE: Predictors of mortality and recurrence after hospitalized cerebral infarction in an urban community: the Northern Manhattan Stroke Study. Neurology 44: 626–634 (1994).

Sacco RL: Risk factors, outcomes, and stroke subtypes for ischemic stroke. Neurology 49: S39–S44 (1997).

Shelton JE, Gaines KJ. Patients' attitudes towards TIA. Va Med Q 122: 24–28 (1995).

Tan KT, Blann AD: To stroke or not to stroke. Is ICAM-1 or CRP the answer? [Editorial]. Neurology. 60: 1884–1885 (2003).

Toole JF, Chambless LE, Heiss G et al.: Prevalence of stroke and and transient ischemia attacks in the Atherosclerosis Risk in Communities (ARIC) Study. Ann Epidemiol 3: 500–503 (1993).

Toole JF: Transient ischemic attack: awareness and prevalence in the community. Health Rep 6: 121–125 (1994).

Toole JF: Medical and surgical management of carotid stenosis. In: Toole JF, ed. Cerebrovascular Disorders. 5thEd. Philadelphia: Lippincott Williams & Wilkins 40–59 (1998).

Tu JV, Hannan EL, Anderson GM et al.: The fall and rise of carotid endarterectomy in the United States and Canada. N Engl J Med 339: 1441–1447 (1998).

van Zuilen EV, Moll FL, Vermeulen FE et al.: Detection of cerebral microemboli by means of transcranial Doppler monitoring before and alter carotid endarterectomy. Stroke 26: 210–213 (1995).

Vitek JJ, Roubin GS, Al-Mubarek N et al.: Carotid artery stenting: technical considerations. AJNR Am J Neuroradiol 21: 1736–1743 (2000).

Wardlaw C. Endarterectomy for asymptomatic carotid stenosis? Lancet 345: 1254–1255 (1995).

Wardlaw JM, Lewis SC, Humphrey P et al.: How does the degree of stenosis affect the accuracy and interobserver variability of magnetic resonance angiography? J Neurol Neurosurg Psychiatry 71: 155–160 (2001).

Waxman SG, Toole JF: Temporal profile resembling TIA in the setting of cerebral infarction. Stroke 14: 433–437 (1983).

Westwood ME, Kelly S, Berry E et al.: Use of magnetic resonance angiography to select candidates with recently symptomatic carotid stenosis for surgery: systematic review. Br Med J 324: 198–202 (2002).

Wiebers DO, Whisnant JP: In: Warlow C, Morris PJ (eds): Transient Ischemic Attacks. New York: Marcel Dekker, p 8 (1982).

THERAPY AND CAROTID ARTERY IMAGING

Chapter 4.1

IMAGING OF EXTRACRANIAL TO INTRACRANIAL BYPASS

H. J. N. Streefkerk, C. A. F. Tulleken, J. Hendrikse, and C. J. M. Klijn

University Departments of Neurology (CJMK), Neurosurgery (HJNS, CAFT), and Radiology (JH), University Medical Center Utrecht and the Rudolf Magnus Institute of Neuroscience, Utrecht, The Netherlands. H. J. N. Streefkerk is currently at the Department of Otorhinolaryngology, St Radboud University Medical Center Nijmegen, The Netherlands

Introduction

Extracranial to intracranial (EC-IC) bypass surgery can be applied to achieve revascularization of the brain in patients in whom the normal pathway of blood flow to the brain is obstructed. Patients who may benefit from revascularization can be divided into two main groups. The first group consists of patients with a giant aneurysm of one of the cerebral arteries, which can not be clipped or coiled and for whom temporary or permanent occlusion of the artery is the only treatment option. The second group comprises patients with recurrent transient ischaemic attacks (TIAs) and stroke associated with occlusion of the internal carotid artery (ICA) at high risk of recurrent ischaemic stroke. The treatment with EC-IC bypass is based on the notion that in some patients with ICA occlusion ischaemic stroke is caused by failure of blood flow towards the brain rather than by embolism [36]. In such "haemodynamically compromised" patients augmentation of blood flow towards the symptomatic hemisphere by means of an EC-IC bypass might theoretically be beneficial.

In this chapter we will concentrate on imaging of the EC-IC bypass in patients with symptomatic ICA occlusion. First, clinical aspects will be discussed. Subsequently, imaging of the EC-IC bypass will be addressed. This will include imaging of the EC-IC bypass with respect to patency and measurements of flow through the bypass, imaging of the effect of the EC-IC bypass on the flow state of the brain, and imaging of the flow territory of the EC-IC bypass. Finally, we will discuss future perspectives.

Clinical aspects of symptomatic ICA occlusion

In patients with occlusion of the ICA symptoms may vary widely in frequency, severity, and duration. Symptoms may involve the eye or the brain. Also the risk of recurrent stroke in patients with symptomatic ICA occlusion may vary widely. A meta-analysis of 44 studies, comprising 3457 patients (including 2902 patients with extracranial ICA occlusion, 224 with intracranial ICA stenosis or occlusion, 293 with middle cerebral artery (MCA) stenosis or occlusion patients and 38 patients in whom the location of the lesion was unknown) showed that the average risk of recurrent stroke is 5.5% (95% confidence interval (CI), 5.1 to 6.0%) with a very large range of 0 to 27% [35]. The annual risk of recurrent ipsilateral stroke was 3.6% (95% CI, 3.1 to 4.2) and the annual risk of vascular death 4.0% (95% CI, 3.5 to 4.5).

Patients who have had only retinal symptoms but no symptoms of cerebral ischaemia are at relatively low risk of stroke. In two separate studies, none of such patients had an ischaemic stroke during a follow up period of more than two years [16], [40]. In these patients collateral pathways are probably sufficient to sustain the blood flow to the brain. Furthermore, patients who only have suffered symptoms of cerebral ischaemia before the occlusion of the ICA was found, have a relatively low risk of ischaemic stroke in comparison with patients who continue to have TIAs in the presence of a documented ICA occlusion [40]. In such patients natural collateral pathways probably can maintain sufficient cerebral blood flow.

If symptoms continue also after the ICA occlusion has been documented and despite antiplatelet therapy, certain so-called haemodynamic features of symptoms may further distinguish patients who are at a relatively high risk of ischaemic stroke. Patients with limb-shaking or with precipitation of symptoms by rising or exercise or by a documented low blood pressure, have a five times higher risk of recurrent ischaemic stroke than patients without these clinical characteristics (HR 5.0; 95% confidence interval (CI) 1.4 to 17.2) [40]. However, the negative predictive value of these specific haemodynamic features of symptoms is low because they occur in only about 14 to 20% of patients with symptomatic ICA occlusion [37], [40].

Also the number and type of collateral pathways that are present in patients with symptomatic ICA occlusion may carry prognostic information. Leptomeningeal pathways that are visible on angiography have been associated with a worse outcome in one study [40] but not in another [16]. In yet another study the number of collateral pathways was inversely related to the risk of recurrent ischaemic stroke [84].

In the last two decades, studies have focused on the measurement of the haemodynamic state of the hemisphere at risk of ischaemic stroke. Several studies, using a variety of techniques including positron emission tomography (PET) [53], magnetic resonance angiography (MRA) [35], [55], electroencephalography (EEG) [10], ^{133}Xe computer tomography (CT) [21], stable Xe CT [49], ultrasonic Doppler [51] have shown that patients with a compromised cerebral blood supply or autoregulation thereof, have a high risk of recurrent ischaemic stroke, probably in the order of 9 to 18% per year [16], [33], [84], [87], [89], [94]. Other studies could not confirm these findings [40], [97].

Identification of patients who are at high risk of recurrent stroke is most important when revascularization surgery is considered as the risk of ischaemic stroke with maximal non-surgical treatment should be weighed against the risk of any revascularization operation. Revascularization surgery may consist of endarterectomy or angioplasty of a severe stenosis in cerebropetal arteries that are important as collateral pathway in patients with symptomatic ICA occlusion, such as the contralateral ICA, the ipsilateral external carotid artery, or the vertebral arteries, or of EC-IC bypass surgery. Only the EC-IC bypass operation has been studied in a randomized controlled trial for it's efficacy in the prevention of recurrent stroke. In 1985, the results of the EC-IC Bypass Study showed that the superficial temporal artery (STA) to middle cerebral artery (MCA) bypass procedure was not more effective than medical treatment alone in reducing stroke in the patient with symptomatic ICA occlusion in general [1]. One of the main points of critique on this trial has been that measurements of cerebral haemodynamics were not performed to select patients who might specifically benefit from the operation.

As a result of the negative results of the EC-IC Bypass Study the operation was largely abandoned throughout the world [8]. However, in recent years interest in the EC-IC bypass procedure has continuously increased. This interest is not only fuelled by the possibility to select patients at high risk of stroke by haemodynamic measurements but also by developments in the techniques of EC-IC bypass surgery which may improve safety as well as increase the flow through the EC-IC bypass. Whether EC-IC bypass surgery can prevent ischaemic stroke in a subgroup of patients with symptomatic ICA occlusion who are at high risk of recurrent ischaemic stroke because there is clinical or technical evidence for a haemodynamically compromised hemisphere on the side of the ICA occlusion, is still unclear. Currently, two studies are underway that address this important question; the American Carotid Occlusion Study (COSS) [17] and the Japanese EC-IC bypass trial (JET study) [50].

EC-IC bypass, the procedure

STA-MCA bypass

In 1967, the first EC-IC bypass in man was performed by the neurosurgeon Yasargil. Using the operating microscope he created an anastomosis between the STA and a cortical branch of the MCA [96]. This procedure is still performed today. After a relatively small temporolateral trephination the STA is

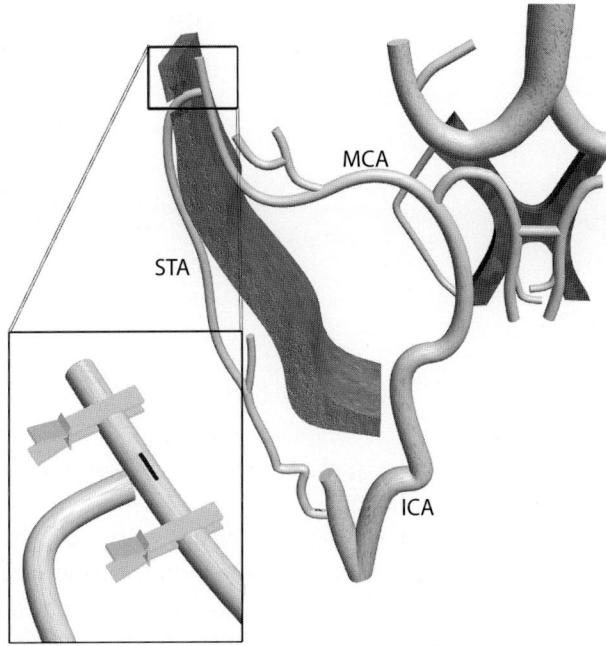

Fig. 1. Schematic representation of a conventional superficial temporal artery to middle cerebral artery anastomosis. After a small craniotomy, the conventional STA-MCA anastomosis is made by temporarily occluding a small cortical branch of the MCA, arteriotomy of the MCA, and suturing of the proximal stump of the STA to the MCA.

connected as an end-to-side anastomosis to one of the cortical branches of the MCA. During the time the surgeon needs to make the anastomosis, the MCA branch is temporarily clipped. A schematic representation of the procedure is shown in Fig. 1.

Over the years surgeons have started to connect the STA to larger third or even second generation MCA branches under the assumption that by choosing a branch with a larger diameter the EC-IC bypass could potentially be more effective for revascularization of the brain. However, the necessity to temporarily clip the recipient vessel exposes the patient to the risk of developing an ischaemic stroke during the operation.

Excimer laser-assisted non-occlusive anastomosis (ELANA)

Since the publication of the negative results of the EC-IC bypass trial, one of us (CAFT) has developed a new technique, now known as the ELANA that allows the construction of a bypass with a recipient artery of a large calibre proximal in the vascular tree. With this technique it is not necessary to temporarily clamp the recipient artery because the distal anastomosis is made with an Excimer laser [69], [81].

Figure 2 shows the schematic representation of the ELANA.

In summary (see right inset of Fig. 2), a saphenous vein graft is identified and harvested from the leg after which it is cut in two parts. One part is connected to the STA with a conventional end-to-side technique. The second part is used for an ELANA anastomosis on the recipient artery, either the distal, intracranial ICA or the proximal MCA. A platinum ring with a diameter of 2.8 or 3.0 mm is stitched into the end of the graft. This ring with the graft is then stitched onto the surface of the artery at the anastomosis site. Subsequently, the Excimer laser catheter is introduced into the free end of the graft until the tip touches the wall of the artery within the graft within the platinum ring. Vacuum suction is applied through the catheter in order to firmly fixate the laser fibres to the vessel wall. After the Excimer laser has been activated, a full thickness disc of the recipient artery wall ("flap") is cut out by the tip of the Excimer laser catheter. When the catheter is withdrawn, the flap is also withdrawn due to the continued vacuum suction and the ELANA anastomosis is complete. The final step then involves the end-to-end connections of the two parts of the grafts.

Figure 3 shows an example of an ELANA on angiography in a 76-year old man who was operated on because of recurrent left hemisphere TIAs.

Follow up studies of patients who underwent an ELANA for the prevention of recurrent ischaemic stroke in patients with symptomatic ICA occlusion are still scarce [38], [39]. The ELANA appears to be a promising type of EC-IC bypass for patients with symptomatic ICA occlusion who are at high risk of recurrent stroke as the amount of flow through an ELANA is larger than through a STA-MCA bypass (see also under 'Flow measurements in the EC-IC bypass') [82]. As a result the haemodynamic effect

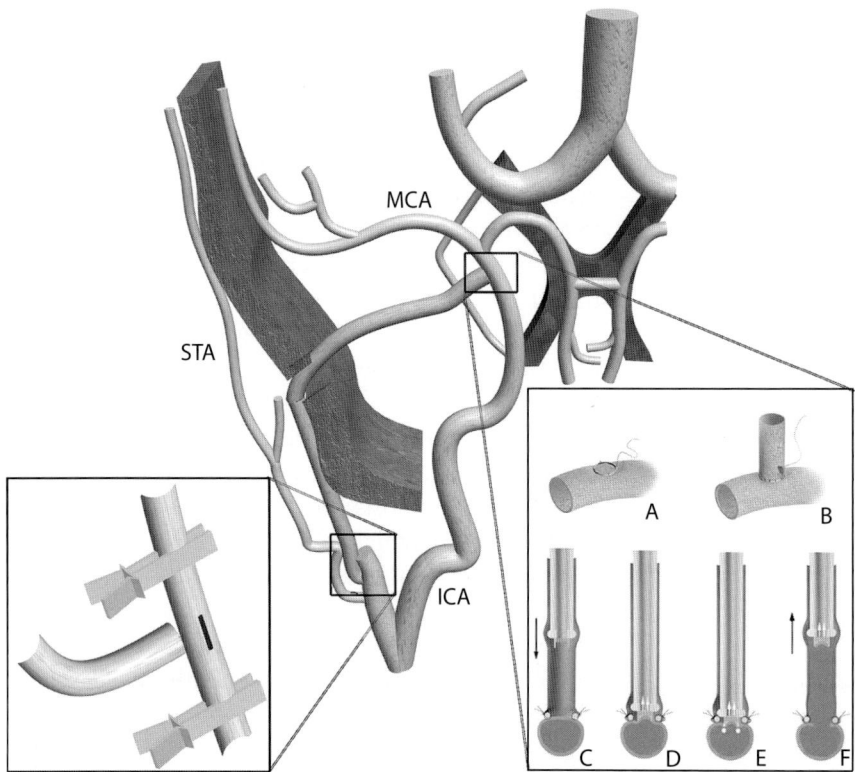

Fig. 2. Schematic representation of high flow revascularization using the ELANA technique. The saphenous graft is cut in two parts. The upstream part is connected using a conventional end-to-side anastomosis to the ECA or a branch of the ECA (left inset). The downstream part is connected to the intracranial ICA using the ELANA technique (right inset). First a platinum ring is connected to the wall of the ICA (A). Then the graft is sutured to both ring and wall (B). The Excimer laser is inserted into the open end of the graft (C) until the tip touches the wall of the ICA within the ring (D). When the laser is activated (E), a small disc of arterial wall ("flap") is excised. Upon withdrawal of the catheter (F), that flap is also removed due to continuing vacuum suction through the catheter. When the ELANA procedure is completed, the upstream part of the graft is connected to the downstream part just outside the skull in an oblique end-to-end anastomosis to facilitate correct entrance of the graft into the skull.

of the ELANA on the blood flow to the hemisphere at risk may also be larger than that of the STA-MCA bypass, but direct comparisons of such measures are not yet available.

Imaging of the EC-IC bypass

Patency of an EC-IC bypass and the amount of flow that will go through it are dependent on several factors, including collateral blood supply [24], choice of and surgical handling of an interposed graft [4], [5], [56], [66], the selection of the donor and recipient artery [59], [71], the suturing technique [19], [71], [72] valvotomy [71] and the use of intraoperative heparin [71], [72]. Also, intra- and postoperative surgical complications may influence the patency [34], [71]. Graft occlusion is almost invariably due to thrombosis as a result of the above mentioned causes [72]. Prolonged cerebral ischemia during the anastomosis procedure may also be of influence [66], [71]. Whereas in the early days of EC-IC bypass surgery measurements were limited to postoperative assessment of patency, currently multiple techniques are available to the neurosurgeon to evaluate not only patency of a bypass but also quantitatively measure the amount of flow through the bypass during the operation. This allows intra-operative recognition of a decrease in flow (for example due to kinking of the EC-IC bypass) and allows revision prior to closure [82].

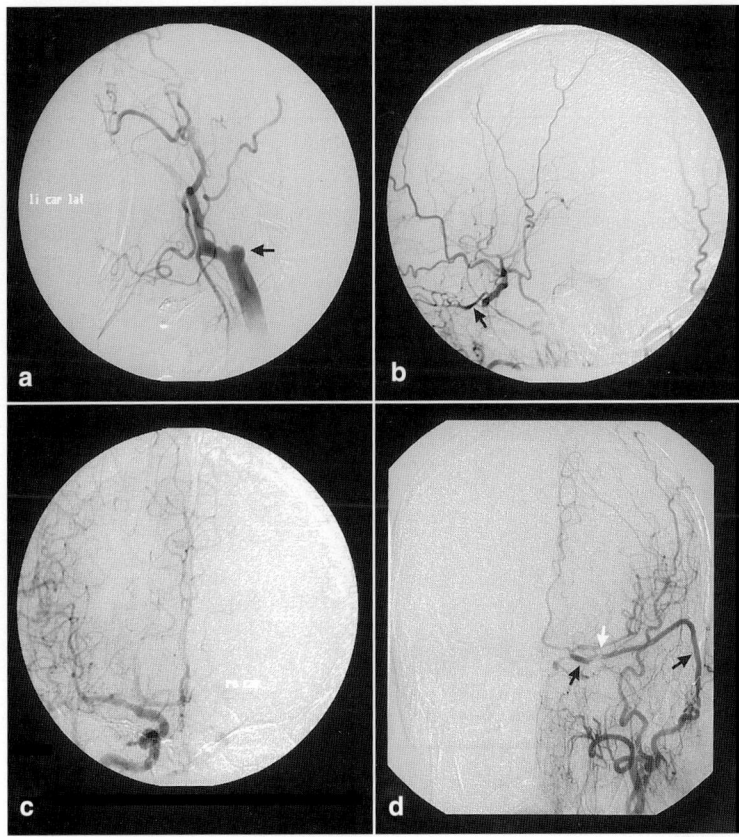

Fig. 3. Angiogram of a 76-year-old right-handed man who had recurrent attacks of expressive dysphasia, right-sided hemiparesis and hypalgesia and transient monocular blindness of the left eye, most of the time occurring immediately after rising from a sitting or lying position. The attacks occurred one to six times a day despite treatment with oral anticoagulants and low-dose aspirin. Selective catheterization of the left common carotid artery showed occlusion of the left ICA (**a**) and filling of the left MCA via the ophthalmic artery (**b**, arrow). Selective catheterization of the right common carotid artery showed filling of the left anterior cerebral artery but not of the left MCA (**c**). The angiography one month postoperatively demonstrated the patent ELANA (**d**, black arrows; white arrow points to a clip artefact) between the STA and the distal, intracranial ICA. After the operation the patient had no further TIAs. Reproduced from [38] by courtesy of S. Karger AG, Basel.

Patency of the EC-IC bypass

In the EC-IC bypass trial in 1995 a patency rate of 96% was found with conventional angiography performed at a median time of 32 days after the operation [1]. Other studies have shown equally high patency rates on angiography [88]. Patency of an EC-IC bypass can also be demonstrated with non-invasive techniques. Using postoperative Doppler ultrasound flow velocity measurements patency rates between 93 and 97% have been found [6], [88], [92]. Postoperative magnetic resonance angiography has evolved since the early nineties and can now confirm patency using quantitative flow measurements with 2D cine phase contrast techniques [42], [43], [83]. Two other recent studies used postoperative computed tomographic angiography and found patency rates of 100% in a series of 11 patients in each study [75], [79].

Patency can also be evaluated during the operation, which makes immediate correction of an anastomosis possible if necessary. Spetzler introduced intra-operative electromagnetic flow measurements in 1976 for confirmation of bypass patency [67]. Later, intra-operative angiography has been demonstrated to show patency but also the location of a bypass stenosis. One study claimed improvement of patency from 90% to 98% using intra-operative angiography [66]. Another study showed a patency rate of 100% in 41 cases with the use of intra-operative angiography [95]. Recently, indocyanine green (ICG) angiography has been developed to verify patency of an EC-IC bypass during the operation [91]. After intravenous administration of ICG, the operating field is illuminated with infrared excitation light which visualizes the intravascular fluorescence and thus can demonstrate patency of the bypass. In this way cath-

Table 1. Effect of EC-IC Bypass on cerebral haemodynamics

Author	Year	Study design (postop period)	Technique	Challenge	Pts	Controls	CBF	CVR	OEF
De Weerd [10]	1982	P (10 d–3 m)	^{133}Xe CT	–	10	10*	+	np	np
Meyer [49]	1982	P (1–3 w)	Stable Xe CT and ^{133}Xe CT	CO_2	33	13*	+	+	np
Karnik [30]	1992	P (2–6 w)	TCD	ACZ	14	14*	nd	+	np
Yonas [98]	1985	R (nd)	Stable Xe CT	–	8	17*	+	np	np
Tanahashi† [74]	1985	P (28 m)	^{133}Xe CT	–	38	22*	–	np	np
Holzschuh [26]	1991	R (5.4 y)	^{133}Xe CT	ACZ	18	29*	–	–	np
Leblanc [48]	1987	R (3–6 m)	PET	CO_2	6	5*	–	nd	–
Thomas [76]	1984	R (2–5 y)	Xe SPECT	–	5	6*	+	np	np
Sunada [70]	1989	P (nd)	^{133}Xe SPECT	ACZ$^{\oplus}$	9	10**	–	np	np
Sasoh [61]	2003	R (6 w)	PET	CO_2	25	10**	+	+	+
Samson [60]	1985	R (1–4 m)	PET	CO_2	11	15**	+	nd	–
Hartmann [22]	1987	R (4–8 w)	^{133}Xe CT	–	25	16**	+	np	np
Neff [55]	2004	R (2–3 m)	MRA	–	25	16**	+	np	np
Anderson [2]	1992	R (1–7 y)	^{133}Xe SPECT	CO_2	13	20**	+	+	np
Yamashita [93]	1991	R (1 m)	Stable Xe CT	ACZ	15	8**	+	+	np
Di Piero [14]	1987	R (12 m)	^{123}IMP SPECT	–	14	0	–	np	np
Iwama [29]	1997	R (19–66 m)	^{123}IMP SPECT	ACZ	44	0	–	+	np
Kume [44]	1998	R (2–4 w)	^{123}IMP SPECT	ACZ	30	0	+	+	np
Kawaguchi [31]	1999	R (1 m)	^{123}IMP SPECT	ACZ	19	0	+	+	np
Schmiedek [63], [64]	1976	R (6.5 m)	^{133}Xe CT	CO_2	33	0	+	+	np
Laurent [47]	1982	R (3–8 w)	^{133}Xe CT	–	35	0	+	np	np
Yonekura [99]	1982	R (2 y)	^{133}Xe CT	–	107	0	–	np	np
Halsey [20]	1982	R (0–26 w)	^{133}Xe CT	CO_2	19	0	–	+	np
Vorstrup [86]	1985	R (> 3 m)	^{133}Xe CT	–	22	0	–	np	np
Bishop [7]	1987	R (3 m)	^{133}Xe CT	CO_2	8	0	–	+	np
Vorstrup [85]	1986	P (2–6 m)	^{133}Xe SPECT	ACZ	18	0	–	+	np
Piepgras [57]	1994	R (2 y)	^{133}Xe SPECT	ACZ	9	0	nd	+	np
Schmiedek [65]	1994	R (4–79 m)	^{133}Xe SPECT	ACZ	28	0	–	+	np
Ishikawa [28]	1995	R (1–3 m)	^{133}Xe SPECT	ACZ	28	0	–	+	np
Grubb [18]	1979	R (2 m)	PET	–	9	0	+	np	np
Powers [58]	1984	R (7d–4 w)	PET	–	17	0	+	np	+
Gibbs [15]	1987	R (1–6 m)	PET	–	12	0	–	np	–
Nagata [53]	1991	R (nd)	PET	–	7	0	+	np	+
Muraishi [52]	1993	R (nd)	PET	–	6	0	+	np	+
Kawamura [32]	1994	R (1–2 m & 1–5 y)	PET	–	13	0	+	np	+
Takagi [73]	1997	R (3–5 m)	PET	CO_2	12	0	+	nd	+
Kuwabara [45]	1998	R (nd)	PET	ACZ	7	0	–	+	+
Kobayashi [41]	1999	R (1.5 m)	PET	CO_2	10	0	+	nd	+
Heilbrun [23]	1975	R (3 m)	Stable Xe CT	–	16	0	+	np	np
Tsuda [80]	1984	R (1–2 m)	Stable Xe CT	CO_2	10	0	+	+	np
Touho [77]	1990	R (nd)	Stable Xe CT	ACZ	16	0	–	+	np
Touho [78]	1990	P (nd)	Stable Xe CT	ACZ	27	0	+	+	np
Schick [62]	1996	R (5.6 y)	Tc SPECT	ACZ, CO_2	47	0	–	+	np
Klijn [38]	2002	R (6 m)	TCD	CO_2	15	0	np	+	np
Hirai [25]	2005	P (2 w)	Xe SPECT	ACZ	40	0	+	+	np

P, prospective; R, retrospective; d, days; w, weeks; m, months; y, years; nd, not described; np, not performed; PET, positron emission tomography; CT, computer tomography; Xe, xenon, SPECT, single photon emission computed tomography; MRA, magnetic resonance angiography; ACZ, acetazolamide; CO_2, carbondioxide; Tc, Technetium; IMP, N-isopropyl-I-123-p-iodoamphetamine; *medically treated patients; **healthy controls; $^{\oplus}$only pre-operative ACZ-challenge; †including the study of Meyer[49]; + indicates improvement; – indicates no improvement.

eter angiography which requires a specialized team as well as specific equipment in the operating room and significantly prolongs surgery can be avoided.

Also, intra-operative Doppler ultrasound flow velocity measurements can be used as a quick and reliable way to assess changes in flow velocity both in the cortical MCA branches as well as in the STA [3], [51].

Flow measurements in the EC-IC bypass

Several techniques have been developed to quantitatively measure flow through an EC-IC bypass. With his intra-operative electromagnetic flow measurement Spetzler measured a flow of 25 ml/min after STA-MCA bypass and subsequent occlusion of the ICA as treatment of a giant ICA aneurysm [67]. Later, the use of intra-operative ultrasound volume flow measurements has been published by several authors [54], [82]. One of them used this technique to measure the flow difference in the STA before and after a STA-MCA bypass operation. During the operation the flow in the STA increased from 13 to 46 ml/min [54]. In eight patients with symptomatic ICA occlusion who underwent an ELANA we found a mean intra-operative flow of 111 ml/min [82]. After a mean interval of 26 days the average post-operative flow in seven of these patients increased to 128 ± 48 ml/min. This increase in flow in the EC-IC bypass is most likely the result of flow adaptation of the EC-IC bypass. Flow adaptation may occur both in the short term (during the procedure) [9], [82] and in the long term (postoperatively) [82]. The flow through an EC-IC bypass may also decrease over time and eventually the EC-IC bypass may occlude. If a patient remains asymptomatic one could presume that the collateral blood supply via the other pathways than the EC-IC bypass has become sufficient to maintain adequate blood flow in the previously symptomatic hemisphere on the side of the ICA occlusion [62]. In such patients the EC-IC bypass may still play a role in the prevention of ischaemic stroke in the acute phase when the patient first presented with TIAs or mildly disabling ischaemic stroke and occlusion of the ICA and had a compromised cerebral blood flow.

Horn recently described the angiographic classification of bypass filling as grade I (poor intracranial opacification of selective external carotid artery injection), grade II (moderate opacification), or grade III (extensive opacification) [27]. In this study, the amount of flow through an EC-IC bypass as measured with MR-based volume flow techniques was shown to correspond to the angiographic grade of filling. Grade I (n = 6) was shown to correspond to a flow of 39.2 ± 9.8 ml/min, Grade II (n = 15) to 73.6 ± 16.7 ml/min, and Grade III (n = 20) to 97.2 ± 26.6 ml/min.

Imaging the effect of EC-IC bypass

Measurements of haemodynamic compromise have not only been used to predict the risk of stroke in patients with symptomatic ICA occlusion [11] but have also been applied to study the effect of EC-IC bypass surgery on the flow state of the brain. A comparative overview of brain perfusion imaging techniques has recently outlined the characteristics of the different techniques with their inherent advantages and disadvantages [90]. Classically, haemodynamic impairment has been classified into two stages [13]. In stage 1 there is autoregulatory vasodilatation. This was defined as an increase in cerebral blood volume (CBV) or an increase in mean vascular transit time (equivalent to the CBV/CBF ratio), with normal CBF, OEF, and oxygen metabolism ($CMRO_2$). In stage 2 autoregulation fails resulting in reduced CBF and increased OEF with normal oxygen metabolism. However, later studies have shown that this model of two stages of haemodynamic impairment may be too simple. Patients with an increased OEF may have normal CBV and slight decreases in CBF may lead to an increased OEF [13]. Whereas stage 2 haemodynamic compromise can only be measured by PET, stage 1 can also be assessed by measurement of so-called cerebrovascular reactivity (CVR) by paired measurements of CBF or blood flow velocity before and after a vasodilatory stimulus such as acetazolamide, carbogen inhalation, or breathholding.

Table 1 summarizes the results of 45 studies that investigated changes in the haemodynamic state of the brain after EC-IC bypass surgery in patients with ICA occlusion. Case reports and series smaller than the arbitrarily chosen number of five patients were not included. In none of the 45 studies patients who underwent EC-IC bypass surgery were compared with patients who were not operated on in a randomized fashion. In the only randomised controlled trial investigating EC-IC bypass surgery haemodynamic measurements were not performed [1]. In eight studies patients who underwent EC-IC bypass surgery were compared with patients who were not operated on [10], [26], [30], [48], [49], [74], [76], [98]. In seven other studies operated patients were compared with haemodynamic measurements in healthy controls [2], [22], [55], [60], [61], [70], [93].

Of the 45 studies of haemodynamic measurements before and after EC-IC bypass surgery, information on pre- and post-operative measurements of CVR was available in 23 studies. All but one study [26] reported improvement in CVR after EC-IC bypass surgery. Some studies reported improvement in vascular reactivity only in a specific subgroup of patients [28], [86], e.g., in patients with collateral blood supply via leptomeningeal vessels and decreased reactivity to ACZ [29]. Of the 23 studies that reported measurements of CVR 20 studies also reported CBF measurements before and after EC-IC bypass surgery. In nine of these no improvement in CBF was observed whereas CVR improved after EC-IC bypass [7], [20], [28], [29], [45], [62], [65], [77], [85]. Of a total of 42 of the 45 studies that reported on CBF, improvement of CBF after EC-IC bypass was

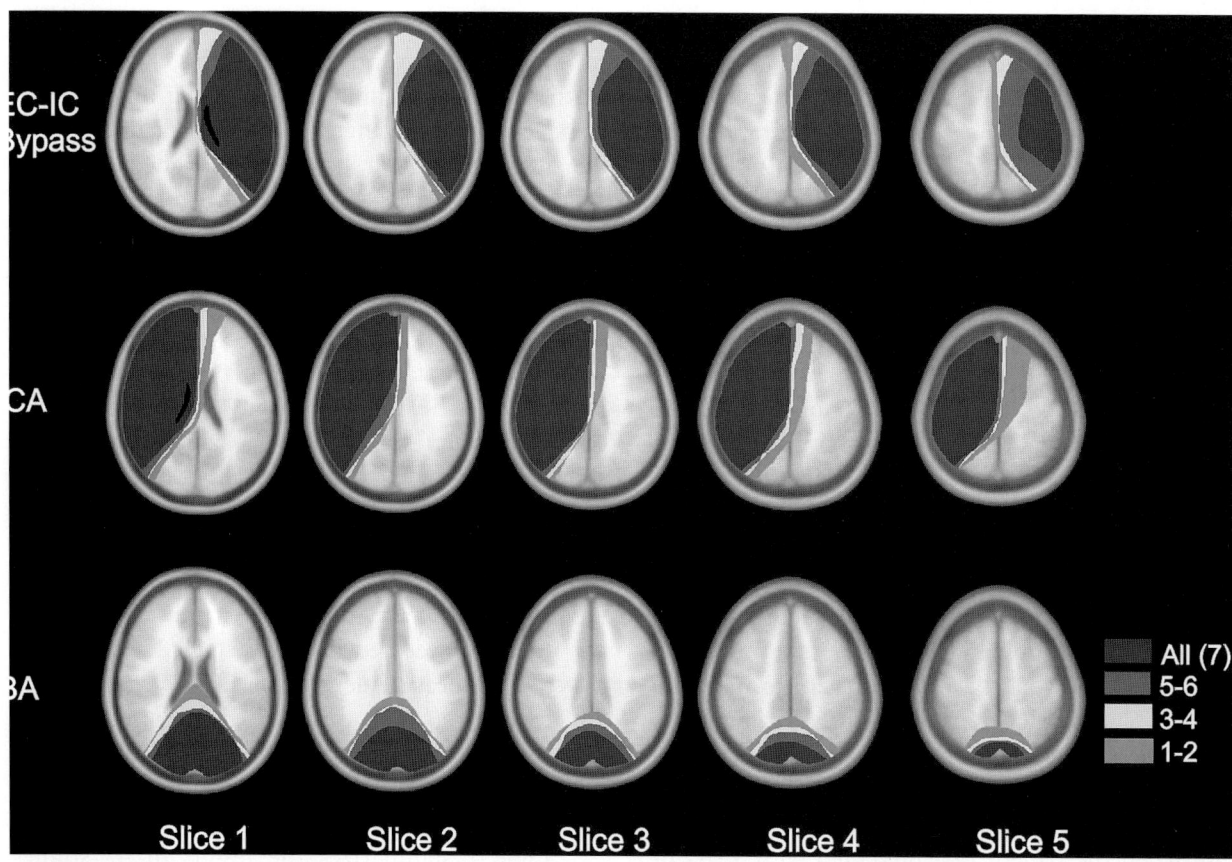

Fig. 4. Average flow territory maps of the EC-IC bypass, contralateral ICA and posterior circulation for the seven patients. Flow territory maps are projected to a standard Talarach brain. The maps of the top, middle and bottom row indicate the overlap of the flow territories of respectively the EC-IC bypass, contralateral ICA and posterior circulation. The dark grey area indicates maximal overlap flow territory present in all seven patients. BA, Basilar artery [24].

observed in 25 studies. In seventeen studies no such improvement was found. Of the 11 studies that contained information of the effect of EC-IC bypass on an increased OEF, eight reported a decrease in OEF after surgery, whereas no amelioration of OEF was found in three other studies [15], [48], [60].

Most postoperative haemodynamic assessments were performed at a relatively short time after the operation that is a few weeks to a few months. In only very few studies long term effects were studied [26], [29], [62], [65], [74], [99]. In three of these six studies EC-IC bypass did not improve CBF or CVR [26], [74], [99] in two studies CVR but not CBF improved after the operation [62], [65] and in the remaining study CVR improved in a small subgroup only [29]. One group first showed postoperative improvement of both CBF, but not CVR in 33 operated patients one to three weeks after the operation [49]. After a mean long-term follow-up of 28 months of this group of patients and five additional patients the improvement in CBF was no longer found [74].

In conclusion, many studies using various techniques have reported improvement of cerebral haemodynamics after STA-MCA bypass, but comparisons with similar patients who were not operated on are lacking. Some studies have shown that improvement in the haemodynamic state of the brain may only occur in a subset of patients [28], [29], [86], may be most prominent in those in whom those measures were most disturbed before operation [47], [58], [99] and improvement that was observed relatively shortly after the EC-IC bypass procedure may not last over time [14], [74], [99]. One study showed that collateral circulation through the bypass developed well and cerebrovascular reactivity improved in patients who had extensive leptomeningeal anastomoses preoperatively in combination with a decreased cerebrovascular reactivity [29]. When interpreting the results of these studies, it is important to realize that cerebral haemodynamic compromise in patients with symptomatic ICA occlusion has also been observed to improve spontaneously without revascularization operation [12], [89], [97]. For these reasons and despite the combined evidence suggesting that in patients with symptomatic ICA occlusion a compromised flow state of the brain can be improved by revascularization with an EC-IC bypass, definite conclusions cannot be drawn.

Imaging the flow territory of the EC-IC bypass

Recently, our group demonstrated the feasibility of selective arterial spin labelling magnetic resonance imaging (ASL-MRI) for follow-up of patients after EC-IC bypass of the ELANA type, providing information on the flow territory of the EC-IC bypass and on regional cerebral blood flow [24]. In this study seven patients underwent an ELANA-operation, four because of recurrent TIAs in the presence of ICA occlusion and impaired TCD CO_2-reactivity and three other patients because of a giant aneurysm of the ICA for which the ICA had to be occluded.

The study showed that the average flow territory of the EC-IC bypass in the seven patients was 15% smaller than the flow territory of the contralateral ICA (p-value, 0.018), whereas the mean CBF of the hemisphere on the side of the EC-IC bypass was similar to the CBF in healthy controls (on average 69.1 ± 17.5 ml/min/100 g brain tissue in healthy controls and 70.4 ± 11.6 ml/min/100 g brain tissue in the four patients with symptomatic ICA occlusion and 71.6 ± 10.6 ml/min/100 g brain tissue in the three patient operated because of a giant aneurysm). On average the volume flow through the EC-IC bypass was lower (169 ± 58 ml/min) than the volume flow through the contralateral ICA (254 ± 88 ml/min; p-value <0.05). This suggests that other collateral pathways than the EC-IC bypass also contributed to the blood supply of the hemisphere ipsilateral to the ICA occlusion. Unfortunately, pre-operative CBF measurements were not available. Fig. 4 shows the average flow territory maps of the EC-IC bypass, of the contralateral ICA and the basilar artery for all seven patients.

The major advantage of ASL-MRI over the imaging of an EC-IC bypass by angiography is that there is no need to use contrast which makes the procedure completely non-invasive and without risk. Another advantage is that apart from the information on the flow territory of the EC-IC bypass, also quantitative CBF and volume flow measurements in the major cerebropetal arteries can be obtained with the same study in one patient. In the future, assessment of cerebrovascular reactivity with this technique may provide even more information.

Future perspectives

Technical advances in EC-IC bypass surgery

The ELANA technique has been continuously improved upon over the years and preliminary evidence from further developments in the laboratory show that it may be possible to further simplify the procedure which will shorten the duration of the operation [68].

Clinical studies

Currently, a new randomized controlled trial is ongoing in North-America, the carotid occlusion surgery study (COSS) [17]. This study investigates whether the STA-MCA anastomosis is better than best medical therapy alone for prevention of recurrent ischaemic stroke in patients with symptomatic ICA occlusion and stage II haemodynamic compromise as indicated by an increased OEF in the hemisphere at risk. It is unclear when the results of this trial can be expected as the inclusion rate has been far slower than expected.

The results of the Japanese EC-IC bypass trial (JET study) are expected in the near future [50].

Further studies should clarify whether the ELANA differs from the STA-MCA bypass in its effect on the blood flow to the hemisphere at risk and its ability to prevent recurrent ischaemic stroke in patients with symptomatic ICA occlusion. The fact that the ELANA technique has now been adopted by neurosurgeons in Finland, Germany, Italy, Russia, the UK and the USA will facilitate the collection of this valuable information [46], [69].

Take home messages

The EC-IC bypass procedure is regaining interest as possible treatment for prevention of ischaemic stroke in patients with ICA occlusion and proven haemodynamic compromise. Trials are currently under way.

Development of the ELANA has allowed the construction of an EC-IC bypass with a recipient artery of large calibre proximal in the vascular tree. The efficacy of this high flow ELANA for prevention of ischaemic stroke in patients with ICA occlusion remains to be determined.

Developments in imaging of the EC-IC bypass have resulted in the possibility to non-invasively assess the EC-IC bypass during the procedure, measure its effect on the flow state of the brain and quantify its flow territory.

Acknowledgements

C. J. M. Klijn is supported by the Netherlands Heart Foundation (grant 2003B263) and by The Netherlands Organisation for Health Research and Development (grant 907-00-103). The comments of L. J. Kappelle, MD, on an earlier version of the chapter are gratefully acknowledged.

References

[1] The EC/IC Bypass Study Group: Failure of extracranial-intracranial arterial bypass to reduce the risk of ischemic stroke. Results of an international randomized trial. N Engl J Med 313: 1191–1200 (1985).
[2] Anderson DE, McLane MP, Reichman OH, Origitano TC: Improved cerebral blood flow and CO2 reactivity after microvascular anastomosis in patients at high risk for recurrent stroke. Neurosurgery 31: 26–33 (1992).
[3] Badie B, Lee FT Jr., Pozniak MA, Strother CM: Intraoperative sonographic assessment of graft patency during extracranial-intracranial bypass. AJNR Am J Neuroradiol 21: 1457–1459 (2000).
[4] Bandyk DF, Towne JB, Schmitt DD, Seabrook GR, Bergamini TM: Therapeutic options for acute thrombosed in situ saphenous vein arterial bypass grafts. J Vasc Surg 11: 680–687 (1990).
[5] Bergamini TM, Towne JB, Bandyk DF, Seabrook GR, Schmitt DD: Experience with in situ saphenous vein bypasses during 1981 to 1989: determinant factors of long-term patency. J Vasc Surg 13: 137–147 (1991).
[6] Berry PR: Cerebral occlusion: Extracranial-intracranial anastomosis. AORN J 41: 901–905, 907 (1985).
[7] Bishop CC, Burnand KG, Brown M, Russell RR, Browse NL: Reduced response of cerebral blood flow to

hypercapnia: restoration by extracranial-intracranial bypass. Br J Surg 74: 802–804 (1987).
[8] Caplan LR, Piepgras DG, Quest DO, Toole JF, Samson D, Futrell N, Millikan C, Flamm ES, Heros RC, Yonekawa Y, Eguchi T, Yonas H, Rothbart D, Spetzler RF: EC-IC bypass 10 years later: is it valuable? Surg Neurol 46: 416–423 (1996).
[9] Charbel FT, Misra M, Clarke ME, Ausman JI: Computer simulation of cerebral blood flow in moyamoya and the results of surgical therapies. Clin Neurol Neurosurg 99 Suppl 2: S68–S73 (1997).
[10] de Weerd AW, Veering MM, Mosmans PC, van Huffelen AC, Tulleken CA, Jonkman EJ: Effect of the extra-intracranial (STA-MCA) arterial anastomosis on EEG and cerebral blood flow: a controlled study of patients with unilateral cerebral ischemia. Stroke 13: 674–679 (1982).
[11] Derdeyn CP, Grubb RL Jr., Powers WJ: Cerebral hemodynamic impairment: methods of measurement and association with stroke risk. Neurology 53: 251–259 (1999).
[12] Derdeyn CP, Videen TO, Fritsch SM, Carpenter DA, Grubb RL Jr., Powers WJ: Compensatory mechanisms for chronic cerebral hypoperfusion in patients with carotid occlusion. Stroke 30: 1019–1024 (1999).
[13] Derdeyn CP, Videen TO, Yundt KD, Fritsch SM, Carpenter DA, Grubb RL, Powers WJ: Variability of cerebral blood volume and oxygen extraction: stages of cerebral haemodynamic impairment revisited. Brain 125: 595–607 (2002).
[14] Di P, V, Lenzi GL, Collice M, Triulzi F, Gerundini P, Perani D, Savi AR, Fieschi C, Fazio F: Long-term non-invasive single photon emission computed tomography monitoring of perfusional changes after EC-IC bypass surgery. J Neurol Neurosurg Psychiatry 50: 988–996 (1987).
[15] Gibbs JM, Wise RJ, Thomas DJ, Mansfield AO, Russell RW: Cerebral haemodynamic changes after extracranial-intracranial bypass surgery. J Neurol Neurosurg Psychiatry 50: 140–150 (1987).
[16] Grubb RL Jr., Derdeyn CP, Fritsch SM, Carpenter DA, Yundt KD, Videen TO, Spitznagel EL, Powers WJ: Importance of hemodynamic factors in the prognosis of symptomatic carotid occlusion. JAMA 280: 1055–1060 (1998).
[17] Grubb RL Jr., Powers WJ, Derdeyn CP, Adams HP Jr., Clarke WR: The Carotid Occlusion Surgery Study. Neurosurg Focus 14: e9 (2003).
[18] Grubb RL Jr., Ratcheson RA, Raichle ME, Kliefoth AB, Gado MH: Regional cerebral blood flow and oxygen utilization in superficial temporal-middle cerebral artery anastomosis patients: an exploratory definition of clinical problems. J Neurosurg 50: 733–741 (1979).
[19] Gundry SR, Jones M, Ishihara T, Ferrans VJ: Optimal preparation techniques for human saphenous vein grafts. Surgery 88: 785–794 (1980).
[20] Halsey JH Jr., Morawetz RB, Blauenstein UW: The hemodynamic effect of STA-MCA bypass. Stroke 13: 163–167 (1982).
[21] Halsey JH Jr., Nakai K, Wariyar B: Sensitivity of rCBF to focal lesions. Stroke 12: 631–635 (1981).
[22] Hartmann A, Rommel T, Winter R, Tsuda Y, Menzel J: Measurements of regional cerebral blood flow in patients following superficial temporal artery-middle cerebral artery anastomosis. Acta Neurochir (Wien) 89: 106–111 (1987).
[23] Heilbrun MP, Reichman OH, Anderson RE, Roberts TS: Regional cerebral blood flow studies following superficial temporal-middle cerebral artery anastomosis. J Neurosurg 43: 706–716 (1975).
[24] Hendrikse J, van der ZA, Ramos LM, van Osch MJ, Golay X, Tulleken CA, van der GJ: Altered flow territories after extracranial-intracranial bypass surgery. Neurosurgery 57: 486–494 (2005).
[25] Hirai Y, Fujimoto S, Toyoda K, Inoue T, Uwatoko T, Makihara N, Yasumori K, Ibayashi S, Iida M, Okada Y: Superficial temporal artery duplex ultrasonography for improved cerebral hemodynamics after extracranial-intracranial bypass surgery. Cerebrovasc Dis 20: 463–469 (2005).
[26] Holzschuh M, Brawanski A, Ullrich W, Meixensberger J: Cerebral blood flow and cerebrovascular reserve 5 years after EC-IC bypass. Neurosurg Rev 14: 275–278 (1991).
[27] Horn P, Vajkoczy P, Schmiedek P, Neff W: Evaluation of extracranial-intracranial arterial bypass function with magnetic resonance angiography. Neuroradiology 46: 723–729 (2004).
[28] Ishikawa T, Houkin K, Abe H, Isobe M, Kamiyama H: Cerebral haemodynamics and long-term prognosis after extracranial-intracranial bypass surgery. J Neurol Neurosurg Psychiatry 59: 625–628 (1995).
[29] Iwama T, Hashimoto N, Takagi Y, Tsukahara T, Hayashida K: Predictability of extracranial/intracranial bypass function: a retrospective study of patients with occlusive cerebrovascular disease. Neurosurgery 40: 53–59 (1997).
[30] Karnik R, Valentin A, Ammerer HP, Donath P, Slany J: Evaluation of vasomotor reactivity by transcranial Doppler and acetazolamide test before and after extracranial-intracranial bypass in patients with internal carotid artery occlusion. Stroke 23: 812–817 (1992).
[31] Kawaguchi S, Sakaki T, Uranishi R: Effects of bypass on CO_2 cerebrovascular reactivity in ischaemic cerebrovascular diseases - based on the intra-operative LCBF and CO_2 cerebrovascular reactivity studies. Acta Neurochir (Wien) 141: 369–374 (1999).

[32] Kawamura S, Sayama I, Yasui N, Uemura K: Haemodynamic and metabolic changes following extra-intracranial bypass surgery. Acta Neurochir (Wien) 126: 135–139 (1994).
[33] Kleiser B, Widder B: Course of carotid artery occlusions with impaired cerebrovascular reactivity. Stroke 23: 171–174 (1992).
[34] Kletter G: The Extra-Intracranial Bypass Operation for Prevention and Treatment of Stroke. New York – Wien, Springer Verlag (1979).
[35] Klijn CJ, Kappelle LJ, Algra A, van Gijn J: Outcome in patients with symptomatic occlusion of the internal carotid artery or intracranial arterial lesions: a meta-analysis of the role of baseline characteristics and type of antithrombotic treatment. Cerebrovasc Dis 12: 228–234 (2001).
[36] Klijn CJ, Kappelle LJ, Tulleken CA, van Gijn J: Symptomatic carotid artery occlusion. A reappraisal of hemodynamic factors. Stroke 28: 2084–2093 (1997).
[37] Klijn CJ, Kappelle LJ, van der Grond J, Algra A, Tulleken CA, van Gijn J: Magnetic resonance techniques for the identification of patients with symptomatic carotid artery occlusion at high risk of cerebral ischemic events. Stroke 31: 3001–3007 (2000).
[38] Klijn CJ, Kappelle LJ, van der Grond J, van Gijn J, Tulleken CA: A new type of extracranial/intracranial bypass for recurrent haemodynamic transient ischaemic attacks. Cerebrovasc Dis 8: 184–187 (1998).
[39] Klijn CJ, Kappelle LJ, van der Zwan A, van Gijn J, Tulleken CA: Excimer laser-assisted high-flow extracranial/intracranial bypass in patients with symptomatic carotid artery occlusion at high risk of recurrent cerebral ischemia: safety and long-term outcome. Stroke 33: 2451–2458 (2002).
[40] Klijn CJ, van Buren PA, Kappelle LJ, Tulleken CA, Eikelboom BC, Algra A, van Gijn J: Outcome in patients with symptomatic occlusion of the internal carotid artery. Eur J Vasc Endovasc Surg 19: 579–586 (2000).
[41] Kobayashi H, Kitai R, Ido K, Kabuto M, Handa Y, Kubota T, Yonekura Y: Hemodynamic and metabolic changes following cerebral revascularization in patients with cerebral occlusive diseases. Neurol Res 21: 153–160 (1999).
[42] Kodama T, Ueda T, Suzuki Y, Yano T, Watanabe K: MRA in the evaluation of EC-IC bypass patency. J Comput Assist Tomogr 17: 922–926 (1993).
[43] Kodoma T, Suzuki Y, Yano T, Watanabe K, Ueda T, Asada K: Phase-contrast MRA in the evaluation of EC-IC bypass patency. Clin Radiol 50: 459–465 (1995).
[44] Kume N, Hayashida K, Iwama T, Cho I, Matsunaga N: Use of 123I-IMP brain SPET to predict outcome following STA-MCA bypass surgery: cerebral blood flow but not vasoreactivity is a predictive parameter. Eur J Nucl Med 25: 1637–1642 (1998).
[45] Kuwabara Y, Ichiya Y, Sasaki M, Yoshida T, Fukumura T, Masuda K, Fujii K, Fukui M: PET evaluation of cerebral hemodynamics in occlusive cerebrovascular disease pre- and postsurgery. J Nucl Med 39: 760–765 (1998).
[46] Langer DJ, Vajkoczy P: ELANA: Excimer Laser-Assisted Nonocclusive Anastomosis for extracranial-to-intracranial and intracranial-to-intracranial bypass: a review. Skull Base 15: 191–205 (2005).
[47] Laurent JP, Lawner PM, O'Connor M: Reversal of intracerebral steal by STA-MCA anastomosis. J Neurosurg 57: 629–632 (1982).
[48] Leblanc R, Tyler JL, Mohr G, Meyer E, Diksic M, Yamamoto L, Taylor L, Gauthier S, Hakim A: Hemodynamic and metabolic effects of cerebral revascularization. J Neurosurg 66: 529–535 (1987).
[49] Meyer JS, Nakajima S, Okabe T, Amano T, Centeno R, Len YY, Levine J, Levinthal R, Rose J: Redistribution of cerebral blood flow following STA-MCA by-pass in patients with hemispheric ischemia. Stroke 13: 774–784 (1982).
[50] Mizumura S, Nakagawara J, Takahashi M, Kumita S, Cho K, Nakajo H, Toba M, Kumazaki T: Three-dimensional display in staging hemodynamic brain ischemia for JET study: objective evaluation using SEE analysis and 3D-SSP display. Ann Nucl Med 18: 13–21 (2004).
[51] Moritake K, Handa H, Yonekawa Y, Nagata I: Ultrasonic Doppler assessment of hemodynamics in superficial temporal artery-middle cerebral artery anastomosis. Surg Neurol 13: 249–257 (1980).
[52] Muraishi K, Kameyama M, Sato K, Sirane R, Ogawa A, Yoshimoto T, Hatazawa J, Itoh M: Cerebral circulatory and metabolic changes following EC/IC bypass surgery in cerebral occlusive diseases. Neurol Res 15: 97–103 (1993).
[53] Nagata S, Fujii K, Matsushima T, Fukui M, Sadoshima S, Kuwabara Y, Abe H: Evaluation of EC-IC bypass for patients with atherosclerotic occlusive cerebrovascular disease: clinical and positron emission tomographic studies. Neurol Res 13: 209–216 (1991).
[54] Nakayama N, Kuroda S, Houkin K, Takikawa S, Abe H: Intraoperative measurement of arterial blood flow using a transit time flowmeter: monitoring of hemodynamic changes during cerebrovascular surgery. Acta Neurochir (Wien) 143: 17–24 (2001).
[55] Neff KW, Horn P, Dinter D, Vajkoczy P, Schmiedek P, Duber C: Extracranial-intracranial arterial bypass surgery improves total brain blood supply in selected symptomatic patients with unilateral internal carotid artery occlusion and insufficient collateralization. Neuroradiology 46: 730–737 (2004).
[56] Okada Y, Shima T, Nishida M, Yamane K: Retroauricular subcutaneous Dacron tunnel for extracranial-in-

tracranial autologous vein bypass graft. Technical note. J Neurosurg 81: 800–802 (1994).
[57] Piepgras A, Leinsinger G, Kirsch CM, Schmiedek P: STA-MCA bypass in bilateral carotid artery occlusion: clinical results and long-term effect on cerebrovascular reserve capacity. Neurol Res 16: 104–107 (1994).
[58] Powers WJ, Martin WR, Herscovitch P, Raichle ME, Grubb RL Jr: Extracranial-intracranial bypass surgery: hemodynamic and metabolic effects. Neurology 34: 1168–1174 (1984).
[59] Regli L, Piepgras DG, Hansen KK: Late patency of long saphenous vein bypass grafts to the anterior and posterior cerebral circulation. J Neurosurg 83: 806–811 (1995).
[60] Samson Y, Baron JC, Bousser MG, Rey A, Derlon JM, David P, Comoy J: Effects of extra-intracranial arterial bypass on cerebral blood flow and oxygen metabolism in humans. Stroke 16: 609–616 (1985).
[61] Sasoh M, Ogasawara K, Kuroda K, Okuguchi T, Terasaki K, Yamadate K, Ogawa A: Effects of EC-IC bypass surgery on cognitive impairment in patients with hemodynamic cerebral ischemia. Surg Neurol 59: 455–460 (2003).
[62] Schick U, Zimmermann M, Stolke D: Long-term evaluation of EC-IC bypass patency. Acta Neurochir (Wien) 138: 938–942 (1996).
[63] Schmiedek P, Gratzl O, Spetzler R, Steinhoff H, Enzenbach R, Brendel W, Marguth F: Selection of patients for extra-intracranial arterial bypass surgery based on rCBF measurements. J Neurosurg 44: 303–312 (1976).
[64] Schmiedek P, Gratzl O, Steinhoff H: Regional blood flow measurement in extra-intracranial anastomoses for cerebral ischemia. Methodologic aspects. Acta Radiol Suppl 347: 247–251 (1976).
[65] Schmiedek P, Piepgras A, Leinsinger G, Kirsch CM, Einhupl K: Improvement of cerebrovascular reserve capacity by EC-IC arterial bypass surgery in patients with ICA occlusion and hemodynamic cerebral ischemia. J Neurosurg 81: 236–244 (1994).
[66] Sekhar LN, Bucur SD, Bank WO, Wright DC: Venous and arterial bypass grafts for difficult tumors, aneurysms, and occlusive vascular lesions: evolution of surgical treatment and improved graft results. Neurosurgery 44: 1207–1223 (1999).
[67] Spetzler R, Chater N: Microvascular bypass surgery. Part 2: physiological studies. J Neurosurg 45: 508–513 (1976).
[68] Streefkerk HJ, Bremmer JP, Tulleken CA: The ELANA technique: high flow revascularization of the brain. Acta Neurochir Suppl 94: 143–148 (2005).
[69] Streefkerk HJ, Wolfs JF, Sorteberg W, Sorteberg AG, Tulleken CA: The ELANA technique: constructing a high flow bypass using a non-occlusive anastomosis on the ICA and a conventional anastomosis on the SCA in the treatment of a fusiform giant basilar trunk aneurysm. Acta Neurochir (Wien) 146: 1009–1019 (2004).
[70] Sunada I: [Measurement of cerebral blood flow by single photon emission computed tomography in cases of internal carotid artery occlusion]. Neurol Med Chir (Tokyo) 29: 496–502 (1989).
[71] Sundt TM Jr., Piepgras DG, Marsh WR, Fode NC: Saphenous vein bypass grafts for giant aneurysms and intracranial occlusive disease. J Neurosurg 65: 439–450 (1986).
[72] Sundt TM, III, Sundt TM Jr: Principles of preparation of vein bypass grafts to maximize patency. J Neurosurg 66: 172–180 (1987).
[73] Takagi Y, Hashimoto N, Iwama T, Hayashida K: Improvement of oxygen metabolic reserve after extracranial-intracranial bypass surgery in patients with severe haemodynamic insufficiency. Acta Neurochir (Wien) 139: 52–56 (1997).
[74] Tanahashi N, Meyer JS, Rogers RL, Kitagawa Y, Mortel KF, Kandula P, Levinthal R, Rose J: Long-term assessment of cerebral perfusion following STA-MCA by-pass in patients. Stroke 16: 85–91 (1985).
[75] Teksam M, McKinney A, Truwit CL: Multi-slice CT angiography in evaluation of extracranial-intracranial bypass. Eur J Radiol 52: 217–220 (2004).
[76] Thomas M, Hennerici M, Marshall J: Cerebral blood flow after carotid occlusion and extracranial-intracranial bypass. J Neurol Neurosurg Psychiatry 47: 148–152 (1984).
[77] Touho H, Karasawa J, Shishido H, Morisako T, Yamada K, Shibamoto K: Hemodynamic evaluation in patients with superficial temporal artery-middle cerebral artery anastomosis – stable xenon CT-CBF study and acetazolamide. Neurol Med Chir (Tokyo) 30: 1003–1010 (1990).
[78] Touho H, Karasawa J, Shishido H, Yamada K, Shibamoto K: Hemodynamic evaluation before and after the STA-MCA anastomosis – with special reference to measurement of regional transit time with intra-arterial digital subtraction angiography. Neurol Med Chir (Tokyo) 30: 663–669 (1990).
[79] Tsuchiya K, Aoki C, Katase S, Hachiya J, Shiokawa Y: Visualization of extracranial-intracranial bypass using multidetector-row helical computed tomography angiography. J Comput Assist Tomogr 27: 231–234 (2003).
[80] Tsuda Y, Kimura K, Iwata Y, Hayakawa T, Etani H, Fukunaga R, Yoneda S, Abe H: Improvement of cerebral blood flow and/or CO_2 reactivity after superficial temporal artery-middle cerebral artery bypass in patients with transient ischemic attacks and watershed-zone infarctions. Surg Neurol 22: 595–604 (1984).
[81] Tulleken CA, Verdaasdonk RM, Beck RJ, Mali WP: The modified excimer laser-assisted high-flow bypass operation. Surg Neurol 46: 424–429 (1996).

[82] van der ZA, Tulleken CA, Hillen B: Flow quantification of the non-occlusive excimer laser-assisted EC-IC bypass. Acta Neurochir (Wien) 143: 647–654 (2001).

[83] van Everdingen KJ, Klijn CJ, Kappelle LJ, Mali WP, van der GJ: MRA flow quantification in patients with a symptomatic internal carotid artery occlusion. The Dutch EC-IC Bypass Study Group. Stroke 28: 1595–1600 (1997).

[84] Vernieri F, Pasqualetti P, Matteis M, Passarelli F, Troisi E, Rossini PM, Caltagirone C, Silvestrini M: Effect of collateral blood flow and cerebral vasomotor reactivity on the outcome of carotid artery occlusion. Stroke 32: 1552–1558 (2001).

[85] Vorstrup S, Brun B, Lassen NA: Evaluation of the cerebral vasodilatory capacity by the acetazolamide test before EC-IC bypass surgery in patients with occlusion of the internal carotid artery. Stroke 17:1 291–1298 (1986).

[86] Vorstrup S, Lassen NA, Henriksen L, Haase J, Lindewald H, Boysen G, Paulson OB: CBF before and after extracranial-intracranial bypass surgery in patients with ischemic cerebrovascular disease studied with 133Xe-inhalation tomography. Stroke 16: 616–626 (1985).

[87] Webster MW, Makaroun MS, Steed DL, Smith HA, Johnson DW, Yonas H: Compromised cerebral blood flow reactivity is a predictor of stroke in patients with symptomatic carotid artery occlusive disease. J Vasc Surg 21: 338–344 (1995).

[88] Weinstein PR, Baena R, Chater NL: Results of extracranial-intracranial arterial bypass for intracranial internal carotid artery stenosis: review of 105 cases. Neurosurgery 15: 787–794 (1984).

[89] Widder B, Kleiser B, Krapf H: Course of cerebrovascular reactivity in patients with carotid artery occlusions. Stroke 25: 1963–1967 (1994).

[90] Wintermark M, Sesay M, Barbier E, Borbely K, Dillon WP, Eastwood JD, Glenn TC, Grandin CB, Pedraza S, Soustiel JF, Nariai T, Zaharchuk G, Caille JM, Dousset V, Yonas H: Comparative overview of brain perfusion imaging techniques. Stroke 36: e83–e99 (2005).

[91] Woitzik J, Horn P, Vajkoczy P, Schmiedek P: Intraoperative control of extracranial-intracranial bypass patency by near-infrared indocyanine green videoangiography. J Neurosurg 102: 692–698 (2005).

[92] Wood JH, Polyzoidis KS, Kee DB Jr., Prats AR, Gibby GL, Tindall GT: Augmentation of cerebral blood flow induced by hemodilution in stroke patients after superficial temporal-middle cerebral arterial bypass operation. Neurosurgery 15: 535–539 (1984).

[93] Yamashita T, Kashiwagi S, Nakano S, Takasago T, Abiko S, Shiroyama Y, Hayashi M, Ito H: The effect of EC-IC bypass surgery on resting cerebral blood flow and cerebrovascular reserve capacity studied with stable XE-CT and acetazolamide test. Neuroradiology 33: 217–222 (1991).

[94] Yamauchi H, Fukuyama H, Nagahama Y, Nabatame H, Ueno M, Nishizawa S, Konishi J, Shio H: Significance of increased oxygen extraction fraction in five-year prognosis of major cerebral arterial occlusive diseases. J Nucl Med 40: 1992–1998 (1999).

[95] Yanaka K, Fujita K, Noguchi S, Matsumaru Y, Asakawa H, Anno I, Meguro K, Nose T: Intraoperative angiographic assessment of graft patency during extracranial-intracranial bypass procedures. Neurol Med Chir (Tokyo) 43: 509–512 (2003).

[96] Yasargil MG: Microsurgery applied to Neurosurgery. New York, Academic Press (1969).

[97] Yokota C, Hasegawa Y, Minematsu K, Yamaguchi T: Effect of acetazolamide reactivity on [corrected] long-term outcome in patients with major cerebral artery occlusive diseases. Stroke 29: 640–644 (1998).

[98] Yonas H, Gur D, Good BC, Latchaw RE, Wolfson SK Jr., Good WF, Maitz GS, Colsher JG, Barnes JE, Colliander KG: Stable xenon CT blood flow mapping for evaluation of patients with extracranial-intracranial bypass surgery. J Neurosurg 62: 324–333 (1985).

[99] Yonekura M, Austin G, Hayward W: Long-term evaluation of cerebral blood flow, transient ischemic attacks, and stroke after STA-MCA anastomosis. Surg Neurol 18: 123–130 (1982).

IMAGING AFTER SURGICAL THROMBENDARTERECTOMY OF THE CAROTID ARTERY

H. Katano and K. Yamada

Departments of Neurosurgery and Restorative Neuroscience and Medical Informatics and Integrative Medicine, Nagoya City University Graduate School of Medical Sciences, Nagoya, Japan

Introduction

Though there have been many descriptions of the preoperative evaluation of carotid stenosis and responsible plaques using digital subtraction angiography (DSA), computed tomography (CT), magnetic resonance imaging (MRI), and the like, few reports can be found concerning postoperative evaluation. For postoperative studies in cases of carotid endarterectomy (CEA), the following factors should be considered. First, for the depiction of amelioration of carotid stenosis and the reduction or diminishment of carotid plaques in comparison with preoperative pictures, it is thought to be necessary to delineate and evaluate the lesions correctly before surgery. Second, for repeat examinations in an outpatient clinic, diagnostic modalities should be less invasive and non-discomforting as well as cost-effective for patients during postoperative follow-up. Third, high performance and high-resolution imaging should be used in order to depict and detect restenosis of the carotid artery, which may occur within several years postoperatively.

In this chapter, imaging after CEA with DSA, 3D-CTA, MRA, and duplex US is presented, discussing advantages and disadvantages of the modalities in focus with these points. We particularly stress the current usefulness of 3D-CTA by multi-detector helical CT (MDCT) with fine reconstruction and promising future in MR angiography.

Digital subtraction angiography (DSA)

Conventional arterial angiography has been the gold standard in evaluating the extent of carotid stenosis (Fig. 3a), the presence of ulceration and collateral flow to the affected cerebral hemisphere. However, this approach is invasive, relatively expensive and discomforting to patients. Complications with conventional angiography using a catheter were reported to arise with an incidence of 1.2% preoperatively and 2.7% in the whole perioperative course in a study of asymptomatic carotid atherosclerosis [2], [3]. These figures cannot be overlooked, considering that the risk of stroke morbidity and mortality from CEA itself is 1.52% (11/724, ACAS). Some authors have argued that the stroke risk due to conventional angiography in recently symptomatic patients is probably only about 0.5%, because most studies classified all strokes that occurred within 24 hours of angiography as procedural complications [9], [28]. However, even 0.5% can be considered clinically meaningful, because aspirin is routinely given after acute ischemic stroke to save approximately 1% of patients [9]. Moreover, conventional angiography provides poor information preoperatively about the presence of calcification on vessel walls and the composition of plaques.

Therefore, regarding postoperative evaluation, except in special cases (e.g., where some factors might make the use of alternate modalities impossible), the routine use of conventional angiography may not be appropriate as a first choice in follow-up studies for patients after CEA, who are usually free from symptoms.

3D-CT angiography

Three-dimensional computed tomography angiography (3D-CTA) has been developed and utilized in the visualization of various cerebral lesions, especially after the advent of multidetector helical CT (MDCT) [16], [18]. Some authors have found it very useful for the depiction of carotid lesions, with advantages over selective angiography [8], [24], [26], [31], MRA and ultrasound sonography (US) [7], [29]. Patients are subjected to minimal discomfort and remarkable spatial representation is possible. The technique thus allows information to be rapidly obtained about the vessel lumen, wall and surrounding structures, with low radiation exposure and at relatively little cost. Recently, neck-clipping operations for ruptured aneurysms have been performed solely with aid of 3D-CTA in many institutes [22].

If 3D-CTA is to be promoted as an alternative to conventional angiography, it is necessary to confirm the match in information gained from the two approaches. In fact, 3D-CTA allows better visualization of structures, facilitating spatial comprehension by three-dimensional reconstruction. Cumming et al. [8] compared images of 3D-CTA by single detector helical CT with conventional images, and found the degree of carotid artery stenosis to correlate with that shown in conventional angiograms. Corti et al. [7] demonstrated the utility of 3D-CTA as a complementary diagnostic tool to duplex US. Sameshima et al. [29] similarly described the benefits

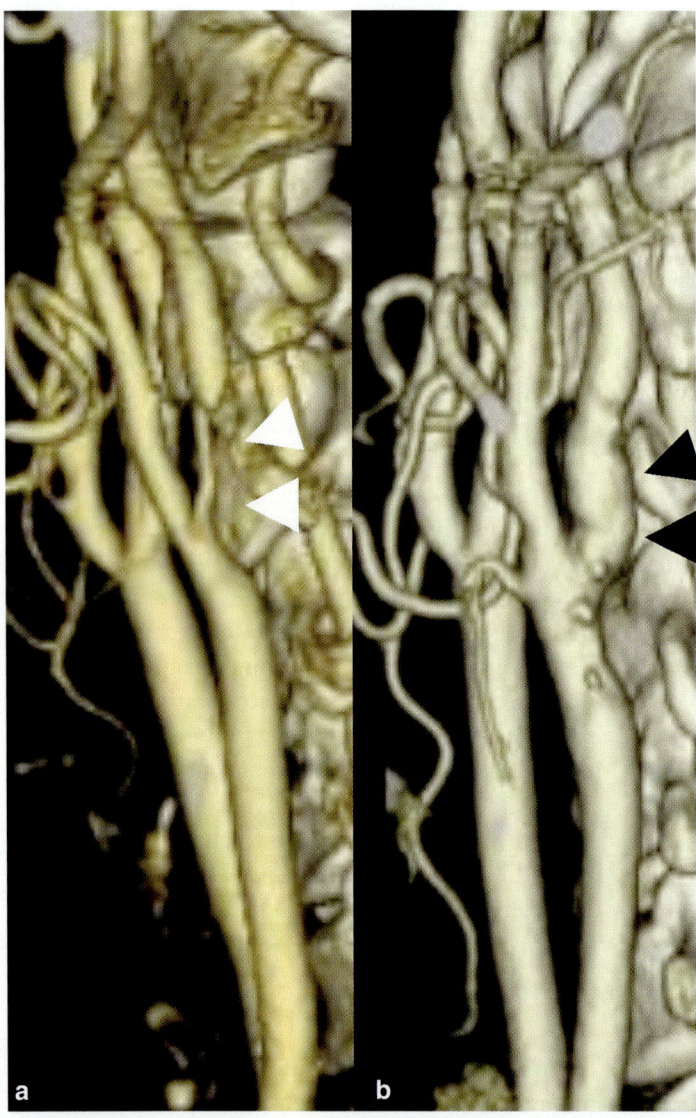

Fig. 1. a Representative 3D-CTA volume rendering (VR) image obtained by multi-detector helical (MD) CT reconstructed with a high-performance workstation showing a severe left carotid stenosis (arrowheads); **b** Representative VR image after CEA showing remarkable improvement of stenosis (arrowheads).

of 3D-CTA in combination with duplex US, MR and conventional angiography. The authors of this paper have employed a high-performance workstation to produce sophisticated reconstructed color images [15] (Fig. 1).

In addition to the accuracy of images, advantages of 3D-CTA as an alternative to conventional angiography are that it is non-invasive and non-discomforting for patients, and that examination is rapid and relatively low in cost. Recent 32 or 64-row MDCT enables rapid scans to be made with low radiation doses and less contrast medium at higher spatial resolution and over a wider scanning area.

In our own postoperative evaluation, amelioration of stenosis of carotid arteries (Figs. 1b, 3d, 4b) and disappearance of calcifications on walls were clearly and unambiguously depicted in 3D images.

It is still a matter of some controversy what imaging technique is most suitable for depiction of carotid stenosis in 3D-CTA. Maximal intensity projection (MIP) displays an angiogram-like image, and Sameshima et al. [29] described a high correlation between the degrees of stenosis estimated by MIP images done with 3D-CTA and conventional angiography. Some investigators have reported that MIP is also useful in the delineation of calcification and ulceration on vessel walls [26], [31]. Corti et al. [7] recently documented that curvilinear reconstructed multiplanar reconstruction (MPR) images allow vessel wall calcification to be ignored, rendering precise definition of the lumen. Hirai et al. [13] applied cross-sectional MPR images perpendicular to the longitudinal axis of the carotid artery and showed the benefits of obtaining information about luminal morphology. Tarján et al. [32] stressed the importance of the calcification-removal process in luminal evaluation and sufficient visualization by Raysum (transparent pseudoradiograph) but not MIP images. Leclerc et al. [20] reported that MIP images enabled correct classification of most stenoses but that mural calcification constitutes a drawback, while the volume rendering (VR) technique may be useful when dense calcifications were located around the residual lumen. A vessel phantom study revealed that MIP, MPR, shaded surface display (SSD), VR and axial views all accurately display vessels and stenoses greater than 4 mm in diameter, whereas with smaller diameters VR tended to be more accurate [4]. In our cases, VR images were useful for evaluating the degree of stenosis and for the detection of calcification and ulceration. However, in a severe stenotic case that showed discontinuities on VR images, MIP was useful in confirming continuity and estimating the degree of stenosis. With both techniques, observation with continuous rotation of images for 360º was of great assistance in selecting the strongest stenotic image. A case of inverted internal and external carotid artery misdiagnosed as common carotid artery stenosis by conventional angiography could thereby be clarified. It is possible that even conventional angiography might have provided the correct diagnosis if examination had been performed from various angles using additional contrast media and radiation. In 3D-CTA, however, a mere 10-cm movement of the computer mouse can facilitate a correct diagnosis. MIP was useful in detecting calcification, especially when it was located dorsally to the carotid bifurcation and when coloring resulted in an appearance similar to that of enhanced vessels due to the density of contrast media in the lumen. Evaluation of carotid stenosis by 3D-CTA should optimally be achieved with complementary usage of VR, MIP, MPR and axial images. Motion and metallic artifacts are problems to be considered in applying 3D-CTA instead of conventional angiography. A dental apparatus may induce artifacts and interfere with evaluation of carotid bifurcations, especially when the location is high. This can be overcome, however, by tilting the head back in the supine position during CT scanning.

A few concerns remain in using 3D-CTA based CEA without selective angiography. The necessity of using contrast media, as with conventional angiography, is still a problem. Allergic reactions may occur and injecting 90 ml of contrast media in 3–4 ml/sec may be hazardous to patients at risk of heart or renal failure. Though evaluation with alternative modalities such as MRA is needed in such cases, most postoperative examinations with 3DCTA seemed to provide excellent information and be sufficient as the sole follow up study.

MR imaging and angiography

While MR angiography itself can be applied in the assessment of carotid stenosis, there is a tendency for overestimation, and good depiction of calcification is not possible, though a recent study using 3D-FISP (fast imaging with steady-state free precession) showed better axial delineation of the content of atheromatous plaques [6]. Three-D acquisitions have much better resolution due to the small partition thickness, while 2D acquisition is more sensitive to slow flow [30]. Usually the white blood technique is based on time of flight (TOF) or phase contrast methods, while black-blood MR imaging techniques [33], [35] depicting the character of the plaque clearly with phase array carotid coils employs 2D fast spin echo (FSE). Contrast-enhanced MR angiography (CEMRA [11] or DSA-MRA [21]) may also augment the accuracy in the assessment of the degree of carotid artery stenosis. Hathout et al. [12] reported that increasing severity of stenosis as measured by CEMRA corresponded to increasing severity at DSA, while Nederkoorn et al. [23] demonstrated in a systematic review of published studies that MRA had more than 70% more discriminatory power compared with duplex US in diagnosing severe stenosis. Thus, techniques in MR angiography (both acquisition techniques and high magnetic field) are constantly advancing, and considering its advantages in enabling exploration without X-ray, it may surpass CTA in the near future as an appropriate tool for postoperative serial follow-up studies (Figs. 2b, c, 3b).

Duplex ultrasound sonography

Duplex US is a handy, non-invasive technique ideal for a postoperative follow up study in outpa-

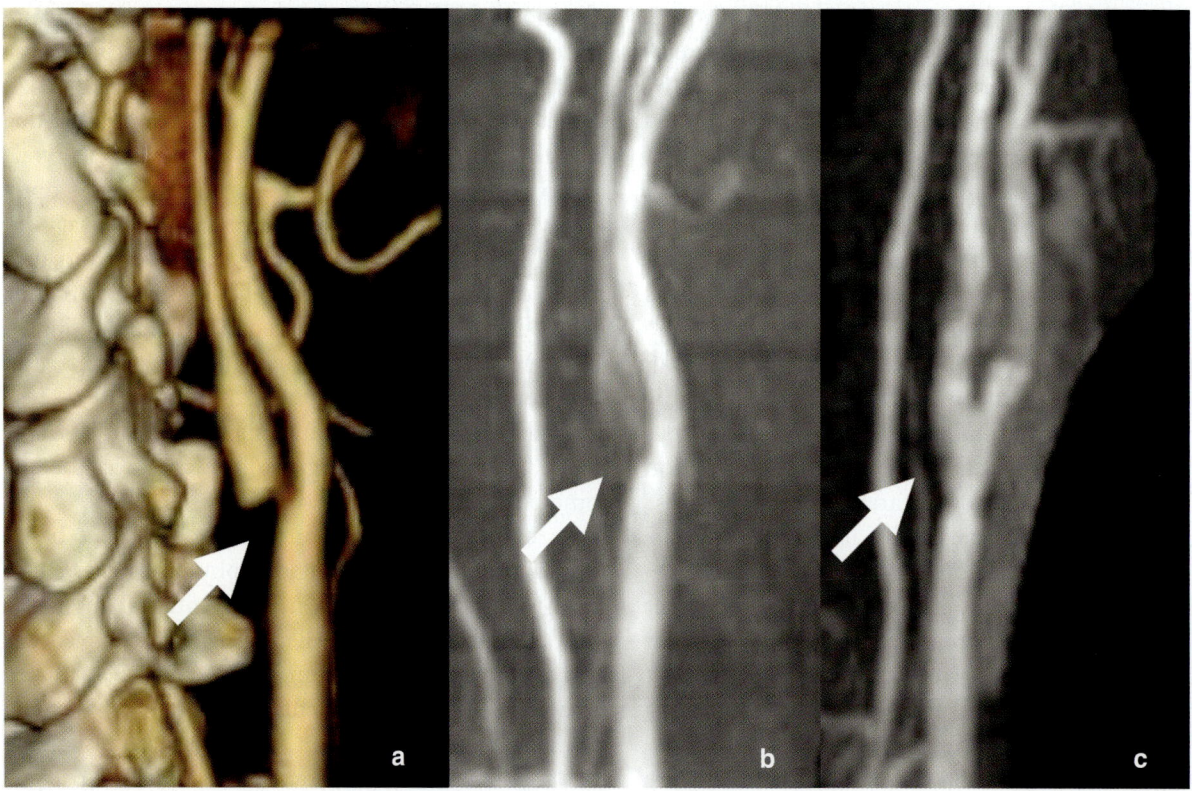

Fig. 2. a Representative VR image of a right carotid stenosis by MDCT demonstrating severe stenosis at carotid bifurcation (arrow); **b** Maximal intensity projection (MIP) image of MRA showing stenosis (arrow); **c** Postoperative MRA depicting amelioration of stenosis (arrow).

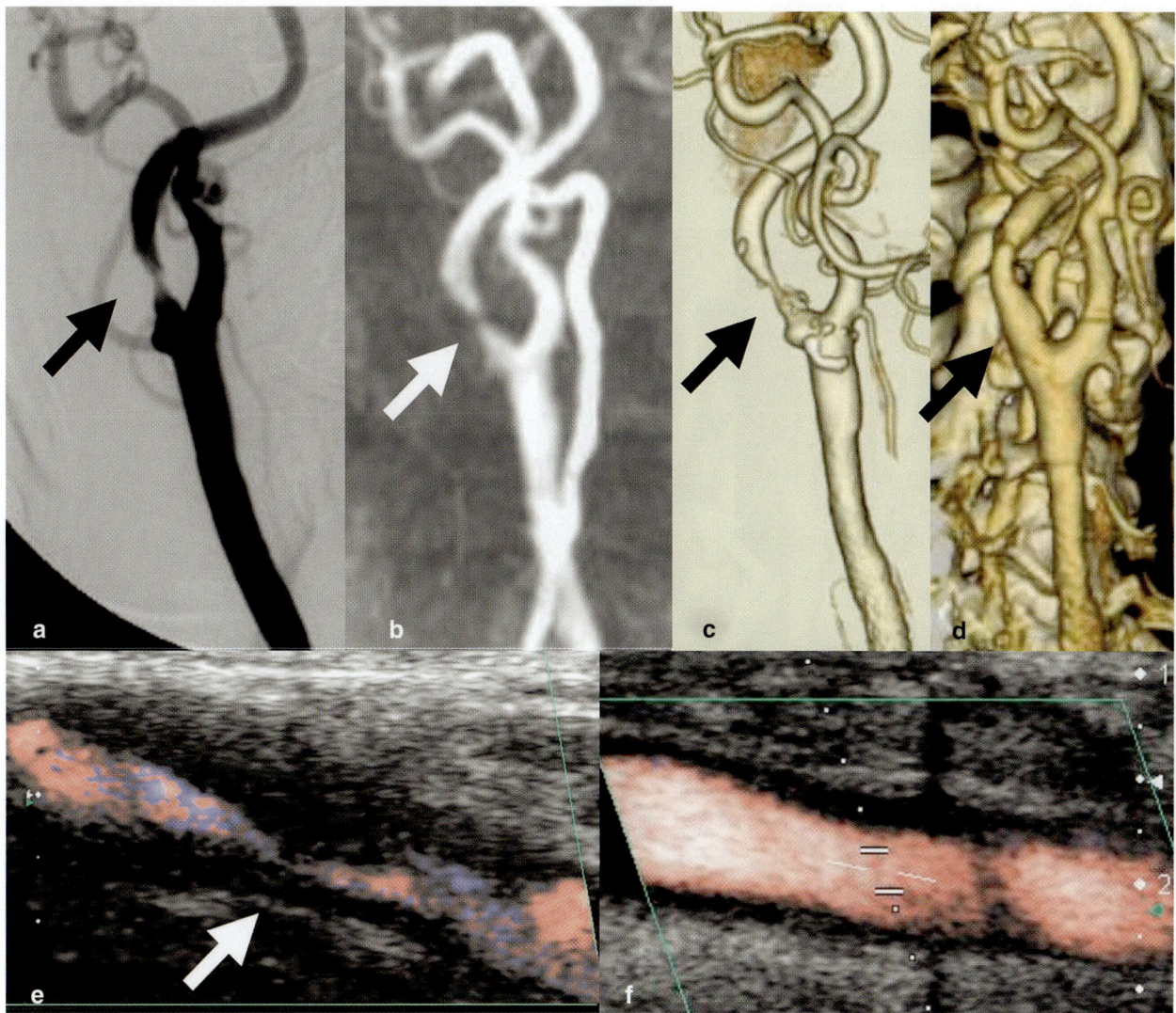

Fig. 3. a Representative conventional angiography of a right carotid bifurcation showing stenosis of the internal carotid artery (arrow); **b** MIP image of MRA of the same case showing stenosis (arrow); **c** VR image of 3D-CTA clearly showing internal carotid artery stenosis (arrow); **d** VR image of 3D-CTA after CEA showing dilation of the stenotic portion (arrow); **e** Power color doppler duplex ultrasound (US) showing apparent stenosis. CEA showing dilation of the stenotic portion (arrow); **f** Power color doppler duplex ultrasound (US) showing apparent stenosis. CEA showing dilation of the stenotic portion.

tient clinics. No other modality can detect floating thrombus or characterize plaque containing hemorrhage and ulceration in real time, and recent color-coded duplex US has remarkably improved the identification of vascular structures [30] (Fig. 3e, f). This ultrasound method, however, seems technician- and machine-dependent, and its representation has relatively low spatial resolution, especially in cases with short neck and high carotid bifurcation [7]. Duplex US also presents difficulties in the precise depiction of vessels with calcified lesions, due to shadowing. Rothwell [28] documented the results of a metaanalysis and concluded that duplex US could not substitute for conventional angiography as the sole modality for pre-CEA imaging [27], [28], since 28% of the decisions about CEA based on duplex US alone were inappropriate. Nevertheless, in postoperative evaluation, improvement of stenosis can be observed by duplex US, at least in preoperatively well-depicted cases. Naturally, complementary usage of duplex US with other modalities would enhance the accuracy. Nonent et al. [25] reported that the concordance rate for the degree of carotid stenosis of duplex US/CEMRA was significantly higher than that with other combinations of noninvasive imaging

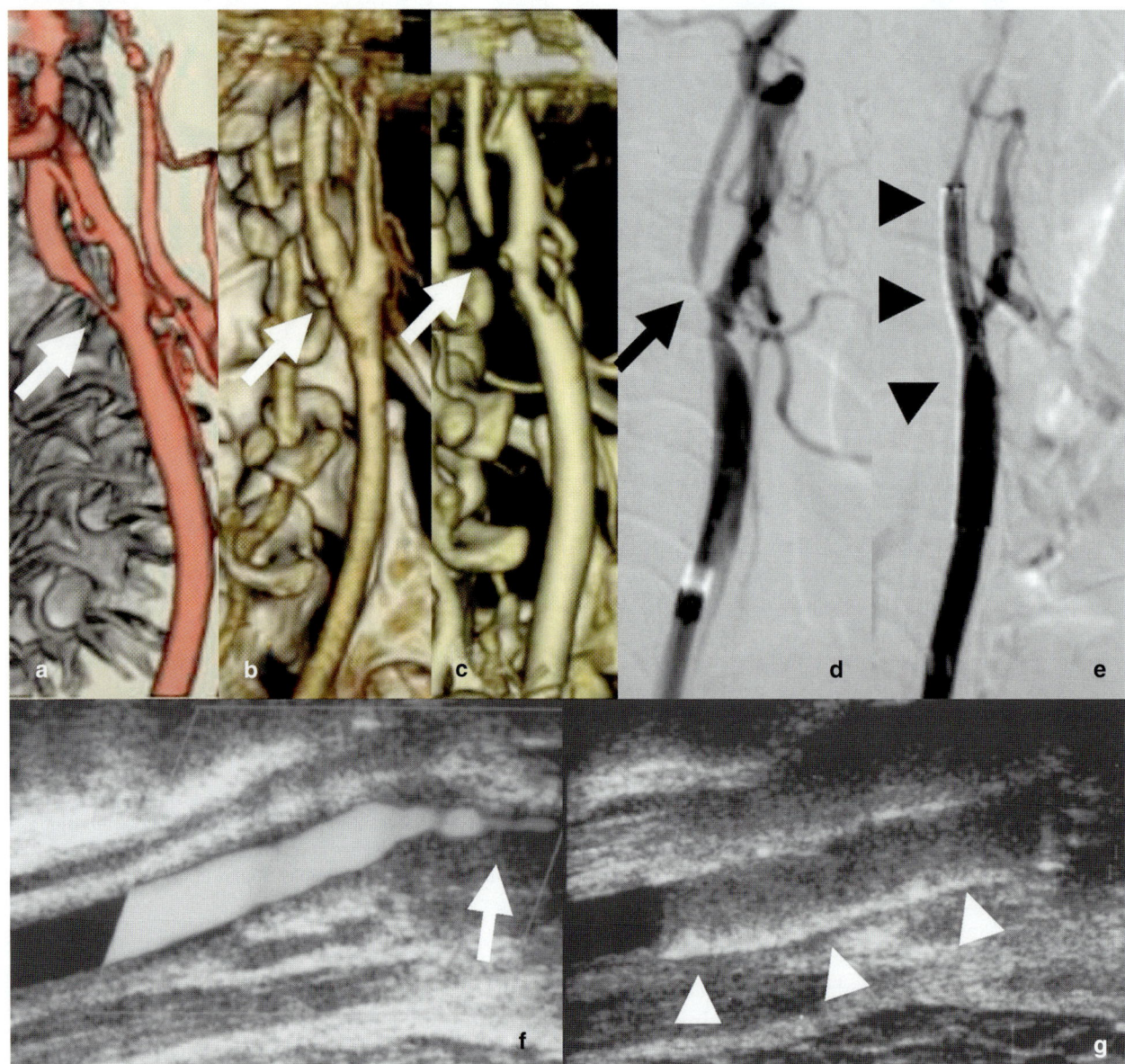

Fig. 4. a Preoperative VR image of right carotid stenosis showing severe stenosis at the bifurcation (arrow); **b** VR image of the same case after CEA showing improvement of stenosis (arrow); **c** VR image of carotid stenosis 10 months after CEA demonstrating re-stenosis (arrow); **d** Conventional angiography showing re-stenosis of internal carotid artery; **e** Conventional angiography depicting improvement of re-stenosis of internal carotid artery with carotid artery stenting (arrowheads); **f** Duplex US image of carotid stenosis 10 months after CEA showing re-stenosis; **g** Duplex US image of carotid artery after stenting showing amelioration of the re-stenosis (arrowheads).

techniques, though they did not employ MDCT for 3DCTA.

Detection of restenosis of carotid artery

Restenoses of carotid arteries after CEA are usually divided into two groups; those experienced within a few years after CEA due to myointimal hyperplasia and others within several postsurgical years due to the relapse of atherosclerotic plaques [19]. Reoperations are reported to range from 1.8 to 8.9% of all CEA cases [1], [10], [27]. Kogure et al. [17] reported that restenosis occurred in 6.7% of 135 CEA cases, while Yamada et al. [34] experienced 5 restenoses in 122 CEAs (4.1%). Restenoses are often observed at the edges of original plaques, especially on the proximal side of the common carotid artery, rather than at the site of the initial stenosis. It is well known that restenoses are more often encountered with women [1]. Patients with slight to moderate restenoses tend to be followed up with non-invasive imagings such as duplex US, MRA and 3DCTA in outpatient clinics, and severe and symptomatic stenoses lead to surgical re-intervention. In such cases, 3DCTA is also useful in providing a clear and accurate view of carotid arteries, either with VR or MIP images. As tissue adhesion makes re-CEA difficult, with relatively high morbidity, carotid angioplasty and stenting (CAS) is currently preferred and applied for the treatment of restenosis (Fig. 4e,g). Since depiction after stenting is also excellent with 3DCTA, it can be a powerful tool for the evaluation of re-stenosis, regardless of surgical options.

Conclusions (Take home messages)

Though DSA remains the gold standard in some facilities in follow up studies after CEA, its use is declining due to the complications it presents and to the development of other diagnostic modalities. Three-D CTA with a high-performance workstation provides detailed images with satisfactory information, though it also presents the problems of X-ray exploration and allergic reaction to contrast media. Duplex US is a handy, non-invasive, real-time technique, but is limited due to its operator dependency and low resolution. MR angiography is promising, though it is still being developed at present. By providing greater accuracy both in the assessment of the degree of stenoses and in the characterization of plaque contents, and with the important advantage of being less invasive, since it is a non-X-ray examination, MRA may well obtain preeminence in the postoperative follow up study of carotid endarterectomy.

References

[1] AbuRahma AF, Snodgrass KR, Robinson PA et al.: Safety and durability of redo carotid endarterectomy for recurrent carotid artery stenosis. Am J Surg 168: 175–178 (1994).

[2] Executive Committee for the Asymptomatic Carotid Atherosclerosis (ACAS) Study: Endarterectomy for asymptomatic carotid artery stenosis. JAMA 273: 1421–1428 (1995).

[3] The Asymptomatic Carotid sclerosis Study Group: Clinical advisory: endarterectomy for patients with asymptomatic internal carotid artery stenosis. Stroke 25: 2523–2524 (1994).

[4] Addis KA, Hopper KD, Lyriboz TA et al.: CT angiography: In vitro comparison of five reconstruction methods. AJR 177: 1171–1176 (2001).

[5] Blakeley DD, Oddone EZ, Hasselblad V, Simel DL, Matchar DB: Noninvasive carotid artery testing. Ann Intern Med 122: 360–365 (1995).

[6] Coombs BD, Rapp JH, Ursell PC et al.: Structure of plaque at carotid bifurcation. High-resolution MRI with histological correlation. Stroke 32: 2516–2521 (2001).

[7] Corti R, Ferrari C, Roberti M et al.: A novel diagnostic approach for investigation of the extracranial cerebral arteries and its complementary role in duplex ultrasonography. Circulation 98: 984–989 (1998).

[8] Cumming MJ, Morrow IM: Carotid artery stenosis: A prospective comparison of CT angiography and conventional angiography. AJR 163: 517–523 (1994).

[9] Davis SM, Donnan GA: Is carotid angiography necessary? Editors disagree. Stroke 34: 1819 (2003).

[10] Gagne PJ, Riles TS, Jacobowits GR et al.: Long-term followup of patients undergoing reoperation for recurrent carotid artery disease. J Vasc Surg 18: 991–1001 (1993).

[11] Goyal M, Nicol J, Gandhi D: Evaluation of carotid artery stenosis: contrast-enhanced magnetic resonance angiography compared with conventional digital sub-

traction angiography. Can Assoc Radiol J 55: 111–119 (2004).
[12] Hathout GM, Duh MJ, El-Saden M: Accuracy of contrast-enhanced MR angiography in predicting angographic stenosis of the internal carotid artery: Linear regression analysis. AJNR 24: 1747–1756 (2003).
[13] Hirai T, Korogi Y, Ono K et al.: Maximum stenosis of extracranial internal carotid artery: Effect of luminal morphology on stenosis measurement by using CT angiography and conventional DSA. Radiology 221: 802–809 (2001).
[14] Johnston DC, Goldstein LB: Clinical carotid endarterectomy decision making: noninvasive vascular imaging versus cerebral angiography. Neurology 56: 1009–1015 (2001).
[15] Katano H, Kato K, Umemura A et al.: Perioperative evaluation of carotid endarterectomy by 3D-CT angiography with refined reconstruction: Preliminary experience of CEA without conventional angiography. Br J Neurosurg 18: 138–148 (2004).
[16] Kato Y, Nair S, Sano H et al.: Multi-slice 3D-CTA-an improvement over single slice helical CTA for cerebral aneurysms. Acta Neurochir 144: 715–722 (2002).
[17] Kogure S, Sakai N, Murao K et al.: Restenosis after CEA: Pathogenesis and treatment. No Shinkei Geka 30: 1303–1312 (2002).
[18] Korogi Y, Takahashi M, Katada K et al.: Intracranial aneurysms: Detection with three-dimensional CT with volume rendering; comparison with conventional angiographic and surgical findings. Radiology 211: 497–506 (1999).
[19] Lattimer CR, Burnand KG: Recurrent carotid stenosis after carotid endarterectomy. Br J Surg 84: 1206–1219 (1997).
[20] Leclerc X, Godefroy O, Lucas C et al.: Internal carotid arterial stenosis: CT angiography with volume rendering. Radiology 210: 673–682 (1999).
[21] Levy R, Prince MR: Arterial-phase three-dimensiional contrast-enhanced MR angiography of the carotid arteries. Am J Roentgenol 167: 211–215 (1996).
[22] Matsumoto M, Sato M, Nakano M: Three-dimensional computerized tomography angiography-guided surgery of acutely ruptured cerebral aneurysms. J Neurosurg 94: 718–727 (2001).
[23] Nederkoorn PJ, van der Graaf Y, Hunink M: Duplex ultrasound and magnetic resonance angiography compared with digital subtraction angiography in carotid arter stenosis. A systematic review. Stroke 34: 1324–1332 (2003).
[24] Nomura M, Katada K, Anno H et al.: Clinical usefulness of helical-scanning CT for the evaluation of arteriosclerotic carotid lesions. Nippon Acta Radiologica 55: 878–884 (1995).
[25] Nonent M, Serfaty J-M, Nighoghossian N et al.: Concordance rate differences of 3 noninvasive imaging techniques to measure carotid stenosis in clinical routine practice. Results of the CARMEDAS multicenter study. Stroke 35: 682–686 (2004).
[26] Ohtaki M, Tanabe S, Uede T et al.: Evaluation of carotid artery stenosis with three-dimensional CT angiography and surgical revascularization. Neurol Surg 24: 995–1002 (1996).
[27] Ouriel K, Green RM: Appropriate frequency of carotid duplex testing following carotid endarterectomy. Am J Surg 170: 144–147 (1995).
[28] Rothwell PM: For severe carotid stenosis found on ultrasound, further arterial evaluation prior to carotid endarterectomy is unnecessary: The argument against. Stroke 34: 1817–1819 (2003).
[29] Sameshima T, Futami S, Morita Y et al.: Clinical usefulness of and problems with three-dimensional CT angiography for the evaluation of arteriosclerotic stenosis of the carotid artery: comparison with conventional angiography, MRA, and ultrasound sonography. Surg Neurol 51: 300–309 (1999).
[30] Simonetti G, Bozzao A, Floris R et al.: Non-invasive assessment of neck-vessel pathology. Eur Radiol 8: 691–697 (1998).
[31] Takamura Y, Tanooka A, Morimoto S: Usefulness of three-dimensional CT angiography (3D-CTA) with a single bolus injection of contrast material for the examination of intracranial and cervical arteries in cerebrovascular disease screening. Neurol Surg 29: 401–406 (2001).
[32] Tarján Z, Mucelli FP, Frezza F et al.: Three-dimensional reconstructions of carotid bifurcation from CT images: evaluation of different rendering methods. Eur Radiol 6: 326–333 (1996).
[33] U-King-Im JM, Trivedi RA, Sala E et al.: Evaluation of carotid stenosis with axial high-resolution black-blood MR imaging. Eur Radiol 14: 1154–1161 (2004)
[34] Yamada K, Kishiguchi T, Ito M et al.: Restenosis following carotid endarterectomy. Clinical profiles and pathological findings. Neurol Med Chir (Suppl) (Tokyo) 38: 284–288 (1998).
[35] Zhang S, Hatsukami TS, Polissar NL et al.: Comparison of carotid vessel wall area measurements using three different contrast-weighted black blood MR imaging techniques. Magn Reson Imaging 19: 795–802 (2001).

Chapter 4.3

IMAGING AFTER CAROTID STENTING

G. M. Biasi, A. Froio, and G. Deleo

Department of Surgical Sciences and Intensive Care, University of Milano-Bicocca, Vascular Surgery Unit, San Gerardo Hospital, Monza, Italy

Introduction

The effectiveness of carotid endarterectomy (CEA) in the prevention of stroke in symptomatic and asymptomatic patients with carotid stenosis has been demonstrated by several randomized studies (Ferguson et al. 1999; Halliday et al. 2004; MRC European Carotid Surgery Trial 1991; ECACAS 1995). Carotid artery stenting (CAS) is an alternative technique that gives favorable results when associated with the use of brain protection devices (BPD) (Cremonesi et al. 2003).

Recent randomized studies tend to demonstrate the non-inferiority of carotid artery stenting (CAS) compared to carotid endarterectomy for the treatment of carotid stenosis [65]. Nevertheless, a review of the randomized evidence does not support changes in clinical practice, apart from recommending carotid endarterectomy as the treatment of choice for suitable carotid artery stenosis [13].

Several ongoing randomized trials are now comparing CEA with CAS in order to establish the gold standard in the prevention of stroke and the results are expected to be published in 4 or 5 years time [28].

Even though it is generally accepted that the composition and the characteristics of the plaque may influence the outcome of CEA and CAS, especially in the case of CAS in which the plaque is not removed but remodeled, indications for either one of the two procedures are mostly based (both in trial and in clinical practice) on the percentage of stenosis and the presence or absence of pre-procedural neurological symptoms, whereas the features of the plaque are somehow disregarded if not ignored. The reason for this is related to the fact that the percentage of stenosis, as well as the presence or absence of symptoms is easy to identify and quantify, whereas the plaque is usually defined as soft, lipidic, fibrolipidic, hemorrhagic, colliquated, ulcerated, pretty homogeneous, etc., which makes the parameter rather undetermined and unreliable.

The advent of high-resolution B-mode scanners and the use of a quantitative, computer-assisted index of echogenicity (such as gray scale median [GSM]) introduced by our team, have greatly improved the correlation between plaque characterization and clinical features [7], [8]. Only after the introduction of the image normalization did the GSM become an objective index of the echogenicity of carotid plaques [18], [50].

Several studies recently indicated that echogenicity is related to the histological components of carotid plaque [17], [26] and that carotid plaque echolucency (low echogenicity) is associated with the development of neurologic events [47], [25], [39], [42] and with an increased number of emboli following CEA and CAS [46], [57], [27].

Based on these assumptions, our group demonstrated in the ICAROS study that carotid plaque echolucency measured by GSM increases the risk of stroke during CAS [6]. For the first time an ultra-sonographic characteristic of the plaque has been correlated to the clinical outcome *during* CAS.

Two issues concerning ultrasound and CAS remain unsolved:

1. Are there echographic characteristics of the carotid plaque that can be recognized before the procedure and that modify the clinical outcome *after* the procedure?
2. Is the duplex scanner accurate for the follow-up of patients treated with carotid stenting?

Clinical knowledge

Surveillance after CAS: Why?

The incidence of restenosis after CAS has been recently reviewed [26]. The incidence of restenoses within 2 years after CAS was 7.5% using a restenosis threshold ≥ 50% and 4% using a cut-off point of 70%. The risk of recurrent stenosis after CAS seems to be greater in the first year after the procedure and then decreases over time. Neointimal proliferation prevailed up to 12 months after CAS in a recent prospective duplex ultrasound study, whereas no further relevant changes in the neointima were observed during the second year [62].

Surveillance after CAS: How?

The analysis of in-stent restenosis has been performed using several approaches, including digital subtraction angiography (DSA), computed tomography angiography (CTA), magnetic resonance angiography (MRA) and duplex ultra-sound.

DSA provides the most reliable analysis of carotid stenosis, both in primitive and in restenotic lesions but the effectiveness of this diagnostic tool is limited by three factors:

- A peri-procedural risk of neurological complications. Patients in ACAS who underwent DSA before carotid endarterectomy were exposed to an additional 1.2% risk of stroke [1].
- DSA is related to silent embolism, as demonstrated by 23% of new lesions at diffusion-weighted magnetic resonance imaging after DSA, without any neurological complication [4]. Due to relationship between silent embolism and late neurological sequelae, DSA could be a cause of late cognitive dysfunction in patients with a history of vasculopathy [60].
- The economical impact: a cost-effectiveness analysis showed that arteriogram accounted for an increase of 43% in total charges [21].

The presence of these issues and the availability of new diagnostic tools pushed some Authors to consider DSA as a low-efficacy diagnostic tool [32], [11]. The debate is still open [15].

CTA is an emerging technique for the evaluation of carotid arterial stenosis [35]. For detection of a 70% to 99% stenosis, the sensitivity was 85% and the specificity was 93%. For detection of an occlusion, the sensitivity and specificity were 97% and 99%, respectively. Only a few papers have analyzed the role of multi-slice CTA in the detection of post-CAS restenosis [12], [38]. Further study is required to confirm the accuracy of this emerging technique.

MRA has the potential to replace diagnostic DSA, due to elevated sensitivity, specificity, positive predictive value and negative predictive value in the diagnosis of carotid stenosis [3], [22], [63]. Nevertheless, the effectiveness of MRA after CAS might be limited by technical issues: stent-related artifacts on contrast-enhanced MR angiography caused an artificial lumen narrowing and a reduction of the signal intensity within the stent. Both of these effects were identified in MR angiogram of nitinol stents and stainless steel stents [58]. Several months after stent implantation, visibility of the stent lumen was improved and diagnostic reliability of contrast-enhanced MR angiography was markedly increased. A probable explanation for this phenomenon might be the formation of a neointimal layer covering the stent struts and thereby reducing stent-related artifacts [9].

Systolic and diastolic flow parameters in the internal carotid artery (ICA) and common carotid artery (CCA) should be measured, as well as carotid ratios. This hemodynamic evaluation of carotid stenosis based on velocity cut-off points, should be used to calculate the degree of stenosis corresponding to the NASCET angiographic criteria [44], [45], [23].

The placement of a stent alters the biomechanical properties of the artery and reduces its compliance, leading to elevated velocity. Robbin studied the use of US in the follow-up of stented carotid arteries and noted that US sensitivity in the detection of intrastent stenosis is promising but further study is required [49]. Similarly, Ringer reviewed their experience with US immediately after carotid stent placement, and concluded that strict US criteria for restenosis after CAS are less reliable than change in velocity over time. An immediate post-stenting Doppler study should be obtained to serve as a reference value for future follow-up evaluation [48].

Lal demonstrated that US velocity measurements are elevated in many patients after stent placement and that velocity criteria designed to evaluate disease in native unstented arteries should be revised for application in these patients [36]. It has been shown that PSV 150 cm/s or greater in combination with an ICA/CCA ratio 2.16 or greater provides optimal sensitivity (100%), specificity (97.6%), PPV (75%), NPV (100%), and accuracy (97.7%) for differentiating 0% to 19% and 20% or greater ICA in-stent residual stenosis after CAS.

The US thresholds used to identify a restenosis were different: 50%, 70% or 80%. The ultrasound criteria to identify these thresholds were different:

- Modified University of Wisconsin criteria [19]: peak systolic velocity (PSV) less than 130 cm/s, 0% to 39%; PSV 130 to 210 cm/s, 40% to 59%; PSV 210 to 300 cm/s with end-diastolic velocity less than 120 cm/s, 60% to 79%; PSV greater than 300 cm/s and end- diastolic velocity greater than 120 cm/s, or internal carotid to common carotid artery systolic velocity ratio greater than 3.2, 80% to 99% [37].
- PSV > 140 cm/s to define > 50% stenosis by carotid ultrasound [33].
- A combination of PSV_{ICA} greater than 1.5 m/sec and a PSV_{ICA}/PSV_{CCA} ratio greater than 2.5 to identify an in-stent restenosis of 50% or greater [52].
- $PSV \geq 120$ cm/s and PSV_{ICA}/PSV_{CCA} ratio ≥ 1.5 for stenoses > 50%. Stenoses > 70% were diagnosed by $PSV \geq 220$ cm/s and PSV_{ICA}/PSV_{CCA} ratio ≥ 3.3 [5].
- $PSV \geq 130$ cm/s for stenoses > 50%. $PSV \geq 210$ cm/s and PSV_{ICA}/PSV_{CCA} ratio ≥ 4.0 for stenoses > 70% [43].

Morevoer, echographic examination allows to perform a morphological analysis. The following clinical case will shed light on this issue.

A 77-year-old asymptomatic man with a sub-occlusive ulcerated plaque of the right internal carotid artery underwent a stenting procedure under general anesthesia in a neuro-radiologist center (Fig. 1a and b).

The procedure was completed without neurological complications and with a technical success, as evidenced at the post-operative angiogram (Fig. 1c).

One month after the procedure an ultrasound examination was performed in our vascular lab. (Fig. 1d) The peak systolic velocity (PSV) was in the normal range, the ratio of the PSV of the ICA compared to that of the CCA was nearly 1. No restenosis could be demonstrated according to the velocitometric criteria. A physician could be satisfied looking at this data.

The morphological analysis allowed us to identify some technical issues, neither visible at the post-procedural angiogram nor using the velocity cut-off points of the duplex scanner examination. The stent diameter at the proximal end was lower than the diameter of the common carotid artery, this undersizing of the stent did not allow to cover the entire plaque. The consequence is that the plaque, with its inflammatory burden, is still there, prone to embolization.

A similar case is represented in Fig. 2a and b. In Fig. 3a–d it is clearly shown why carotid plaque calcification has been considered a contraindication to endovascular treatment. All these details could not be recognized by conventional angiography. Carotid ultrasound allows to see both inside (the "angiography point of view") and outside the vessel, where the plaque is remodeled.

Negative and positive remodeling are important predictors of clinical outcome after coronary stenting [14], [51], [29]. Only ultrasound can accurately quantify these parameters [10].

Surveillance after CAS: Who?

It has been demonstrated that patients with excessive neointimal formation more frequently suffered major adverse cardiovascular events (MACE, including myocardial infarction, stroke and death) compared to those with normal neointimal formation (61% vs. 16% at 24 months after CAS) [53]. Moreover, C-reactive protein levels were associated both with MACE as well as with excessive neointimal formation during follow-up. This might reflect a state of exaggerated vascular reactivity in response to injury in these patients. Vascular inflammation, which correlated both with neointimal hyperplasia and cardiovas-

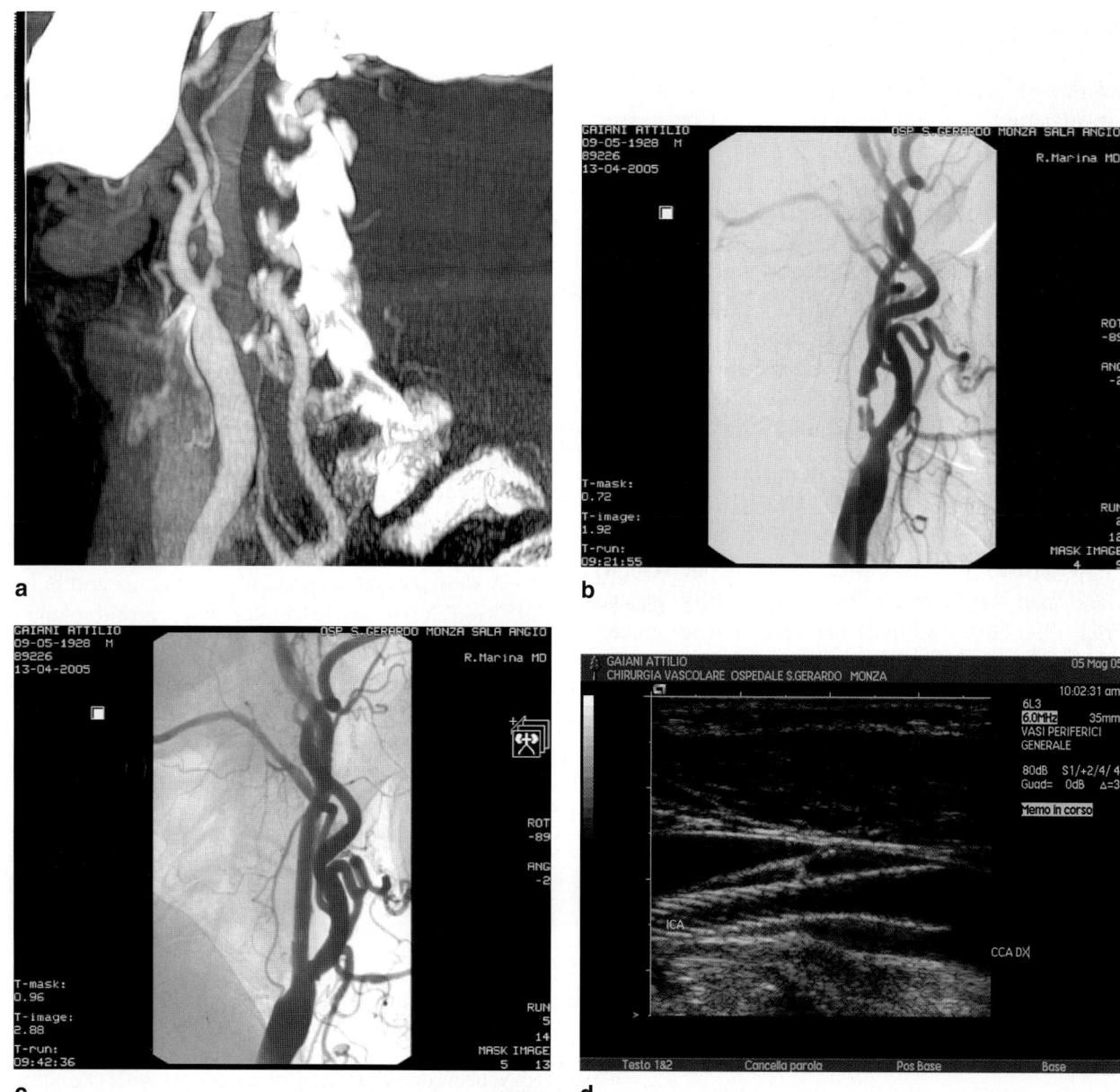

Fig. 1. a Preoperative CT scan; b preoperative angiogram; c postoperative angiogram; d ultrasound evaluation 2 months after the procedure.

cular events, potentially represents a common characteristic among different vascular pathologies. Patients with higher CRP levels need closer surveillance both with respect to restenosis as well as late MACE.

A follow-up after carotid stent deployment is required in order to identify patients with restenoses, which are more liable to develop neurological and cardiac complications.

Several predictors of restenosis have been identified. It has been demonstrated that older age, female sex, diabetes, implantation of multiple stents and post-procedural percent stenosis were associated with increased incidence of restenosis [33], [62].

Patients with a 6-month restenosis had significantly higher post-intervention serum levels of acute-phase reactants compared with the levels in patients

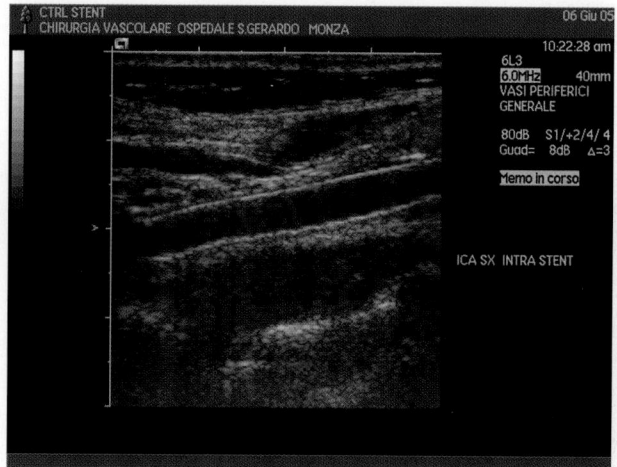

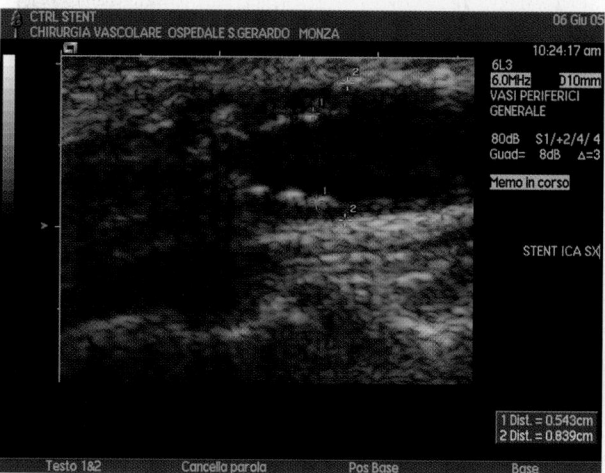

Fig. 2. Ultrasound evaluation 3 months after carotid stent deployment. Please note the non-perfect deployment of the stent in the proximal edge.

without restenosis. 48-hour post-intervention CRP level was independent clinical predictors of post-angioplasty outcome [52]. Setacci et al. evidenced that post-operative fever was a predictive factor for the development of in-stent restenosis [56].

It has been recently demonstrated that the incidence of carotid plaque echolucency is higher in patients with restenosis compared to those without (93% vs. 32%) [55]. IL-6 and CRP concentrations were negatively correlated with carotid plaque echogenicity. Higher IL-6 levels, in addition to CRP levels, appear to be associated with lower echogenicity of carotid plaques, suggesting a link between inflammation and echolucency [66].

Carotid plaque echolucency can be considered as the ultrasonographic manifestation of the inflammatory state linked to atherosclerosis. Carotid echolucency evaluation is very useful to understand better the pathogenesis of restenosis, the inflammatory state of carotid plaque and the correlation between the embolic potential of carotid atherosclerosis, and the development of neurological complications [24], [39], [42].

Aspects to the future: GSM calculation

The GSM is a computer-assisted grading of the echogenicity of carotid plaques. It is a measure of the overall plaque echogenicity, which is a quantitative index of the echoes registered from the plaque.

The following conditions are needed to ensure the reliability of the GSM.

Duplex scanner setup

Every duplex scanner allows to collect images with the characteristics required for the computer-assisted analysis of echogenicity. For GSM calculation there are no unsuitable duplex scanners. A 7 MHz linear array single or multi-frequency transducer should be used.

The dynamic range is the range in acoustic power (in decibels) between the faintest and the strongest signals that can be displayed on the screen. The decrease of the dynamic range increases the apparent contrast in the image. For GSM calculation the maximum dynamic range should be used in order to have the greatest possible display of gray scale values (greyer and flatter image). The frame rate, which means the number of scanning that the probe does producing the images, must be positioned at the maximum level, ensuring good temporal resolution.

The persistence is the number of frames which are mathematically added to produce each image. Higher persistence tends to suppress noise, but it is always done at the expense of time resolution, and it

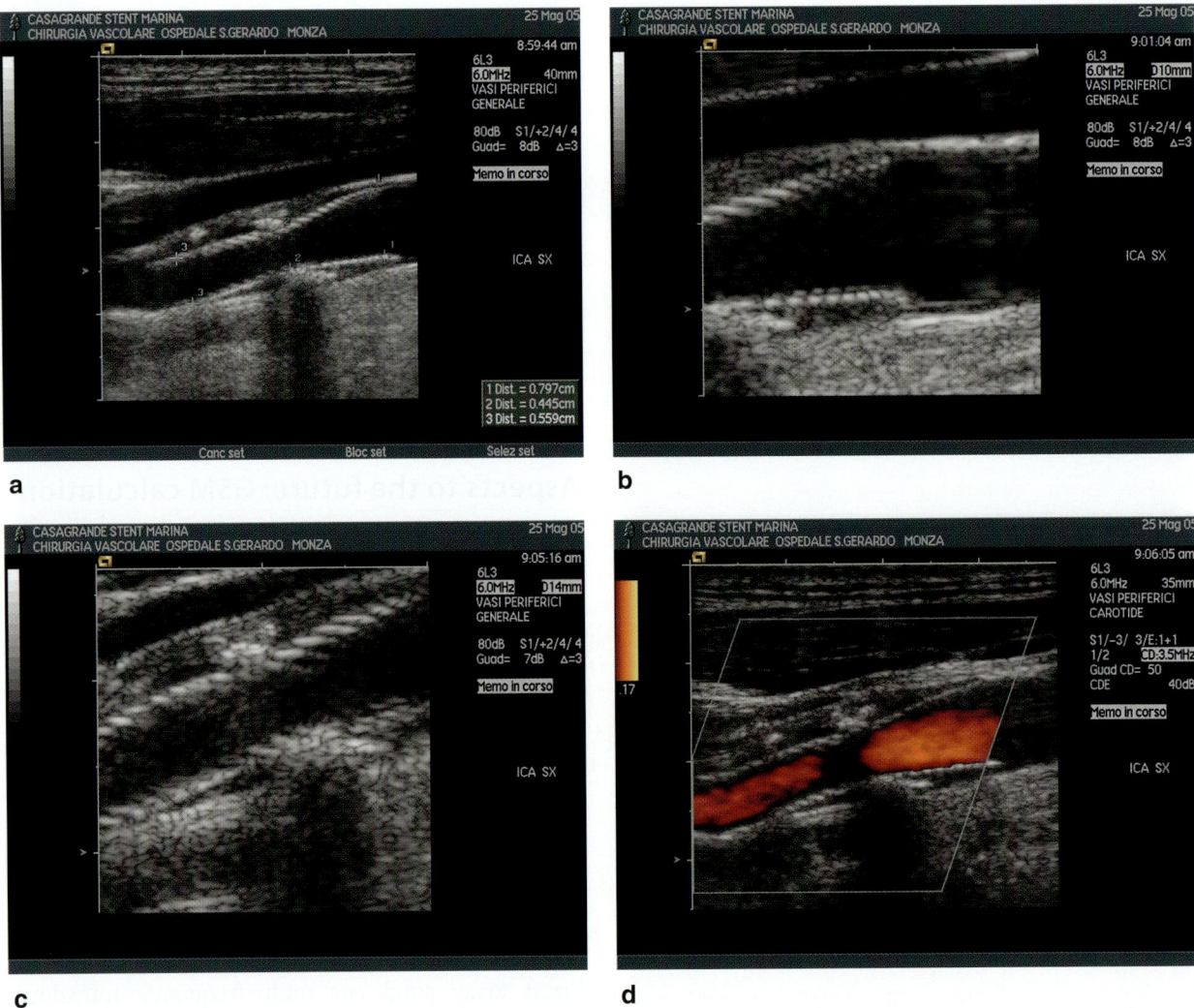

Fig. 3. Ultrasound evaluation 3 months after carotid stent deployment. Please note the non-perfect deployment of the stent due to a calcified plaque.

may blur real targets. The persistence is displayed on the screen device as a series of numbers from 1 to 5 and the right persistence would be 2 or 3 (medium to low level).

A linear post-processing curve is used because image normalization is achieved with linear scaling.

The overall gain should be increased until the plaque can be easily recognized and noise appears within the lumen. It should then be decreased to obtain a lumen free of noise (black).

The time gain compensation (TGC) curve is adjusted (gently sloping) with the aim of obtaining images where the far and near wall of the artery produce the same echogenicity. At the level of the arterial lumen no gains of the TGC-curve must be done. This is essential for normalization of carotid plaques with anterior and posterior components. The consequence of this is that the ultrasound beam should be at 90° to the arterial wall, with a horizontal adventitia.

Image recording

The patient should be in supine position. The carotid vessels are analyzed using different longitudinal views (anterolateral, lateral and posterolateral). The minimum depth should be used, so that the plaque occupies a large part of the image. Excessive magnification is not required.

In case of acoustic shadow the image can be analyzed only if > 50% of the area depicts acoustic information. The GSM cannot be calculated in plaques without any ultrasound information due to acoustic shadowing. The bigger the section of plaque that can be visualized, more accurate is the information provided by GSM.

Before image recording, the following criteria should be fulfilled:

1. Blood: a noiseless vessel lumen in the vicinity of the plaque.
2. Adventitia: in the proximity of the plaque it should be bright, thick and horizontal.
3. Plaque: well defined and with the maximum thickness.
4. Anterior and posterior walls of the carotid artery should be visible.

The following images (in longitudinal projections) should be recorded:

1. The B-mode (gray scale) image.
2. The color image: may help in the delineation of the luminal margin of the plaque (especially with hypoechoic dark plaques).

Attention should be paid in order to have B-mode and color image in the same plane.

Digital storage media (magneto-optical disk and compact disk) are preferred to analogical video tape requiring video grabber card.

Image normalization and GSM calculation

GSM is calculated using Adobe Photoshop (5.0 or higher). In Adobe Photoshop both the B-mode and the color image should be open. In the B-mode image the color information should be discarded: from the "Image" menu, click on "Mode", then "Grayscale". Using the "Lasso" tool, drag the pointer to outline the plaque. Then, click on "Histogram" in the "Image" menu. The "median" value shown in the panel is the GSM.

Hypoechoic dark (echolucent) regions are associated with a GSM that tended to approach 0, whereas hyperechoic bright (echogenic) regions are associated with a GSM that tended to approach 255.

The GSM calculated in this manner in not standardized and consequently the GSM is influenced by duplex scanner settings. The lack of reproducibility of non-standardized GSM has been demonstrated by our group and by others: the GSM cut-off point for the identification of carotid plaques at increased risk of stroke was 50 in Milan and 32 in London [17], [7].

Normalization (standardization) allows to compare images from different scanners by different ultrasonographers. Thanks to normalization, GSM is highly reproducible index of echogenicity [18], [50].

Image normalization is a gray scale transformation using linear scaling: gray scale values of all pixels in image are adjusted according to 2 reference points, blood and adventitia. Blood and adventitia were selected (in stead of muscles, vertebrae, intima-media complex, etc.) because they are easily and clearly recognizable in the vicinity of the plaque and constitute the two distinct ends of gray scale (blood = dark, adventitia = bright). The process modifies the image such that in the resultant image the GSM of the blood is in the range of 0 to 5 and the GSM of the adventitia in the range of 185–195.

Several steps are required for image normalization.

Using the "Lasso" tool, drag the pointer to select an area in the blood that should be free of noise. To check this, in the "Image" menu click on "Histogram". The "median" value shown in the panel is the GSM. The GSM of the selected area in the blood should be 0. If not, the gain of duplex scanner is not set properly (see above).

Similarly, using the "Lasso" tool, the brightest part of the adventitia on the same arterial wall of the plaque should be selected. It is important to note that:

- Image magnification should be performed before adventitia outlining.
- The selected area should not be too small (area, not a point!).
- The selected area should be horizontal.

The GSM of adventitia should then be obtained using the "Histogram" function. Unlike the

GSM of blood, every GSM value measured in the adventitia is accepted.

To normalize the image, click on 'Image' menu then 'Adjustments' and finally 'Curves'. The straight line shown in the panel represents the relationship between the gray scale of the input (x-axis) image and that of the output (y-axis). Each axis has a black and a white edge: this is the gray scale, ranging from 0 (completely black) to 255 (completely white).

The aim of normalization is to modify the subjectivity related to the echographic examination. This purpose can be achieved using the brightest (adventitia) and the faintest (blood) area of the image: in particular conditions (the duplex scanner settings described above) these areas are independent of the type of duplex scanner and the ultrasonographer. Normalizing the image the faintest point remains unchanged with a GSM value of 0 before and 0 after standardization (a proper gain adjustment is essential for this purpose). On the other hand, the GSM value of the brightest area (adventitia) drives all the normalization process: the adventitial GSM value measured before (input value) is converted arbitrarily to a GSM value of 190 (output value). In the normalized image the GSM value of blood and adventitia is 0 and 190 respectively, independent of the type of duplex scanner and the ultrasonographer.

In Adobe Photoshop, the straight line shown in the panel should be modified so that the new line crosses a new point with the input value corresponding to measured adventitial GSM value and the output value corresponding to 190.

The image is now standardized (Fig. 4a before, Fig. 4b after normalization). Using the "Lasso" tool the plaque should be outlined. In the "Histogram" panel the following measurements are obtained:

a. GSM, defined as the median of overall gray shades of the pixels in the plaque
b. Total percentage of echolucent pixels, defined as the percentage of pixels with GSM < 25 (PEP25).

The reproducibility of this method is high [18], [50].

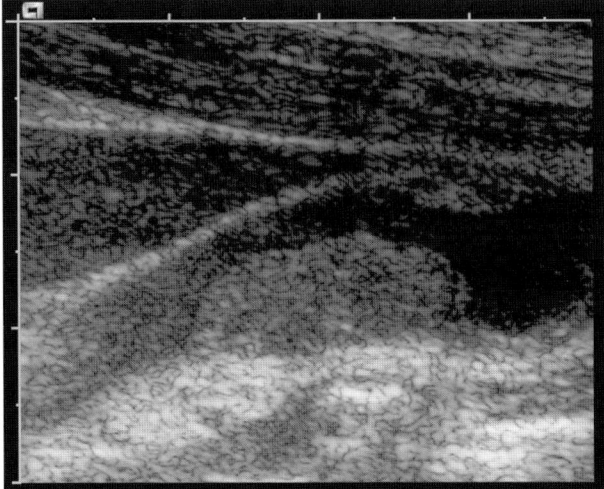

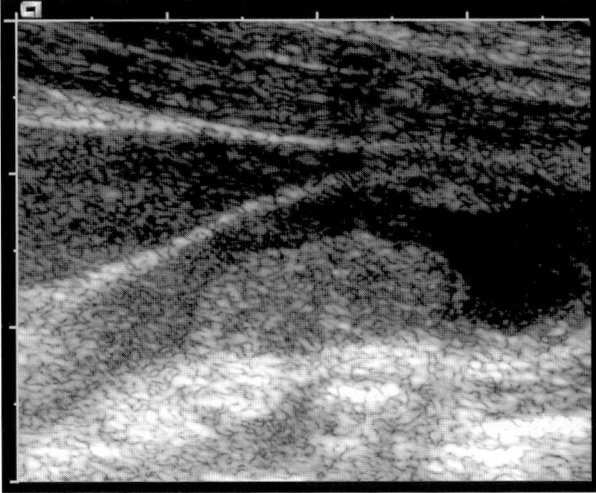

Fig. 4. a B-mode image before normalization; **b** B-mode image after normalization.

Clinical role of GSM before and during carotid stenting

Our group has recently published the results of the ICAROS study [6]. ICAROS was an international multicenter registry, which collected 418 cases of carotid stenting procedures from the 11 participating centers. An echographic evaluation of carotid plaque with GSM measurement was made preprocedurally.

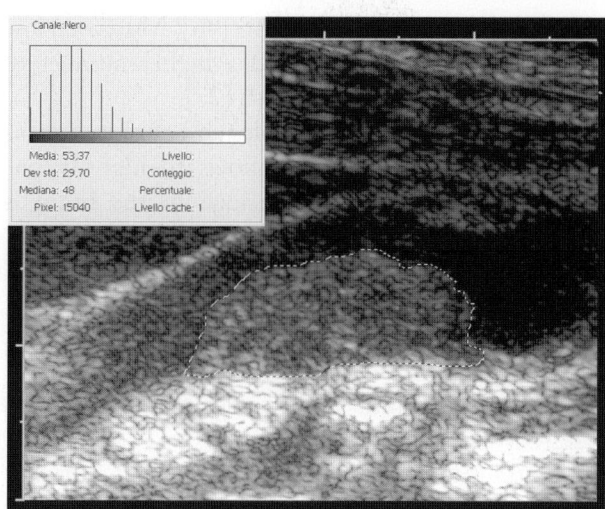

Fig. 5. GSM calculation.

The overall rate of neurological complications was 6.7% (28/418), with transient ischemic attack 3.1% (13/418), minor strokes 2.2% (9/418) and major stroke 1.4% (6/418), while no deaths were observed.

GSM value in complicated patients was significantly lower than in uncomplicated ones, both in the stroke ($p < 0.005$) and in the stroke plus TIA ($p < 0.005$) subset. A receiver operating characteristic (ROC) curve was used to choose the best GSM cutoff value: the most successful threshold value was 25. The prevalence of a GSM value less than 25 (echolucent plaques) is high, we found it in 155/418 (37%) patients. Eleven out of 155 patients with GSM $\leq$ 25 had a stroke (7.1%) compared to 4 out of 263 patients with GSM $>$ 25 (1.5%, $p = 0.005$). The event rates increased to 12.9% and 3.0%, respectively, when both stroke and TIA were counted ($p = 0.002$).

There were 5/219 (2.3%) strokes in protected and 10/199 (5.0%) in unprotected procedures ($p = 0.18$). However, protection gave different results in the GSM subgroups: in patients with GSM $\leq$ 25 BPD tended to increase the risk of stroke (12.5% vs. 5.2%, $p = 0.15$), whereas it had a protective value in the echogenic subgroup (0% vs. 4.8%, $p = 0.01$). Carotid plaque echolucency, as measured by GSMd25, can identify a subset of patients in which the effectiveness of BPD is lower. The overall neurological complication rate was higher in primitive lesions than that in restenosis (5.2% vs. 2.2%, $p = $ ns). This difference was observed also in GSM $>$ 25 patients (4.0% vs. 0%, $p < 0.05$), but not in GSM $\leq$ 25 patients (6.6% vs. 7.8%, $p = $ ns).

The stroke rate was 2.8% for asymptomatic and 5.3% symptomatic patients ($p = $ ns), with similar trend in GSM subsets. The neurological complication rate was 1.5% (3/202) in $<$ 85% carotid stenosis rate subset and 5.6% (12/216) in ?85% ($p < 0.05$). The neurological complication rate was significantly higher in patients with positive cerebral CT than in those with negative CT (7.7% vs. 2.4%, $p < 0.05$).

A multivariate regression analysis revealed that GSM (OR = 7.11, $p = 0.0019$) and degree of stenosis (OR = 5.76, $p = 0.010$) are significant independent predictors of stroke alone, while preprocedural symptomatology (OR = 2.92, $p = 0.061$) and preprocedural brain CT (OR = 2.54, $p = 0.099$) are borderline significant. Similar results were found in the analysis of stroke plus TIA as endpoints.

Carotid restenosis, with a GSM value higher than 25, can be safely treated. Restenoses with GSM $\leq$ 25 should be considered at higher risk of brain embolization: the appropriate type of procedure and brain protection should be chosen.

The clinical impact of GSM relies on the ability to identify a wide number of patients at higher risk of stroke during CAS and to distinguish subsets of patients (with restenosis or with protected procedure) in which the rate of neurological complications is different from the overall population.

Computer-assisted echogenicity evaluation through image normalization and measurement of GSM is a simple method to identify preprocedurally high risk carotid plaques, in which endovascular treatment could be burdened with a higher risk. GSM is one of the parameters that should be mandatory for indication to treatment in order to quantify the individual risk related to the specific procedure. A low GSM value is not an absolute contraindication to CAS, but an index related to a higher risk for the procedure.

Echographic evaluation of carotid plaque through GSM should therefore always be included in the planning of any clinical trial on the endovascular treatment of carotid lesions.

Clinical role of GSM after carotid stenting

What late events can be predicted with the preoperative evaluation of carotid plaque echolucency through GSM?

1. Restenosis. It has been recently demonstrated that the incidence of carotid plaque echolucency is higher in patients with restenosis compared to those without (93% vs. 32%) [55]. Carotid plaque echolucency, as measured by GSM < 25, allows to identify patients in which the risk of restenosis is higher.
2. Major adverse cardiovascular events, including myocardial infarction and stroke. Patients with restenosis more frequently suffered major adverse cardiovascular events (MACE, including myocardial infarction, stroke and death) compared to those with normal neointimal formation (61% vs. 16% at 24 months after CAS) [53]. Carotid plaque echolucency, as measured by GSM < 25, allows to identify patients in which the risk of late cardiac and neurological events is higher.
3. Neurological dysfunction and dementia. Carotid artery stenting is associated with new areas of cerebral ischemia, as detected by using Diffusion-Weighted MR Imaging (DW-MRI) [41], [31], [34]. Around 40% of early DW-MRI lesions are definite brain infarction on follow-up MRI [64]. The presence of silent brain infarcts increased the risk of dementia and 3-year mortality [60], [40]. The use of brain protection devices reduce the rate of stroke and death during CAS, but they do not protect from silent cerebral ischemia: neuroprotected CAS is associated with DW-MRI lesions in significant rate, ranging from 19% to 43%. [30], [54], [59], [20] Neurological dysfunction and dementia should be included as new endpoints in studies concerning the endovascular treatment of carotid lesions.

The reduction of dementia and silent brain infarcts requires a decrease of embolic load to the brain. This purpose can be achieved using 3 strategies: a correct technique of CAS, the use of brain protection devices and the selection of carotid plaques with a lower embolic load. It has been demonstrated that echolucent plaques generated a higher number of embolic particles following CAS [46]. Morevoer, low GSM value plaques generated a higher number of embolic particles following CAS [27].

In conclusion, carotid plaque echolucency, as measured by GSM < 25, allows to identify patients in which the embolic load to the brain is higher [6].

Take home message

- Duplex ultrasound can reliably quantify carotid restenosis after CAS.
- Carotid restenosis is not a frequent event, but...
- ...it is associated with an increased incidence of cardiovascular events (death, stroke and myocardial infarction) following CAS.
- Surveillance after CAS is mandatory for secondary prevention.
- Primary prevention of restenosis should rely on the identification of predictors of intimal hyperplasia.
- Preoperative carotid plaque echolucency is a predictor of carotid restenosis.
- The Gray Scale Median (GSM) is a computer-assisted quantitative objective index of echolucency.
- The GSM can identify patients at increased risk of stroke during carotid stenting.
- The GSM can identify patients at increased risk of restenosis after carotid stenting.
- The GSM can identify patients at increased risk of late cardiac and neurological events after carotid stenting.
- The GSM is a simple, low-cost, effective brain protection device, reducing cardiovascular events before, during and after the procedure.

References

[1] Anonymous: Endarterectomy for asymptomatic carotid artery stenosis. Executive Committee for the Asymptomatic Carotid Atherosclerosis Study. JAMA 273: 1421–1428 (1995).

[2] Anonymous: Carotid revascularization using endarterectomy or stenting systems (CARESS): phase I clinical trial. J Endovasc Ther 10: 1021–1030 (2003).

[3] Back MR, Rogers GA et al.: Magnetic resonance angiography minimizes need for arteriography after inadequate carotid duplex ultrasound scanning. J Vasc Surg 38: 422–430 (2003).

[4] Bendszus M, Koltzenburg M et al.: Silent embolism in diagnostic cerebral angiography and neurointerventional procedures: a prospective study. Lancet 354: 1594–1597 (1999).

[5] Bergeron P, Roux M et al.: Long-term results of carotid stenting are competitive with surgery. J Vasc Surg 41: 213–221 (2005).

[6] Biasi GM, Froio A et al.: Carotid plaque echolucency increases the risk of stroke in carotid stenting: the Imaging in Carotid Angioplasty and Risk of Stroke (ICAROS) study. Circulation 110: 756–762 (2004).

[7] Biasi GM, Mingazzini PM et al.: Carotid plaque characterization using digital image processing and its potential in future studies of carotid endarterectomy and angioplasty. J Endovasc Surg 5: 240–246 (1998).

[8] Biasi GM, Sampaolo A et al.: Computer analysis of ultrasonic plaque echolucency in identifying high risk carotid bifurcation lesions. Eur J Vasc Endovasc Surg 17: 476–479 (1999).

[9] Borisch I, Hamer OW et al.: In Vivo Evaluation of the Carotid Wallstent on Three-dimensional Contrast Material-enhanced MR Angiography: Influence of Artifacts on the Visibility of Stent Lumina. J Vasc Interv Radiol 16: 669–677 (2005).

[10] Briguori C, Tobis J et al.: Discrepancy between angiography and intravascular ultrasound when analysing small coronary arteries. Eur Heart J 23: 247–254 (2002).

[11] Buskens E, Nederkoorn PJ et al.: Imaging of carotid arteries in symptomatic patients: cost-effectiveness of diagnostic strategies. Radiology 233: 101–112 (2004).

[12] Cademartiri F, Mollet N et al.: Images in cardiovascular medicine. Neointimal hyperplasia in carotid stent detected with multislice computed tomography. Circulation 108: e147 (2003).

[13] Coward LJ, Featherstone RL et al.: Safety and efficacy of endovascular treatment of carotid artery stenosis compared with carotid endarterectomy: a Cochrane systematic review of the randomized evidence. Stroke 36: 905–911 (2005).

[14] Dangas G, Mintz GS et al.: Preintervention arterial remodeling as an independent predictor of target-lesion revascularization after nonstent coronary intervention: an analysis of 777 lesions with intravascular ultrasound imaging. Circulation 99: 3149–3154 (1999).

[15] Derdeyn CP: Conventional angiography remains an important tool for measurement of carotid arterial stenosis. Radiology 235: 711–712 (2005).

[16] El-Barghouty, Geroulakos NG et al.: Computer-assisted carotid plaque characterisation. Eur J Vasc Endovasc Surg 9: 389–393 (1995).

[17] El-Barghouty, Levine NMT et al.: Histological verification of computerised carotid plaque characterisation. Eur J Vasc Endovasc Surg 11: 414–416 (1996).

[18] Elatrozy T, Nicolaides A et al.: The effect of B-mode ultrasonic image standardisation on the echodensity of symptomatic and asymptomatic carotid bifurcation plaques. Int Angiol 17: 179–186 (1998).

[19] Faught WE, Mattos MA et al.: Color-flow duplex scanning of carotid arteries: new velocity criteria based on receiver operator characteristic analysis for threshold stenoses used in the symptomatic and asymptomatic carotid trials. J Vasc Surg 19: 818–827 (1994).

[20] Flach HZ, Ouhlous M et al.: Cerebral ischemia after carotid intervention. J Endovasc Ther 11: 251–257 (2004).

[21] Garrard CL, Manord JD et al.: Cost savings associated with the nonroutine use of carotid angiography. Am J Surg 174: 650–653 (1997).

[22] Goyal M, Nicol J et al.: Evaluation of carotid artery stenosis: contrast-enhanced magnetic resonance angiography compared with conventional digital subtraction angiography. Can Assoc Radiol J 55: 111–119 (2004).

[23] Grant EG, Benson CB et al.: Carotid artery stenosis: grayscale and Doppler ultrasound diagnosis – Society of Radiologists in Ultrasound consensus conference. Ultrasound Q 19: 190–198 (2003).

[24] Gronholdt ML, Nordestgaard BG et al.: Ultrasonic echolucent carotid plaques predict future strokes. Circulation 104: 68–73 (2001).

[25] Gronholdt ML, Nordestgaard BG et al.: Echo-lucency of computerized ultrasound images of carotid atherosclerotic plaques are associated with increased levels of triglyceride-rich lipoproteins as well as increased plaque lipid content. Circulation 97: 34–40 (1998).

[26] Groschel K, Riecker A et al.: Systematic review of early recurrent stenosis after carotid angioplasty and stenting. Stroke 36: 367–373 (2005).

[27] Henry M, Henry I et al.: Benefits of cerebral protection during carotid stenting with the PercuSurge GuardWire system: midterm results. J Endovasc Ther 9: 1–13 (2002).

[28] Hobson RW 2nd, Howard VJ et al.: Carotid artery stenting is associated with increased complications in octogenarians: 30-day stroke and death rates in the CREST lead-in phase. J Vasc Surg 40: 1106–1111 (2004).

[29] Hong YJ, Jeong MH et al.: Impact of preinterventional arterial remodeling on in-stent neointimal hyperplasia and in-stent restenosis after coronary stent implantation. Circ J 69: 414–419 (2005).

[30] Jaeger H, Mathias K et al.: Clinical results of cerebral protection with a filter device during stent implantation of the carotid artery. Cardiovasc Intervent Radiol 24: 249–256 (2001).

[31] Jaeger HJ, Mathias KD et al.: Cerebral ischemia detected with diffusion-weighted MR imaging after stent implantation in the carotid artery. AJNR 23: 200–207 (2002).

[32] Kent KC, Kuntz KM et al.: Perioperative imaging strategies for carotid endarterectomy. An analysis of morbidity and cost-effectiveness in symptomatic patients. Jama 274: 888–893 (1995).

[33] Khan MA, Liu MW et al.: Predictors of restenosis after successful carotid artery stenting. Am J Cardiol 92: 895–897 (2003).

[34] Koch C, Kucinski T et al.: Endovascular therapy of high-degree stenoses of the neck vessels-stent-supported percutaneous angioplasty of the carotid artery without cerebral protection. Rofo 174: 1506–1510 (2002).

[35] Koelemay MJ, Nederkoorn PJ et al.: Systematic review of computed tomographic angiography for assessment of carotid artery disease. Stroke 35: 2306–2312 (2004).

[36] Lal BK, Hobson RW 2nd et al.: Carotid artery stenting: is there a need to revise ultrasound velocity criteria? J Vasc Surg 39: 58–66 (2004).

[37] Lal BK, Hobson RW 2nd et al.: In-stent recurrent stenosis after carotid artery stenting: life table analysis and clinical relevance. J Vasc Surg 38: 1162–1168 (2003).

[38] Lell M, Anders K et al.: CTA of carotid artery with different scanner types. Radiologe 44: 967–974 (2004).

[39] Liapis CD, Kakisis JD et al.: Carotid stenosis: factors affecting symptomatology. Stroke 32: 2782–2786 (2001).

[40] Liebetrau M, Steen B et al.: Silent and symptomatic infarcts on cranial computerized tomography in relation to dementia and mortality: a population-based study in 85-year-old subjects. Stroke 35: 1816–1820 (2004).

[41] Loevblad KO, Pluschke W et al.: Diffusion-weighted MRI for monitoring neurovascular interventions. Neuroradiology 42: 134–138 (2000).

[42] Mathiesen EB, Bonaa KH et al.: Echolucent plaques are associated with high risk of ischemic cerebrovascular events in carotid stenosis: the tromso study. Circulation 103: 2171–2175 (2001).

[43] McCabe DJ, Pereira AC et al.: Restenosis after carotid angioplasty, stenting, or endarterectomy in the Carotid and Vertebral Artery Transluminal Angioplasty Study (CAVATAS). Stroke 36: 281–286 (2005).

[44] Moneta GL, Edwards JM et al.: Correlation of North American Symptomatic Carotid Endarterectomy Trial (NASCET) angiographic definition of 70% to 99% internal carotid artery stenosis with duplex scanning. J Vasc Surg 17: 152–157 (1993).

[45] Moneta GL, Edwards JM et al.: Screening for asymptomatic internal carotid artery stenosis: duplex criteria for discriminating 60% to 99% stenosis. J Vasc Surg 21: 989–994 (1995).

[46] Ohki T, Marin ML et al.: Ex vivo human carotid artery bifurcation stenting: correlation of lesion characteristics with embolic potential. J Vasc Surg 27: 463–471 (1998).

[47] Polak JF, Shemanski L et al.: Hypoechoic plaque at US of the carotid artery: an independent risk factor for incident stroke in adults aged 65 years or older. Cardiovascular Health Study. Radiology 208: 649–654 (1998).

[48] Ringer AJ, German JW et al.: Follow-up of stented carotid arteries by Doppler ultrasound. Neurosurgery 51: 639–643 (2002).

[49] Robbin ML, Lockhart ME et al.: Carotid artery stents: early and intermediate follow-up with Doppler US. Radiology 205: 749–756 (1997).

[50] Sabetai MM, Tegos TJ et al.: Reproducibility of computer-quantified carotid plaque echogenicity: can we overcome the subjectivity? Stroke 31: 2189–2196 (2000).

[51] Sahara M, Kirigaya H et al.: Arterial remodeling patterns before intervention predict diffuse in-stent restenosis: an intravascular ultrasound study. J Am Coll Cardiol 42: 1731–1738 (2003).

[52] Schillinger M, Exner M et al.: Acute-phase response after stent implantation in the carotid artery: association with 6-month in-stent restenosis. Radiology 227: 516–521 (2003).

[53] Schillinger M, Exner M et al.: Excessive carotid in-stent neointimal formation predicts late cardiovascular events. J Endovasc Ther 11: 229–239 (2004).

[54] Schluter M, Tubler T et al. Focal ischemia of the brain after neuroprotected carotid artery stenting. J Am Coll Cardiol 42: 1007–1013 (2003).

[55] Setacci C, Donato G de et al.: In-stent Restenosis After Carotid Angioplasty and Stenting: A Challenge for the Vascular Surgeon. Eur J Vasc Endovasc Surg 29: 601–617 (2005).

[56] Setacci C, Pula G et al.: Determinants of in-stent restenosis after carotid angioplasty: a case-control study. J Endovasc Ther 10: 1031–1038 (2003).

[57] Tegos TJ, Sabetai MM et al.: Correlates of embolic events detected by means of transcranial Doppler in patients with carotid atheroma. J Vasc Surg 33: 131–138 (2001).

[58] Teng MM, Tsai F et al.: Three-dimensional contrast-enhanced magnetic resonance angiography of carotid artery after stenting. J Neuroimaging 14: 336–341 (2004).

[59] Terada T, Tsuura M et al.: Results of endovascular treatment of internal carotid artery stenoses with a newly developed balloon protection catheter. Neurosurgery 53: 617–623 (2003).

[60] Vermeer SE, Prins ND et al.: Silent brain infarcts and the risk of dementia and cognitive decline. N Engl J Med 348: 1215–1222 (2003).

[61] Willfort-Ehringer A, Ahmadi R et al.: Neointimal proliferation within carotid stents is more pronounced in diabetic patients with initial poor glycaemic state. Diabetologia 47: 400–406 (2004).

[62] Willfort-Ehringer A, Ahmadi R et al.: Healing of carotid stents: a prospective duplex ultrasound study. J Endovasc Ther 10: 636–642 (2003).

[63] Willinek WA, Falkenhausen M von et al.: Noninvasive detection of steno-occlusive disease of the supra-aortic arteries with three-dimensional contrast-enhanced magnetic resonance angiography: a prospective, intra-individual comparative analysis with digital subtraction angiography. Stroke 36: 38–43 (2005).

[64] Wolf O, Heider P et al.: Microembolic signals detected by transcranial Doppler sonography during carotid endarterectomy and correlation with serial diffusion-weighted imaging. Stroke 35: e373–e375 (2004).

[65] Yadav JS, Wholey MH et al.: Protected carotid-artery stenting versus endarterectomy in high-risk patients. N Engl J Med 351: 1493–1501 (2004).

[66] Yamagami H, Kitagawa K et al.: Higher levels of interleukin-6 are associated with lower echogenicity of carotid artery plaques. Stroke 35: 677–681 (2004).

PROSPECTS TO THE FUTURE

Chapter 5

IMAGING IN CAROTID ARTERY STENOSIS: PROSPECTS TO THE FUTURE

B. J. Schaller and M. Buchfelder

Department of Neurosurgery, University Hospital Göttingen, Germany

In recent years, the clinical impact has emphasized the need for a more detailed analysis of atherosclerotic plaques in carotid artery stenosis. Information beyond the resulting degree of narrowing of the vessel lumen on angiography seems to be desirable. Epidemiologic studies have shown that a large proportion of persons who have sudden ischemic events have no prior ischemic symptoms [43]. More importantly, it has been found that acute coronary syndromes often result from plaque rupture at sites with no or only modest luminal narrowing on angiography [64]; similar observations can be found in the coronary system [26]. Vascular remodelling has often occurred at such sites, which consists of atherosclerosis-associated morphologic and biologic changes of the vessel wall without significant stenosis [27]. Thus there is considerable demand for diagnostic procedures that specifically identify rupture-prone, vulnerable plaques as the most frequent cause of sudden ischemic events [44], [45], also in the cerebrovascular system. To reach this goal, our pathophysiological understanding of cerebrovascular system has to be significantly improved.

Hemodynamic aspects

The mean arterial pressure or perfusion pressure in brain arteries is not routinely measured to identify the presence of hemodynamic impairment. Instead, we rely on physiological imaging studies to identify or infer the presence of normal compensatory mechanisms to reduced cerebral perfusion pressure [16]. When the mean arterial pressure in a cortical artery decreases, two compensatory responses may occur [17]. By means of these two responses, normal oxygen metabolism and brain function are preserved. The first is autoregulatory vasodilatation of the small distal arterioles. This serves to reduce vascular resistance and maintain cerebral blood flow (and the delivery of oxygen and glucose) at near normal rates [18]. The second response occurs when cerebral blood flow decreases. To maintain normal oxygen metabolism and normal neurologic function, neurons may increase the fraction of oxygen extracted from the blood (oxygen extraction fraction) [33]. The average baseline oxygen extraction fraction is approximately 30% and can increase to 80%. These two mechanisms may occur simultaneously [17]: cerebral blood flow decreases slightly through the autoregulatory range, leading to slight but measurable increases in oxygen extraction fraction [65]. When autoregulatory capacity is finally exceeded, blood flow decreases more rapidly and oxygen extraction fraction increases dramatically [40].

Different physiological imaging tests assess different compensatory mechanisms [16]. Paired flow studies compare a baseline measurement of cerebral blood flow or blood velocity with a second measurement after a vasodilatory stimulus. The existence of preexisting autoregulatory vasodilatation is inferred if cerebral blood flow or blood velocity does not increase normally. A second category of studies is also intended to identify autoregulatory vasodilatation. These studies involve measurements of mean transit time directly or by calculation from the ratio of independent measurements of cerebral blood flow and blood volume. The method used in the current study falls into this category. Mean transit time is equal to the ratio of cerebral blood volume over blood flow by the central volume theorem. Mean transit time increases with autoregulatory vasodilatation

[24]. Cerebral blood volume also increases, but this response may be variable for a number of reasons, as described below. The final category of studies uses direct measurements of oxygen extraction fraction.

The relative importance of hemodynamic and embolic mechanisms represents an important point for symptomatic patients with severe carotid stenosis, because the benefit with revascularization is so dramatic, regardless of the mechanism [51]. Determination of hemodynamic status may have great potential for two other patient populations, however: patients with complete carotid occlusion and those with asymptomatic carotid stenosis. Hemodynamic impairment, as identified by some but not all physiological imaging methods, has been proved to be a powerful and independent risk factor for stroke in patients with symptomatic carotid occlusion. A multicenter, randomized clinical trial of surgical revascularization (external to internal carotid artery bypass) for patients with symptomatic carotid occlusion and increased oxygen extraction fraction is underway (Carotid Occlusion Surgery Study, National Institutes of Health, National Institute of Neurological Disorders and Stroke, NS39526). Although bypass surgery for occlusive cerebrovascular disease is still controversial, a recent large retrospective study suggests both an improvement of symptoms and signs and a risk-reduction for future cerebrovascular events after surgery [41].

The prevalence of hemodynamic impairment in patients with asymptomatic carotid occlusive disease seems low [58], [66]. This low prevalence may account in part for the low risk of ischemic stroke with medical treatment and, consequently, the marginal benefit with revascularization. The absolute annual risk reduction for carotid endarterectomy reported in the "Asymptomatic Carotid Atherosclerosis Study" was 1% (ACAS 1995). The presence of hemodynamic impairment may be a powerful predictor of subsequent ischemic stroke in this population [66]. This is one area of research with enormous clinical implications: if a subgroup of asymptomatic patients who are at high risk because of hemodynamic factors could be identified, it would be possible to target surgical or endovascular treatment at those most likely to benefit.

Measurements of relative cerebral blood volume showed little change between middle cerebral artery and other regions at baseline or between baseline and follow-up studies despite the large changes in first moment transit time [17]. First, the relationship between cerebral blood volume and autoregulatory vasodilatation is not linear or direct. The autoregulatory changes occur at the level of small penetrating arterioles. These vessels represent a small fraction of total cerebral blood volume. The largest component of cerebral blood volume is venous, and the degree to which autoregulatory vasodilatation leads to increased cerebral blood volume may be variable. Second, there may be physiological variability between patients in the relationship between cerebral blood volume and autoregulatory vasodilatation. Data regarding cerebral blood volume changes through the autoregulatory range and beyond in animal studies have been variable: some have shown a dramatic increase, others a slight increase, and others no increase [84], [28], [76]. Human studies indicate that individual variability seems to occur [17]. Third, it may be difficult to accurately measure changes in cerebral blood volume due to autoregulatory vasodilatation. Normal cerebral blood volume is approximately 4%. A 25% increase in cerebral blood volume would increase this to 5%, which would be a 1% change in an imaging voxel. This may be difficult to accurately identify. Finally, different imaging methods may be more or less sensitive to these small changes. If the largest changes in cerebral blood volume are seen in pial veins, techniques that are more sensitive to parenchymal vessels would be less sensitive to these changes.

Atherosclerosis

Hemodynamic forces play an active role in vascular pathologies, particularly in relation to the localization of atherosclerotic lesions. It has been established that low shear stress combined with cyclic reversal of flow direction (oscillatory shear stress) affects the endothelial cells and may lead to an initiation of plaque development. Atherosclerosis starts with subendothelial lipid deposition [82]. The initial response to lipid deposition is intimal thickening [68]. This is an adaptive response, associated with mild vascular smooth muscle cell proliferation. Persistence of subendothelial lipid leads to expression of inflammatory markers on surface endothelial cells, which attracts monocytes and macrophages to the site [20], [54]. To provide oxygen for the inflammatory cells, the lesion develops locally increased vasa vasorum [2], [85], [32]. These lesions are referred to as intimal xanthomas or fatty streaks [69], [79]. They subsequently develop pathologic intimal thickening characterized by an extracellular lipid pool without a necrotic core, with a proteoglycan-rich extracellular matrix. Such lesions may lead to acute ischemic syndromes associated with plaque erosion, or stabilize into thin fibrous cap atheromas [68], [79]. During stabilization, the necrotic core is covered by a combination of a collagen and smooth muscle cell-rich cap. However, in the presence of large numbers of inflammatory cells, there is leakage of enzymes, such as matrix metalloproteinases, which digest the collagen and weaken the fibrous cap [26]. These circumstances lead to a thin fibrous cap atheroma, which is often a harbinger of plaque rupture and acute ischemic syndromes. Subclinically eroded or ruptured plaques may heal to reenter at any of the later stages of the atherosclerotic vascular pathology (see Table 1).

Macrophages found in atheroma are derived from circulating monocytes. Monocytes are attracted to sites of inflammation by local expression of integrin receptors and specific cell attractant peptides such as monocyte-chemoattractant peptide 1. After the initial endothelial injury and expression of short-lasting integrin molecules, monocyte adherence is brought about by chemotactic peptides and adhesion molecules [49], [12], [52]. The multifactorial attachment of the monocytes to the endothelium commits monocytes to pass through the interendothelial cell junctions mediated by cadherins. Arrival of the monocytes in the subendothelium is associated with neoexpression of scavenger receptors that allow ingestion of modified low-density lipoprotein (LDL) cholesterol and subsequent transformation into foam cells [35], [34], [71]. Expression of novel receptors on the monocytes during transgression can be targeted with the help of appropriately radiolabeled natural ligands and represents a great hope to visualize atherosclerotic lesion in the carotid artery.

Molecular imaging

Conventional imaging technologies are based on anatomical, physiological, or metabolic heterogeneity to provide image contrast. Conversely, the emerging field of molecular imaging uses targeted and "activatable" imaging agents to exploit specific molecular targets, pathways, or cellular processes to generate image contrast [10], [80], [31]. The underpinning hypothesis of this approach is that most disease processes have a molecular basis that can be exploited to do the following: (i) detect disease earlier; (ii) stratify disease subsets (e.g., active versus inactive); (iii) objectively monitor novel therapies by imaging molecular biomarkers; and (iv) prognosticate disease. Molecular imaging is a multidisciplinary field that aims to provide disease-specific molecular information through diagnostic imaging studies. The primary advantage of magnetic resonance imaging (MRI) as a molecular imaging system is its ability to provide soft tissue and functional information by exploring proton density, perfusion, diffusion, and biochemical contrasts. This feature allows coregistration of molecular information with anatomical information within a single imaging mode.

The molecular imaging has introduced and tested a variety of approaches for specific targeting

Table 1. Conventional pathologic and imaging markers of plaque vulnerability (adapted from [50])

Carotid artery intima/media thickness
Erosion
Ulceration
Thrombus
Intraplaque hemorrhage
Calcification
Status of fibrous cap
Status of lipidic core
Degree of plaque inflammation
Microembolic signals on transcranial Doppler

of molecular features of unstable plaques such as macrophage infiltration [53], proliferating smooth muscle cells [48], matrix metalloproteinase activation [63] apoptosis of macrophages and smooth muscle cells [36], [37], oxidative stress [77], and proangiogenetic factors [62]. Many of these targets are linked with inflammation, which is known to be a key biologic feature of active atherosclerotic plaques that are prone to rupturing [44], [45].

Inflammation itself can be targeted by molecular imaging by use of fluorine 18 deoxyglucose (FDG). The advantage of this approach is that it is based on a tracer that is well established for clinical imaging of tumors and stroke and there widely available. As a consequence, and in contrast to most of the other above-mentioned approaches, FDG's application in human beings is facilitated. Several studies have reported FDG uptake in atherosclerotic lesions-for example, in patients with carotid stenosis [60] or in the systemic vasculature of cancer patients [73]. But will FDG imaging of atherosclerotic lesions ever reach clinical relevance? Several challenges are associated with the identification of tracer accumulation in the vessel wall: First, the small size of the target area requires imaging systems with sufficiently high spatial resolution and detection sensitivity. The size and volume of most atherosclerotic lesions are below the spatial resolution of currently available clinical nuclear imaging systems, but developments in detector technology are ongoing and will help to further increase the resolution of positron emission tomography (PET) and single photon emission computed tomography (SPECT) systems in the future. However, as is the case for other tracers, issues related to biodistribution and blood clearance need to be addressed to achieve sufficiently high target-to-background ratios for stable imaging of plaque inflammation.

It is of note that Tawakol et al. [74] were able to visualize specific FDG uptake in aortic lesions of rabbits using a standard clinical PET scanner. Structures below the spatial resolution of a scanner can be visualized if the target-to-background ratio for the object and sensitivity of the scanner are sufficiently high. Low background activity is an advantage for detection of the target but often makes localization difficult because of lack of visualization of surrounding structures. Tawakol et al. have addressed this issue in a subgroup of their animals by using separately obtained morphologic computed tomography (CT) data for software fusion with PET data. Clearly, the availability of hybrid PET-CT and SPECT-CT systems will greatly facilitate morphologic localization of biologic tracer accumulation in the future.

The key question for biologic imaging of atherosclerotic lesions is whether a sufficiently low detection threshold for accumulation of plaque-targeted tracers can be obtained, as well as whether the imaging signal will be robust and reproducible. FDG seems to be one tracer candidate, but other molecular-targeted probes will need to be evaluated and compared. Only after these methodology-related questions have been addressed can clinical trials be initiated to answer the question of whether detection of plaque activity is truly related to vulnerability and to patient outcome and to establish a clinical role for molecular imaging of atherosclerosis.

Since the receptors for chemo-attractants or adhesion molecules are expressed exclusively by the lesional monocytes, radiolabeled ligands and antibodies to these receptors have been used for the non-invasive detection of atherosclerotic lesions [11]. ^{131}I- and ^{99m}Tc-labeled monocyte chemoattractan protein-1 (MCP-1) has been shown to selectively accumulate in lipid-rich, macrophage-rich regions of an experimental atherosclerosis model in rabbits [32], [69]. The quantitative MCP-1 uptake was directly proportional to the prevalence of immunohistochemically characterized macrophages in the atherosclerotic lesions; MCP-1 uptake was not related to the prevalence of smooth muscle cells. Further, 99mTc-labeled MCP-1 uptake is high enough to be detected by external gamma camera imaging. On the other hand, the adhesion molecules have been targeted with antibodies directed against intracellular adhesion molecule (ICAM) or vascular cell adhesion molecular (VCAM) in murine experimental models of heart and skin transplantation, respectively, which offer a proof of principle that inflammation imaging is possible [79], [26]. Similarly, HLA-DR targeting could also be applied to plaque imaging, having previously been used in the imaging of murine cardiac allograft rejection [49]. HLA-DR is abundantly expressed by the lesional macrophages in vulnerable plaques and plaques undergoing rupture.

After migration to the subendothelial neointimal layer, monocytes develop scavenger receptors including (30) types A I and II, CD36, CD68, and Fc RII [52]. These receptors can be imaged with radiolabeled LDL cholesterol imaging in patients with angiographically confirmed carotid vessel disease [35]. Carotid artery lesions were accurately recognized in patients injected with ^{125}I- or ^{99m}Tc-labeled LDL; no LDL uptake was observed in the vertebral arteries or the carotid arteries of control subjects. The concentration of ^{125}I-LDL in the areas of focal accumulation was up to three times higher than in the surrounding vessel. Other components of the LDL cholesterol complex, such as cholesteryl esters and apolipoprotein B, have also been targeted, but only in experimental atherosclerotic models [34], [71]. Expression of immunoglobulin receptor (Fc RII), which also mediates lipid ingestion, has been targeted with some success by radiolabeled nonspecific immunoglobulin G, in both experimental and clinical settings [46]. Imaging of the peripheral arterial lesions in four patients demonstrated focal uptake of 111In-immunoglobulin in 9 of 12 angiographically documented lesions.

Two related processes contribute to rupture of the fibrous cap: (i) release of metalloproteinases (MMP) in the fibrous cap (most likely by injured macrophages) and (ii) collective death of the macrophages in the cap (most likely due to local hostile conditions, leading to release of the intracellular contents of these cells). Both processes have been targeted by molecular imaging. Davies et al. have used a ^{111}In-labeled broad-spectrum MMP inhibitor to image experimental atherosclerotic lesions in rabbits [11]; this inhibitor avidly binds to MMP-1-3, 7-9, and 13. By non-invasive gamma imaging, the atherosclerotic lesions were visualized best at 3 hours. Preliminary observations suggest that in vivo quantitation of MMP in atherosclerotic plaques is feasible, and correlates with their pathologic distribution in the plaque. The uptake becomes markedly attenuated after dietary modification and statin therapy, which leads to abrogation of MMP activity and histomorphologic stabilization of the atherosclerotic lesions.

The hostile environment in the plaque results in apoptosis of macrophages and smooth muscle cells in the lesion. Oxidized LDL is particularly toxic to these cells [70]. MMP release is associated with death of macrophages at the plaque rupture site. Apoptosis can occur in 50% of macrophages at the site of rupture, while stable plaques have negligible apoptosis of macrophages in the cap [8]. Since apoptosis may contribute to plaque vulnerability, it has been tested the ability of ^{99m}Tc-labeled annexin-V to detect atherosclerosis in vivo in a rabbit model [3], [37]. The atherosclerosis could be clearly identified in these animals 2 h after intravenous administration. In normal vessels there was no localization of radiotracer in the vessel wall. The accumulation of annexin-V in atherosclerotic lesions was approximately nine-fold greater than in the corresponding region. Sections from atherosclerotic animals demonstrated a positive correlation between the overall macrophage burden of the plaque and uptake of radiolabeled tracer; there was no association with the smooth muscle cell burden. Also, the lesional prevalence of apoptosis (of macrophages) was directly proportional to annexin-V uptake.

Efforts to identify vulnerable atherosclerotic plaques by molecular imaging need to be supported. By facing the methodological challenges related to plaque imaging, nuclear neuroscience will expand beyond its present boundaries. If camera technology is refined for the purpose of plaque detection, if understanding of available tracers is improved, and if novel tracers and targets are introduced, the entire field of cerebrovascular imaging will benefit.

Ultrasonic contrast agents have been introduced to improve image resolution and specificity, for example, acoustic liposomes conjugated with monoclonal antibodies or gas-filled phospholipid microbubbles. Using this approach, it has been possible to image a range of targets similar to those described for MRI. Specifically, ICAM-1, vascular cell adhesion molecule 1, P-selectin, fibrin, and integrins have all been imaged with targeted ultrasound probes [9]. Optical techniques offer an interesting approach to functional imaging. Fluorescent probes can be introduced in a quiescent or "quenched" state pending activation (e.g., by enzymatic clivage), at which point fluorescence can increase many hundred-fold. Optical techniques offer excellent spatial and temporal resolution but at the expense of tissue penetration compared, for example, with MRI or positron-emission tomography. In spite of these difficulties, it is possible to image small structures in 3D using multiphoton microscopy. Multiple probes can form part of the same experiment. For example, thrombus formation has been imaged in real time, in vivo using fluorescently labeled antibodies to fibrin, anti-tissue factor (TF), and CD41 (platelet specific). Imaging using near-infrared fluorescent agents has been adapted to protease imaging. After site-specific cleavage by proteolytic enzymes, the probe becomes brightly fluorescent. This technique identified the activity of the macrophage-associated protease cathepsin B in the atherosclerotic plaques of apolipoprotein-E-deficient mice [21].

A vision of the future

Understanding the pathogenesis and biological behavior of atherosclerotic vascular disease has shifted the focus of clinical care from the degree of luminal encroachment by the lesion to the likelihood of progression of the lesion. Although percent stenosis has traditionally been the parameter for treating cerebrovascular artery disease, it does not predict the clinical outcomes such as likelihood of development of acute ischemic syndromes [78], [47]. Luminal obstruction remains important as an explanation of the symptomatic presentation of the disease. Confirmation of the site and extent of cerebrovascular narrowing in these patients will be done by computed tomography (CT) and magnetic resonance imaging, eliminating the need for diagnostic selective cerebrovascular angiography. On the other hand, the prognosis of an atheroma (independent of whether the lesion causes narrowing) is determined by the histopathology of the lesion [78]. Plaques likely to cause a coronary event have a large necrotic core, containing numerous inflammatory cells [12]. The inflamed necrotic core is covered by a rather attenuated fibrous cap, which is also infiltrated with inflammatory cells [38]. When the integrity of this thin inflamed cap is lost, an acute event often occurs [22]. Although techniques such as angioscopy [42], [75], intravascular ultrasonography [29], [57], optical coherence tomography [6], [83], ultrasound elastography [14], [15], and magnetic resonance imaging [67], [61], [81] have been employed to identify these inflamed lesions, they have had limited success. Two techniques that have been successful at identifying the inflammatory components are thermal probes and appropriate nuclear probes [72], [46]. The characterization of vulnerable plaques is particularly important when there is a heightened systemic inflammatory state, such as in patients with diabetes or hyperlipidemia and in chronic smokers. The evidence of systemic inflammation is closely associated with worse outcomes in atherosclerotic disease and has often been identified by peripheral markers of inflammation, including C-reactive protein, myeloperoxidase, glutathione peroxidase-1, and activated circulating leukocytes [4], [5], [55].

A substantial number of the population suffers from symptomatic or otherwise diagnosed cerebrovascular artery disease [1]. These patients represent the tip of the iceberg. A larger number harbor less severe, asymptomatic disease that may present first with an acute coronary event, including sudden death. In two-thirds of the symptomatic patients, thrombotic occlusion of the vessel wall results from rupture of the plaque [7]. Since inflammation plays a pivotal role in plaque rupture, diagnostic targeting strategies should focus on identifying plaque inflammation (see Table 2).

Conclusion

Atherosclerosis is a diffuse and multisystem, chronic inflammatory disorder involving the vascular, metabolic, and immune systems. The traditional risk assessment relies on clinical, biological, and conventional imaging tools. However, these tools fall short in predicting near-future events, particularly in individual clinical practice. At the beginning of the third millennium, it is essential to reconsider the assess-

Table 2. Clinical imaging of the high-risk or vulnerable plaque (adapted from [23]). *IVUS*: Intravascular ultrasound, *OCT*: optical coherence tomography, *US*: ultrasound, *UFCT*: ultrafast computerized tomography, *MRI*: magnetic resonance imaging, *TEE*: transesophageal echocardiography

	Luminal Percentage Stenosis	Wall	Lipid	Fibrous	Thrombus	Calcium
X-ray angiography	+	...	...	...	?	?
IVUS*	−	?	−	?	−	
Angioscopy	...	...	−	...	−	...
Thermography/OCT†/Raman spectroscopy/NIR	...	?	?	?	?	?
US‡	+	+	...	...	...	...
UFCT	?+	...	...	...	...	+
Nuclear scintigraphy	...	...	−	...	+	...
MRI	?+	?+	?+	?+	?+	?+

* *IVUS in carotid arteries is theoretically feasible.*
† *Optical coherence tomography (OCT) is able to image the vessel in very high resolution.*
‡ *TEE may identify some of the plaque components in the aorta.*

ment of vulnerable carotid artery plaques in light of new imaging tools in order to optimize therapeutic management. Accordingly, a new stratification for atherothrombotic risk may involve, in the future, the combination of systemic markers, high-resolution MRI, and molecular imaging that targets the inflammatory and thrombotic components of atherosclerotic plaque.

Take home message

– Atherosclerotis of the carotid artery represents a diffuse, chronic inflammatory disorder that involves the vascular, metabolic and immune system and leads to plaque vulnerability.
– Traditional imaging tools fall short in predicting near-future events in patients with vulnerable carotid artery plaque.
– Multi-modal assessment of plaques vulnerability involving the combination of systematic markers, new imaging methods that target inflammatory and thrombotic components, and the potential of emerging therapies may lead to a new stratification system for atherothrombotic risk and to a better preservation of atherosclerotic stroke.

References

[1] American Heart Association: Heart disease and stroke statistics – 2004 update. Dallas: American Heart Association (2004).
[2] Barger AC, Beeuwkes R III, Lainey LL et al.: Hypothesis: vasa vasorum and neovascularization of human coronary arteries. A possible role in the pathophysiology of atherosclerosis. N Engl J Med 310: 175–177 (1984).
[3] Baumgartener H: Eine neue Methode zur Erzeugung von Thromben durch gezielte Überdehnung der Gefässwand. Zentralbl Gesamte Exp Med 137: 227–249 (1963).
[4] Blankenberg S, Rupprecht HJ, Bickel C et al.: Glutathione peroxidase 1 activity and cardiovascular events in patients with coronary artery disease. N Engl J Med 349: 1605–1613 (2003).
[5] Brennan ML, Penn MS, Van Lente F et al.: Prognostic value of myeloperoxidase in patients with chest pain. N Engl J Med 349: 1595–1604 (2003).
[6] Brezinski ME, Tearney GJ, Bouma BE et al.: Optical coherence tomography for optical biopsy. Properties and demonstration of vascular pathology. Circulation 93: 1206–1213 (1996).
[7] Burke AP, Farb A, Malcom GT, Liang YH, Smialek J, Virmani R: Coronary risk factors and plaque morphology in men with coronary disease who died suddenly. N Engl J Med 336: 1276–1282 (1997).
[8] Carpenter KL, Challis IR, Arends MJ. Mildly oxidised LDL induces more macrophage death than moderately oxidised LDL: roles of peroxidation, lipoprotein-asso-

ciated phospholipase A2 and PPAR gamma. FEBS Lett 553: 145–150 (2003).
[9] Chen J, Tung CH, Mahmood U et al.: In vivo imaging of proteolytic activity in atherosclerosis. Circulation. 105: 2766–2771 (2002).
[10] Choudhury RP, Fuster V, Fayad ZA: Molecular, cellular and functional imaging of atherothrombosis. Nat Rev Drug Disc 3: 913–925 (2004).
[11] Davies MJ, Gordon JL, Gearing AJ et al.: The expression of the adhesion molecules ICAM-1, VCAM-1, PECAM, and E-selectin in human atherosclerosis. J Pathol 171: 223–229 (1993).
[12] Davies MJ, Thomas AC: Plaque fissuring – the cause of acute myocardial infarction, sudden ischaemic death, and crescendo angina. Br Heart J 53: 363–373 (1985)
[13] DeForge LE, Schwendner SW, DeGalan MR et al.: Noninvasive assessment of lipid disposition in treated and untreated atherosclerotic rabbits. Pharm Res 6: 1011–1016 (1989).
[14] de Korte CL, Carlier SG, Mastik F, Doyley MM, van der Steen AF, Serruys PW, Bom N: Morphological and mechanical information of coronary arteries obtained with intravascular elastography; feasibility study in vivo. Eur Heart J 23: 405–413 (2002).
[15] de Korte CL, van der Steen AF, Cespedes EI, Pasterkamp G: Intravascular ultrasound elastography in human arteries: initial experience in vitro. Ultrasound Med Biol 24: 401–408 (1998).
[16] Derdeyn CP, Grubb RL Jr, Powers WJ: Cerebral hemodynamic impairment: methods of measurement and association with stroke risk. Neurology 53: 251–259 (1999).
[17] Derdeyn CP, Videen TO, Yundt KD et al.: Variability of cerebral blood volume and oxygen extraction: stages of cerebral haemodynamic impairment revisited. Brain 125: 595–607 (2002).
[18] Dirnagl U, Pulsinelli W: Autoregulation of cerebral blood flow in experimental focal brain ischemia. J Cereb Blood Flow Metab 10: 327–336 (1990).
[19] Executive Committee for the Asymptomatic Carotid Atherosclerosis Study.: Endarterectomy for asymptomatic carotid artery stenosis. JAMA 273: 1421–1428 (1995).
[20] Faggiotto A, Ross R, Harker L: Studies of hypercholesterolemia in the nonhuman primate. I. Changes that lead to fatty streak formation. Arteriosclerosis 4: 323–340 (1984).
[21] Falati S, Gross P, Merill-Skoloff G et al.: Real time in vivo imaging of platelets, tissue factor and fibrin during arterial thrombus formation in the mouse. Nat Med 8: 1175–1181 (2002).
[22] Falk E: Why do plaques rupture? Circulation 86: III30–III42 (1992).
[23] Fayad ZA, Fuster V: Clinical imaging of the high-risk or vulnerable atherosclerotic plaque. Circ Res 89: 305–316 (2001).
[24] Ferrari M, Wilson DA, Hanley DF et al.: Effects of graded hypotension on cerebral blood flow, blood volume, and mean transit time in dogs. Am J Physiol 262: H1908–H1914 (1992).
[25] Fuster V, Badimon L, Badimon JJ et al.: The pathogenesis of coronary artery disease and the acute coronary syndromes. N Engl J Med 326: 242–250 (1992).
[26] Galis ZS, Sukhova GK, Lark MW et al.: Increased expression of matrix metalloproteinases and matrix degrading activity in vulnerable regions of human atherosclerotic plaques. J Clin Invest 94: 2493–2503 (1994).
[27] Glagov S, Weisenberg E, Zarins CK et al.: Compensatory enlargement of human atherosclerotic coronary arteries. N Engl J Med 316: 1371–1375 (1987).
[28] Grubb RL Jr, Raichle ME, Phelps ME et al.: Effects of increased intracranial pressure on cerebral blood volume, blood flow, and oxygen utilization in monkey. J Neurosurg 43: 385–398 (1975).
[29] Gussenhoven EJ, Essed CE, Lancee CT et al.: Arterial wall characteristics determined by intravascular ultrasound imaging: an in vitro study. J Am Coll Cardiol 14: 947–952 (1989).
[30] Hardoff R, Braegelmann F, Zanzonico P et al.: External imaging of atherosclerosis in rabbits using an 123I-labeled synthetic peptide fragment. J Clin Pharmacol 33: 1039–1047 (1993).
[31] Jaffer FA, Weissleder R: Molecular imaging in the clinical arena. JAMA 293: 855–862 (2005).
[32] Kamat BR, Galli SJ, Barger AC et al.: Neovascularization and coronary atherosclerotic plaque: cinematographic localization and quantitative histologic analysis. Hum Pathol 18: 1036–1042 (1987).
[33] Kety SS, King BD, Horvath SM et al.: The effects of an acute reduction in blood pressure by means of differential spinal sympathetic block on the cerebral circulation of hypertensive patients. J Clin Invest 29: 402–407 (1950).
[34] Khoo JC, Miller E, Pio F et al.: Monoclonal antibodies against LDL further enhance macrophage uptake of LDL aggregates. Arterioscler Thromb 12: 1258–1266 (1992).
[35] Khoo JC, Miller E, McLoughlin P et al.: Enhanced macrophage uptake of low density lipoprotein after self-aggregation. Arteriosclerosis 8: 348–358 (1988)
[36] Kietselaer BL, Reutelingsperger CP, Heidendal GA et al.: Noninvasive detection of plaque instability with use of radiolabeled annexin A5 in patients with carotid-artery atherosclerosis, N Engl J Med 350: 1472–1473 (2004).
[37] Kolodgie FD, Petrov A, Virmani R et al.: Targeting of apoptotic macrophages and experimental atheroma

with radiolabeled annexin V A technique with potential for noninvasive imaging of vulnerable plaque. Circulation 108: 3134–3139 (2003).
[38] Kolodgie FD, Narula J, Burke AP et al.: Localization of apoptotic macrophages at the site of plaque rupture in sudden coronary death. Am J Pathol 157: 1259–1268 (2000).
[39] Lees RS, Lees AM, Strauss HW: External imaging of human atherosclerosis. J Nucl Med 24: 154–156 (1983).
[40] McHenry LC Jr, Fazekas JF, Sullivan JF: Cerebral hemodynamics of syncope. Am J Med Sci 80: 173–178 (1961).
[41] Mendelowitsch A, Taussky P, Rem JA et al.: Clinical outcome of standard extracranial-intracranial bypass surgery in patients with symptomatic atherosclerotic occlusion of the internal carotid artery. Acta Neurochir (Wien). 146: 95–101 (2004).
[42] Mizuno K, Miyamoto A, Satomura K et al.: Angioscopic coronary macromorphology in patients with acute coronary disorders. Lancet 337: 809–812 (1991)
[43] Myerburg RJ, Interian Jr A, Mitrani RM, et al, Frequency of sudden cardiac death and profiles of risk. Am J Cardiol 80: 10F–19F (1997).
[44] Naghavi M, Madjid M, Gul K et al.: Thermography basket catheter In vivo measurement of the temperature of atherosclerotic plaques for detection of vulnerable plaques. Catheter Cardiovasc Interv 59: 52–59 (2003).
[45] Naghavi M, Libby P, Falk E et al.: From vulnerable plaque to vulnerable patient: a call for new definitions and risk assessment strategies: Part I. Circulation 108: 1664–1672 (2003).
[46] Narula J, Virmani R et al.: Radionuclide imaging of atherosclerotic lesions. In: Dilsizian V, Narula J, Braunwald E, eds. Atlas of nuclear cardiology. Philadelphia: Current Medicine 2003.
[47] Narula J, Virmani R, Iskandrian AE: Strategic targeting of atherosclerotic lesions. J Nucl Cardiol 6(1 Pt 1): 81–90 (1999).
[48] Narula J, Petrov A, Bianchi C et al.: Noninvasive localization of experimental atherosclerotic lesions with mouse/human chimeric Z2D3 F(ab')2 specific for the proliferating smooth muscle cells of human atheroma Imaging with conventional and negative charge-modified antibody fragments. Circulation 92: 474–484 (1995).
[49] Nelken NA, Coughlin SR, Gordon D et al.: Monocyte chemoattractant protein-1 in human atheromatous plaques. J Clin Invest 88: 1121–1127 (1991).
[50] Nighoghossian N, Derex L, Douek P.: The vulnerable carotid artery plaque: current imaging methods and new perspectives. Stroke 36: 2764–2772 (2005).
[51] North American Symptomatic Carotid Endarterectomy Trial Collaborators: Beneficial effect of carotid endarterectomy in symptomatic patients with high-grade carotid stenosis. N Engl J Med 325: 445–453 (1991).
[52] O'Brien KD, Allen MD, McDonald TO et al.: Vascular cell adhesion molecule-1 is expressed in human coronary atherosclerotic plaques. Implications for the mode of progression of advanced coronary atherosclerosis. J Clin Invest 92: 945–951 (1993).
[53] Ohtsuki K, Hayase M, Akashi K et al.: Detection of monocyte chemoattractant protein-1 receptor expression in experimental atherosclerotic lesions An autoradiographic study. Circulation 104: 203–208 (2001).
[54] Osterud B, Bjorklid E: Role of monocytes in atherogenesis. Physiol Rev 83: 1069–1112 (2003).
[55] Pearson TA, Mensah GA, Alexander RW et al.: Markers of inflammation and cardiovascular disease: application to clinical and public health practice: a statement for healthcare professionals from the Centers for Disease Control and Prevention and the American Heart Association. Circulation 107: 499–511 (2003)
[56] Peebles CR: Non-invasive coronary imaging: computed tomography or magnetic resonance imaging? Heart 89: 591–594 (2003).
[57] Potkin BN, Bartorelli AL, Gessert JM et al.: Coronary artery imaging with intravascular high-frequency ultrasound. Circulation 81: 1575–1585 (1990).
[58] Powers WJ, Derdeyn CP, Fritsch SM et al.: Benign prognosis of never-symptomatic carotid occlusion. Neurology 54: 878–882 (2000).
[59] Rubin RH, Fischman AJ: The use of radiolabeled non-specific immunoglobulin in the detection of focal inflammation. Semin Nucl Med 24: 169–179 (1994).
[60] Rudd JH, Warburton EA, Fryer TD et al.: Imaging atherosclerotic plaque inflammation with [18F]-fluorodeoxyglucose positron emission tomography. Circulation 105: 2708–2711 (2002).
[61] Ruehm SG, Corot C, Vogt P, Kolb S, Debatin JF: Magnetic resonance imaging of atherosclerotic plaque with ultrasmall superparamagnetic particles of iron oxide in hyperlipidemic rabbits. Circulation 103: 415–422 (2001).
[62] Sadeghi MM, S Krassilnikova S, Zhang J et al.: Detection of injury-induced vascular remodeling by targeting activated alphavbeta3 integrin in vivo. Circulation 110: 84–90 (2004).
[63] Schafers M, Riemann B, Kopka K et al.: Scintigraphic imaging of matrix metalloproteinase activity in the arterial wall in vivo. Circulation 109: 2554–2559 (2004).
[64] Schaller B: Ischemic preconditioning as induction of ischemic tolerance after transient ischemic attacks in human brain: its clinical relevance. Neurosci Lett 377: 206–11 (2005).
[65] Schumann P, Touzani O, Young AR et al.: Evaluation of the ratio of cerebral blood flow to cerebral blood vol-

[65] ume as an index of local cerebral perfusion pressure. Brain 121: 1369–1379 (1998).
[66] Silvestrini M, Vernieri F, Pasqualetti P et al.: Impaired cerebral vasoreactivity and risk of stroke in patients with asymptomatic carotid artery stenosis. JAMA 283: 2122–2127 (2000).
[67] Skinner MP, Yuan C, Mitsumori L, Hayes CE, Raines EW, Nelson JA, Ross R: Serial magnetic resonance imaging of experimental atherosclerosis detects lesion fine structure, progression and complications in vivo. Nat Med 1: 69–73 (1995).
[68] Stary HC, Chandler AB, Dinsmore RE et al.: A definition of advanced types of atherosclerotic lesions and a histological classification of atherosclerosis. A report from the Committee on Vascular Lesions of the Council on Arteriosclerosis, American Heart Association. Circulation 92: 1355–1374 (1995).
[69] Stary HC, Chandler AB, Glagov S et al.: A definition of initial, fatty streak, and intermediate lesions of atherosclerosis. A report from the Committee on Vascular Lesions of the Council on Arteriosclerosis, American Heart Association. Arterioscler Thromb 14: 840–856 (1994).
[70] Steinberg D, Witzum JL: Lipoproteins, lipoprotein oxidation, and atherogenesis. In: Cheien KR, ed. Molecular basis of cardiovascular disease. Philadelphia: Saunders; 458–476 (1998).
[71] Steinberg D, Lewis A: Conner Memorial Lecture. Oxidative modification of LDL and atherogenesis. Circulation 95: 1062–1071 (1997).
[72] Stefanadis C, Diamantopoulos L, Vlachopoulos C et al.: Thermal heterogeneity within human atherosclerotic coronary arteries detected in vivo: a new method of detection by application of a special thermography catheter. Circulation 99: 1965–1971 (1999).
[73] Tatsumi M, Cohade C, Nakamoto Y et al.: Fluorodeoxyglucose uptake in the aortic wall at PET/CT Possible finding for active atherosclerosis. Radiology 229: 831–837 (2003).
[74] Tawakol A, Migrino RQ, Hoffmann U et al.: Noninvasive in vivo measurement of vascular inflammation with F-18 fluorodeoxyglucose positron emission tomography. J Nucl Cardiol. 12: 294–301 (2005).
[75] Thieme T, Wernecke KD, Meyer R et al.: Angioscopic evaluation of atherosclerotic plaques: validation by histomorphologic analysis and association with stable and unstable coronary syndromes. J Am Coll Cardiol 28: 1–6 (1996).
[76] Tomita M: Significance of cerebral blood volume. In: Tomita M, Sawada T, Naritomi H, Heiss W-D, eds. Cerebral Hyperemia and Ischemia: From the Standpoint of Cerebral Blood Volume. Amsterdam: Elsevier Science Publishers BV 1988.
[77] Tsimikas S, Palinski W, Halpern SE et al.: Radiolabeled MDA2, an oxidation-specific, monoclonal antibody, identifies native atherosclerotic lesions in vivo. J Nucl Cardiol 6: 41–53 (1999).
[78] van der Wal AC, Becker AE, van der Loos CM et al.: Site of intimal rupture or erosion of thrombosed coronary atherosclerotic plaques is characterized by an inflammatory process irrespective of the dominant plaque morphology. Circulation 89: 36–44 (1994).
[79] Virmani R, Kolodgie FD, Burke AP et al.: Lessons from sudden coronary death: a comprehensive morphological classification scheme for atherosclerotic lesions. Arterioscler Thromb Vasc Biol 20: 1262–1275 (2000).
[80] Weissleder R, Mahmood U: Molecular imaging. Radiology 40: 219–316 (2001).
[81] Wentzel JJ, Aguiar SH, Fayad ZA: Vascular MRI in the diagnosis and therapy of the high risk atherosclerotic plaque. J Interv Cardiol 16: 129–142 (2003).
[82] Witztum JL: The oxidation hypothesis of atherosclerosis. Lancet 344: 793–795 (1994).
[83] Yabushita H, Bouma BE, Houser SL et al.: Characterization of human atherosclerosis by optical coherence tomography. Circulation 106: 1640–1645 (2002).
[84] Zaharchuk G, Mandeville JB, Bogdanov AA Jr et al.: Cerebrovascular dynamics of autoregulation and hypoperfusion: an MRI study of CBF and changes in total and microvascular cerebral blood volume during hemorrhagic hypotension. Stroke 30: 2197–2205 (1999).
[85] Zamir M, Silver MD: Vasculature in the walls of human coronary arteries. Arch Pathol Lab Med 109: 659–662 (1985).

List of Authors

M. Berg MD PhD, Department of Clinical Radiology, Kuopio University Hospital, Kuopio, Finland

K. Bettermann MD, Department of Neurology, Wake Forest University School of Medicine, Winston-Salem, USA

G. M. Biasi MD, Department of Surgical Sciences and Intensive Care, University of Milano-Bicocca, Vascular Surgery Unit, San Gerardo Hospital, Monza, Italy

M. Buchfelder MD, Department of Neurosurgery, University Hospital, Göttingen, Germany

B. Butz MD, Department of Radiology, University Hospital, Regensburg, Germany

C. Chaves MD, Department of Neurology, Lahey Clinic, Burlington, USA

G. Deleo MD, Department of Surgical Sciences and Intensive Care, University of Milano-Bicocca, Vascular Surgery Unit, San Gerardo Hospital, Monza, Italy

C. P. Derdeyn MD, Mallinckrodt Institute of Radiology and the Departments of Neurology and Neurological Surgery, Washington University School of Medicine, St. Louis, USA

M. P. Dunphy MD, Nuclear Medicine Service, Department of Radiology, Memorial Sloan-Kettering Cancer Center, New York, USA

A. Froio MD, Department of Surgical Sciences and Intensive Care, University of Milano-Bicocca, Vascular Surgery Unit, San Gerardo Hospital, Monza, Italy

J. H. Gillard MD, University Department of Radiology, Addenbrooke's Hospital, Cambridge, UK

M. Goyal MD, Department of Diagnostic Imaging, The Ottawa Hospital, Ottawa, Ontario, Canada

S. P. S. Howarth MD, University Department of Radiology and Department of Neurosurgery, Addenbrooke's Hospital, Cambridge, UK

J. Hendrikse MD, Department of Radiology, University Medical Center Utrecht and the Rudolf Magnus Institute of Neuroscience, Utrecht, The Netherlands

H. Katano MD, Departments of Neurosurgery and Restorative Neuroscience, Nagoya City University Graduate School of Medical Sciences, Japan

W. S. Kerwin, Department of Radiology, University of Washington, Seattle, USA

J. U. King-Im MD, University Department of Radiology, Addenbrooke's Hospital, Cambridge, UK

C. J. M. Klijn MD, Department of Neurology, University Medical Center Utrecht and the Rudolf Magnus Institute of Neuroscience, Utrecht, The Netherlands

B. K. Lal MD, Division of Vascular Surgery, Department of Surgery, University of Medicine and Dentistry of New Jersey-New Jersey Medical School, Newark, New Jersey, USA

G. Lee MD, Department of Neuro-radiology, Lahey Clinic, Burlington, USA

K. O. Lövblad MD, Neuroradiology Unit, Radiology Department, HUG Geneva University Hospital, Geneva, Switzerland

A. D. Mackinnon MD, Department of Clinical Neurology, University College London, The National Hospital for Neurology and Neurosurgery, Queen Square, London, UK

H. Manninen MD, PhD, Department of Clinical Radiology, Kuopio University Hospital, Kuopio, Finland

D. J. C. McCabe MD, Department of Clinical Neurology, University College London, The National Hospital for Neurology and Neurosurgery, Queen Square, London, UK

A. D. Platt MD, Department of Clinical Neurology, University College London, The National Hospital for Neurology and Neurosurgery, Queen Square, London, UK

B. J. Schaller MD, Department of Neuroscience, Karolinska Institute, Stockholm, Sweden

A. Srinivasan MD, Department of Diagnostic Imaging, The Ottawa Hospital Ottawa, Ontario, Canada

H. W. Strauss MD, Nuclear Medicine Service, Department of Radiology, Memorial Sloan-Kettering Cancer Center, New York, USA

H. J. N. Streefkerk MD, Department of Neurosurgery, University Medical Center Utrecht and the Rudolf Magnus Institute of Neuroscience, Utrecht, The Netherlands

J. F. Toole MD, Department of Neurology, Wake Forest University School of Medicine, Winston-Salem, USA

C. A. F. Tulleken MD, Department of Otorhinolaryngology, St. Radboud University Medical Center Nijmegen, The Netherlands

R. Vanninen MD, PhD, Department of Clinical Radiology, Kuopio University Hospital, Kuopio, Finland

K. Yamada MD, Departments of Neurosurgery and Restorative Neuroscience, Nagoya City University Graduate School of Medical Sciences, Japan

SpringerMedicine

Vinko V. Dolenc

Microsurgical Anatomy and Surgery of the Central Skull Base

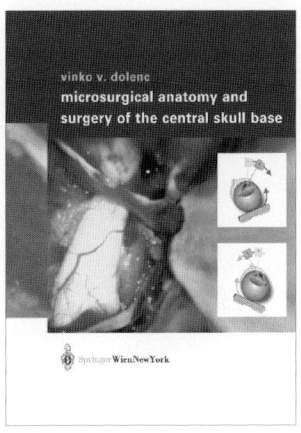

Assisted by L. Rogers.
2003. XI, 304 pages. 189 illustrations.
Hardcover **EUR 198,–**
ISBN-13 978-3-211-83236-3

The atlas covers the normal microsurgical anatomy of the central skull base as well as the pathological anatomy of the tumorous and vascular lesions of this region. The book gives a detailed description of the contemporary approaches to the individual pathologies in the central skull base which have evolved in the last 15 years and represent the summary of the experience gained by the author through continuous neuroanatomy laboratory work as well as in performing over 1500 operations in the region.

Complete or partial resection of the tumorous lesions, the exclusion of aneurysms and preservation of the patency of the internal carotid artery will be presented as well as the cost-benefit ratios of these direct surgical approaches to the central skull base. The large number of operations is a very valuable and unique source of technical data and statistics and allows a careful evaluation of the approaches to the region based on a precise understanding of the underlying anatomy.

SpringerWienNewYork

P.O. Box 89, Sachsenplatz 4–6, 1201 Vienna, Austria, Fax +43.1.330 24 26, books@springer.at, **springer.at**
Haberstraße 7, 69126 Heidelberg, Germany, Fax +49.6221.345-4229, SDC-bookorder@springer-sbm.com, springer.com
P.O. Box 2485, Secaucus, NJ 07096-2485, USA, Fax +1.201.348-4505, service@springer-ny.com, springer.com
All errors and omissions excepted. Recommended retail price. Net-price subject to local VAT.

SpringerMedicine

Henri M. Duvernoy

The Human Brain

Surface, Three-Dimensional Sectional Anatomy with MRI, and Blood Supply

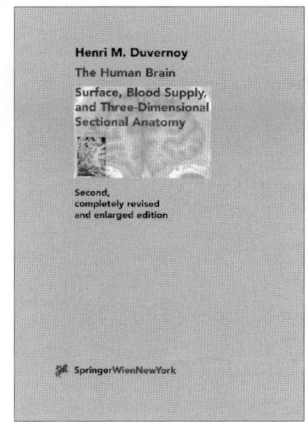

2., completely rev. and enlarged ed.
1999. VII, 491 p. 272 illus.
Hardcover **EUR 298,–**
ISBN-13 978-3-211-83158-8

The recent progress of medical imaging due to CT, MRI, and the three-dimensional reconstruction of cerebral structures calls for a better understanding of the anatomy of the brain. Therefore, this book comprises serial sections – 2 mm thick – of the cerebral hemispheres and diencephalon in the coronal, sagittal, and axial planes. So as to point out the level of the sections more accurately, each section is shown from different angles emphasizing the surrounding hemisphere surfaces.

This three-dimensional approach has proven to be extremely useful to apprehend the difficult anatomy of the gyri and sulci of the brain. Certain complex cerebral structures such as the occipital lobe, the deep grey matter (basal ganglia and thalamus), and the vascularization are demonstrated in greater detail.

The second edition of this successful atlas has been completely revised and updated. 44 serial sections have been added showing the brain in much greater detail. Mostly two MRI views of improved quality are presented with almost every section. A chapter on the vascular anatomy of the brain with beautiful color drawings has been added.

SpringerWienNewYork

P.O. Box 89, Sachsenplatz 4–6, 1201 Vienna, Austria, Fax +43.1.330 24 26, books@springer.at, springer.at
Haberstraße 7, 69126 Heidelberg, Germany, Fax +49.6221.345-4229, SDC-bookorder@springer-sbm.com, springer.com
P.O. Box 2485, Secaucus, NJ 07096-2485, USA, Fax +1.201.348-4505, service@springer-ny.com, springer.com
All errors and omissions excepted. Recommended retail price. Net-price subject to local VAT.

SpringerMedicine

E. L. Feldman, W. Grisold, J. W. Russell, U. A. Zifko

Atlas of Neuromuscular Diseases

A Practical Guideline

2005. X, 474 pages. 200 illus. in color.
Hardcover **EUR 198,–**
ISBN-13 978-3-211-83819-8

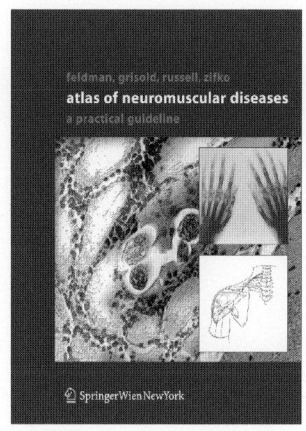

This atlas is a comprehensive outline of neuromuscular diseases, written by experienced American and European authors. It discusses all aspects of neuromuscular disorders including the cranial nerves, spinal nerves, motor neurone disease, the nerve plexus, peripheral nerves, mononeuropathies, entrapment syndromes, polyneuropathies, the neuromuscular junction, and muscle disease. Each chapter is uniformly structured into anatomy, symptoms, signs, pathogentic possibilities, diagnosis and differential diagnosis, therapy and prognosis.

Additionally the diagnostic tools and investigations used in neuromuscular disease are explained and a practical guide is given how to advance from symptoms to syndromes. For each disease the therapeutic options are described. It contains large number of clinical and histologic pictures from the practical experience of the authors and also a number of artists drawings to facilitate the understanding of anatomic structures.

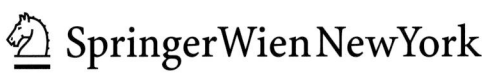

P.O. Box 89, Sachsenplatz 4–6, 1201 Vienna, Austria, Fax +43.1.330 24 26, books@springer.at, springer.at
Haberstraße 7, 69126 Heidelberg, Germany, Fax +49.6221.345-4229, SDC-bookorder@springer-sbm.com, springer.com
P.O. Box 2485, Secaucus, NJ 07096-2485, USA, Fax +1.201.348-4505, service@springer-ny.com, springer.com
All errors and omissions excepted. Recommended retail price. Net-price subject to local VAT.

SpringerMedicine

Walter Hruby (ed.)

Digital (R)Evolution in Radiology

Bridging the Future of Health Care

2., revised and enlarged edition.
2006. XVI, 379 pages. Numerous figures, partly in colour.
Hardcover **EUR 160,–**
ISBN-13 978-3-211-20815-1

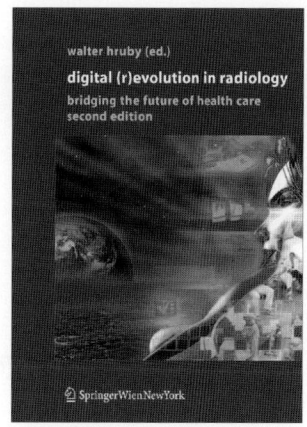

According to a statement of Gordon Moore computer performance doubles every 18 months. So it is not surprising that the "half-time" of modern computers is rapidly decreasing. Increasing demands of public health for radiology together with a rapid development of information technology and innovations result in a digital environment, where thorough guidance is necessary. This book is such a solid guidance for radiologists and other medical staff working in this field.

The second edition has been brought up-to-date, revised and new aspects have been incorporated that focus on the synergy that results from the integration of digital systems used in radiology such as image fusion, "functional" imaging, electronic patient records and health networks, etc. It is intended for radiologists and all other physicians, as well as technicians, scientists, IT-experts, health care providers and health maintenance organisations. The IT-market now has changed so much that Integrated Health Care Enterprise becomes reality.

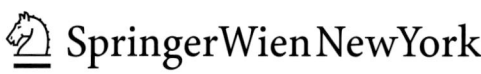

P.O. Box 89, Sachsenplatz 4–6, 1201 Vienna, Austria, Fax +43.1.330 24 26, books@springer.at, springer.at
Haberstraße 7, 69126 Heidelberg, Germany, Fax +49.6221.345-4229, SDC-bookorder@springer-sbm.com, springer.com
P.O. Box 2485, Secaucus, NJ 07096-2485, USA, Fax +1.201.348-4505, service@springer-ny.com, springer.com
All errors and omissions excepted. Recommended retail price. Net-price subject to local VAT.

Springer and the Environment

WE AT SPRINGER FIRMLY BELIEVE THAT AN INTERnational science publisher has a special obligation to the environment, and our corporate policies consistently reflect this conviction.

WE ALSO EXPECT OUR BUSINESS PARTNERS – PRINTERS, paper mills, packaging manufacturers, etc. – to commit themselves to using environmentally friendly materials and production processes.

THE PAPER IN THIS BOOK IS MADE FROM NO-CHLORINE pulp and is acid free, in conformance with international standards for paper permanency.